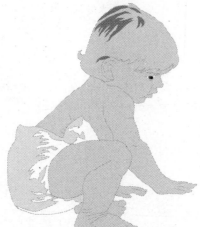

Pediknots–
Pediatric Case Studies

'Don't judge each day by the harvest you reap.
But, by the seeds you plant'.
—Robert Louis Stevenson

The heights of great men reached and kept were not
obtained by sudden flight.
But, they while their companions slept, were toiling
upward in the night.
—Henry Wordsworth Longfellow

Pediknots– Pediatric Case Studies

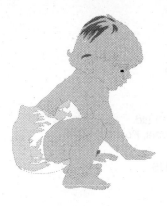

KE Elizabeth
Ph. D, MD, DCH, FIAP
E-mail: elizake@hotmail.com

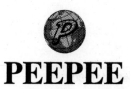

PEEPEE
PUBLISHERS AND DISTRIBUTORS (P) LTD.

Pediknots—Pediatric Case Studies

Published by
Pawaninder P. Vij
Peepee Publishers and Distributors (P) Ltd.
7/31, First Floor, Ansari Road, Daryaganj, Post Box-7243
New Delhi-110002 (India)

Ph: 65195868, 9811156083, 23246245

e-mail: peepee160@yahoo.co.in

e-mail: peepee160@rediffmail.com

e-mail: peepee160@gmail.com

www.peepeepub.com

This book has been published in good faith that the material provided by authors/contributors is original. Every effort is made to ensure accuracy of material, but publisher, printer and author/editor will not be held responsible for any inadvertent errors. In case of any dispute, all legal matters to be settled under Delhi jurisdiction only.

First Edition: **2008**

ISBN: 81-8445-039-7

Printed at
Lordson, C-5/19, Rana Pratap Bagh, Delhi-110 007

With profound and enduring gratitude
to
My parents
My family
My teachers
and
My 'child patients'
Who gave so much of themselves for shaping
and
remodeling me
and
contributing to the well-being
and
welfare of others

FOREWORD

I am happy to record the foreword for this book, **'Pediknots—Pediatric Case Studies'** by Dr. K.E. Elizabeth. I have always admired her academic brilliance, clinical dedication and research capabilities.

The lucid style of presentation is commendable and touches upon all major areas of pediatrics in 16 chapters. The author's extensive experiences in teaching, pediatric practice and research as well as active participation in several social and professional organizations and mass media education programmes have helped to bring out this valuable book.

Several review type of books by different authors are in limelight, but case discussion type of presentations are very few in the discipline of Pediatrics. The chapters on Pediatric case recording, growth, nutrition, developmental Pediatrics, various systemic diseases intensive care and community Pediatrics are packed with information and practical tips. The different charts and tables included in the text and appendix form a 'ready reckoner' to students of UG and PG caliber, researchers and practising doctors.

I am confident that this valuable compilation will encourage contemporary and future Pediatricians to develop a holistic approach for the assessment and management of child related issues.

Dr. MKC Nair
Ph.D, M.Med. Sc., MD, FIAP, FIACAM
(IAP National President 2004)
Professor of Pediatrics and Epidemiology
Director, Child Development Centre
Medical College, Thiruvananthapuram
Email: nairmkc@rediffmail.com

PREFACE

An enquiring analytical mind –
An unquenchable thirst for new knowledge–
And heart felt compassion for the ailing–
These are the prominent traits among the committed clinicians
who have preserved the passion of medicine.
— Louis Debakey

Now, we have almost completed a full circle. The phenomenal development of Modern Scientific Medicine in the turn of the 20th century has made dramatic changes in the quality and quantity of knowledge and applications in the field of health care. Those who have knowledge and information at their fingertips were considered 'genius' earlier, but now these are available at the keyboards. It is only a question of time and interest to retrieve them and apply them optimally. Thus, the whole approach has changed now. Hence, Lawrence Lee remarked, **'The world does not pay for what a person knows. But, it pays for what a person does with what he knows'.**

This compilation of PEDIKNOTS—PEDIATRIC CASE STUDIES, discusses the depths and heights of Pediatrics and the length and breadth of Child Health in 16 Chapters. A simple and unique classroom case discussion style is adopted to target UGs, PGs and practising clinicians. The chapters on Community Pediatrics and Intensive Care are meant for deeply dedicated candidates, who want to pursue preventive and curative services. The appendix is designed as a collection of all what is relevant to the discipline of Pediatrics.

I dedicate this humble effort of mine to my colleagues, friends and students with an optimistic note. My plea is to keep all your 'six senses' open to 'assess, analyze and apply' what you gather. This 'triple A approach' is a sure way to success.

And, I assure you success in both profession and personal life.
'Success is the sum total of small efforts repeated day in and out', remarked Robert Collier
And **'Sweat plus sacrifice equals success',**
said Charles O Finley.

I bow down before God Almighty, who gave me the courage and strength to 'shoot for the star and at least hit the moon, when most don't even shoot'. I also thank Dr. Binoy Thomas, Dr. Prasanth and Dr. Anand N for their help in organising the book.

KE Elizabeth

CONTENTS

APPENDICES

ABBREVIATIONS

Abd	Abdomen
AED	Anti Epileptic Drug
AGN	Acute Glomerulo Nephritis
ANC	Ante Natal Checkup
ATT	Anti TB Treatment
C/F	Clinical Features
CFT	Capillary Filling Time
DD	Differential Diagnosis
DI	Diabetes Insipidus
DM	Diabetes Mellitus
EBM	Expressed Breast Milk
GERD	Gastro-Esophageal Reflux Disease
H/o	History of
I&D	Incision and Drainage
IMS	Infant Milk Substitute
Lt	Left
MAC	Mid Arm Circumference
Max	Maximum
Mini	Minimum
NB	Newborn
NICU	Neonatal Intensive Care Unit
O/E	On Examination
OFC	Occipito Frontal Circumference
PEM	Protein Energy Malnutrition
PICU	Pediatric Intensive Care Unit
PR	Pulse Rate, Per Rectal
PS	Peripheral Smear
R/o	Rule out
RF	Rheumatic Fever
RIF	Right Iliac Fossa
RR	Respiratory Rate
Rt	Right
UTI	Urinary Tract Infection

SUGGESTED READING

RECOMMENDED REFERENCE BOOKS AND JOURNALS

- Behrman Ehrman RE, Kliegman RM, Jenson HB, Stanton BF: Nelson Textbook of Pediatrics.
- Harcourt Asia Pie Ltd., 18th edition, 2008.
- Rudolph AM, Hoffman JIE, Rudolph CD, Rudolph S: Pediatrics, Appletion and Lange, 20th edition, 1996.
- Campbell AGM, McIntosh N, Forfar and Arneil, S: Textbook of Pediatrics, ELBS, 4th edition, 1992.
- Ghai OP, Gupta P, Paul VK: Essential Pediatrics, Interprint, New Delhi.
- IAP, Textbook of Pediatrics.
- Singh M: Pediatrics Clinical Methods, Saga Publications.
- The Harrier Lane Handbook, Mosby and Harcourt India.
- Singh M, Deorari AK, Drug Doses in Children.

Growth and Development
- Illingworth RS: The development of the infant and young child, Normal and abnormal, Churchill Livingstone.

Nutrition
- Alleye GAO, Hay RW, Picou DI, Stanford JP, Whitehead RG: Protein energy malnutrition, Jaypee Brothers, New Delhi.
- WHO Management of severe malnutrition: A manual for physicians and other senior health workers, WHO, Geneva, 1999.
- Suskind RM, Lewinter-Suskind C: The malnourished child, Nestle Nutrition Workshop Series, Volume 19, 1990.
- Elizabeth KE: Nutrition and Child Development, Paras Publishing, Hyderabad, 3rd edition, 2007 (Reprint).
- Suraj Gupte: Textbook of Pediatric Nutrition, Jaypee Brothers, N. Delhi.

Infectious Diseases
- Feigin RD, Cherry ID: Textbook of Pediatric Infectious Diseases, W.B. Saunders.
- Remington JS, Klein JO: Infectious Diseases of the Fetus and Newborn Infant, W.B. Saunders.
- Weatherall DJ, Ledingham JGG, Warrell DA, Oxford Textbook of Medicine, Volume I, Oxford University Press.
- Cook G, Manson S: Tropical diseases, ELBS and W.B. Saunders Co.
- Seth V, Kebra SK: Essential of Tuberculosis in Children, Jaypee Brothers, New Delhi.
- Pizzo PA, Wilfert CM: Pediatric AIDS, Lippincott Williams.

Intensive care
- Singh M: Medical Emergencies in Children, Sagar Publications.
- Nichols DG: Textbook of Pediatric Intensive Care, Williams and Wilkins.
- Neonatal and Pediatric Emergencies, Sachdeva *et al.,* Jaypee Brothers, New Delhi.

Neonatology
- Singh M: Care of the Newborn, Sagar Publication, 2000.
- Avery GB, Fletcher MA, MacDonald MG: Neonatology—Pathophysiology and Management of the Newbron, Lippincott William and Wilkins.

- Cloherty JP, Stark AR: Manual of Neonatal Care, Lippincott—Raven Publishers.
- Kattwinkel I: Textbook of neonatal resuscitation, American Heart Association and American Academy of Pediatrics.

Neurology
- Swaiman B, Kenneth F, Ashwal S: Pediatric Neurology: Principles and Practice, St. Louis Mosby.
- Brett EM: Pediatric Neurology, Churchill Livingstone.
- Menkers JH: Textbook of Childhood Neurology, Lea and Febiger.

Cardiology
- Allen HO, Clark FB, Gutgesell HP, DJ: Moss and Adam S: Heart Disease in Infants, Children and Adolescent, Lippincott Williams and Wilkins.
- Park MK: Pediatric cardiology for practitioners, Mosby-Year Book, Inc.

Gastroenterology
- Suchy FI, Sokol RJ, Balistreri WF: Liver disease in children, Lippincott Williams and Wilkins.
- Bhan MK, Bhatnagar S: Guidelines for management of diarrhoea in children.
- Ministry of Health, GOI and WHO/SEARO, 2000.

Endocrinology
- Lifshitz F: Pediatric Endocrinology Marcel Dekker, Inc.
- Sharma S, Singhal T, Bajpai A: Management protocols in pediatric endocrinology.
- Desai MP, Bhatia B, Menon PSN: Pediatric Endocrine Disorders, Orient Longman, 2001.

Nephrology
- Barratt TM, Avner ED, Harmon WE: Pediatric Nephrology, Baltimore Williams and Wilkins.
- Srivastava RN, Bagga A: Pediatric Nephrology, 3rd edition, Jaypee Brothers, New Delhi, 2001.

Hematology and Oncology
- Nathan DG, Orkin SH, Nathan and Oski S: Hematology of Infancy and Childhood, W.B. Saunders, 5th edition, 1998.

Rheumatology
- Cassidy JT, Petty RE: Textbook of Pediatric Rheumatology W.B. Saunders.

Respiratory Medicine
- Chernick V, Boat TF, Kendig S: Disorders of the Respiratory Tract in Children, WB Saunders.

IMNCI
- Integrated Management of Neonatal and Childhood Illness, Ministry of Health, GOI, New Delhi, 2007.

Preventive and Social Pediatrics
- K. Park: Park's Textbook of Preventive and Social Medicine, 19th edition, M/s. Banarsidas Bhanot Publisher, Jabalpur.

Plate 1

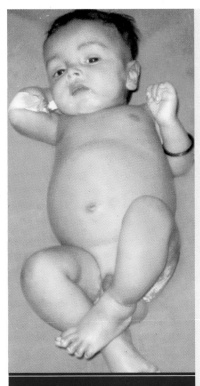

Fig. 1: Kwashiorkor

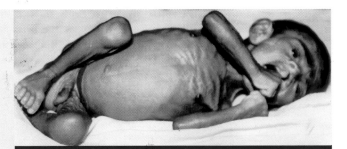

Fig. 2: Marasmus with cleft lip and palate

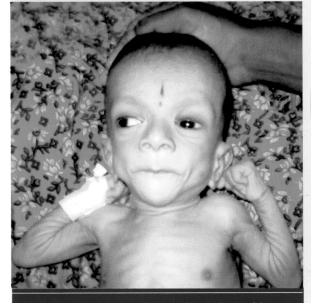

Fig. 3: Marasmus with loss of buccal pad of fat

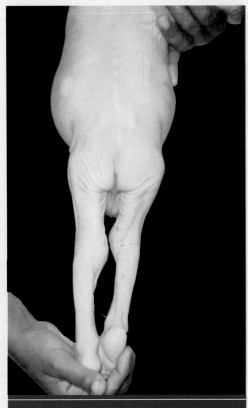

Fig. 4: Marasmus with extreme wasting

Plate   2

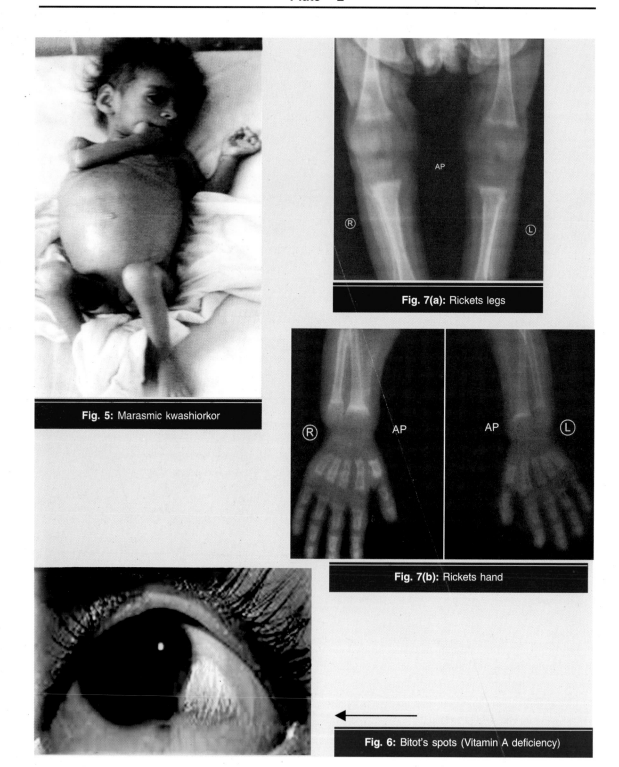

Fig. 5: Marasmic kwashiorkor

Fig. 7(a): Rickets legs

Fig. 7(b): Rickets hand

Fig. 6: Bitot's spots (Vitamin A deficiency)

Plate 3

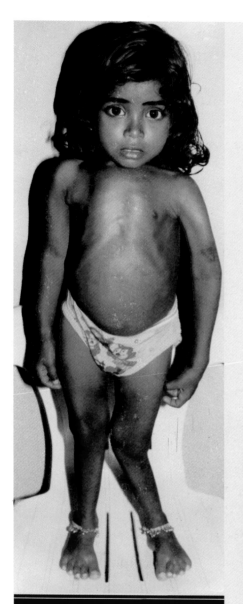

Fig. 8: Refractory rickets

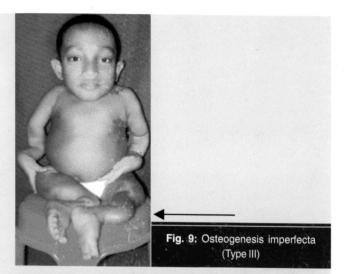

Fig. 9: Osteogenesis imperfecta (Type III)

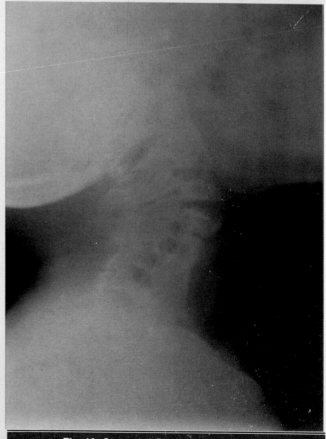

Fig. 10: Congenital 'Block Vetebra' (C4 - C7)

Plate 4

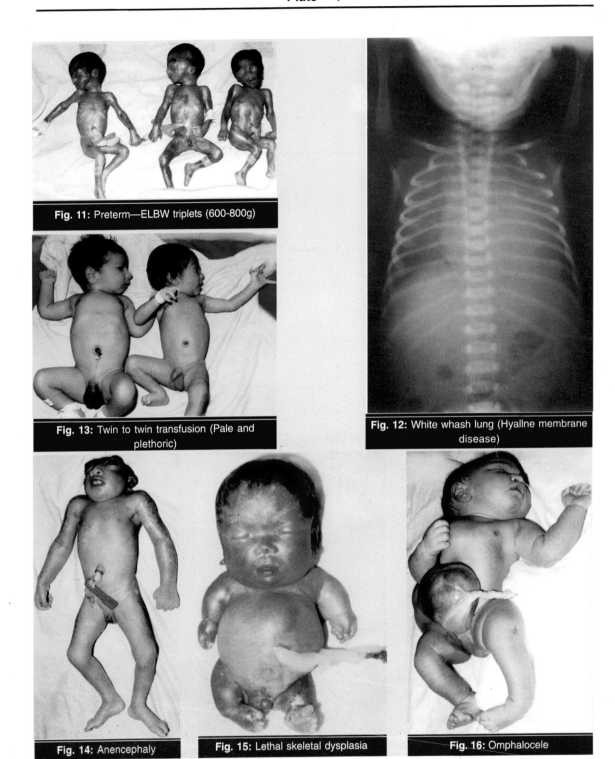

Fig. 11: Preterm—ELBW triplets (600-800g)

Fig. 13: Twin to twin transfusion (Pale and plethoric)

Fig. 12: White whash lung (Hyallne membrane disease)

Fig. 14: Anencephaly

Fig. 15: Lethal skeletal dysplasia

Fig. 16: Omphalocele

Plate 5

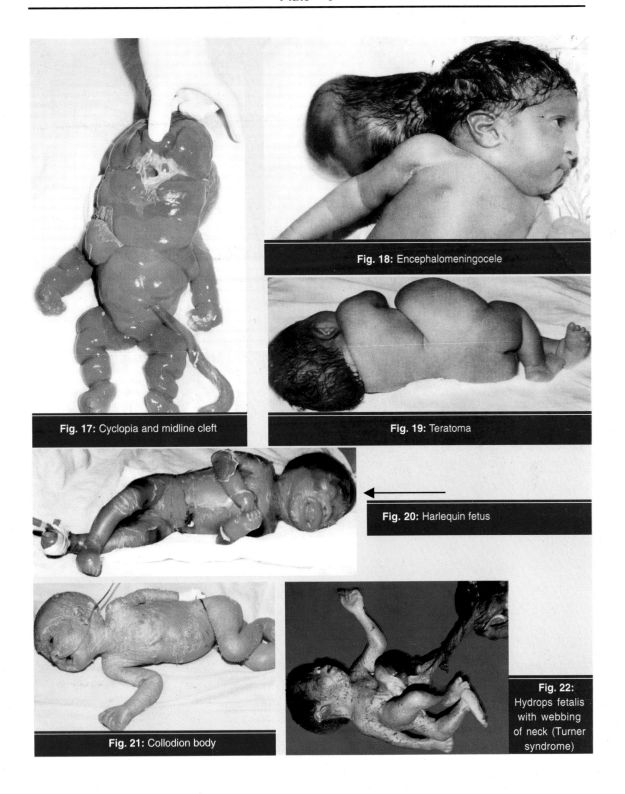

Fig. 17: Cyclopia and midline cleft

Fig. 18: Encephalomeningocele

Fig. 19: Teratoma

Fig. 20: Harlequin fetus

Fig. 21: Collodion body

Fig. 22: Hydrops fetalis with webbing of neck (Turner syndrome)

Plate 6

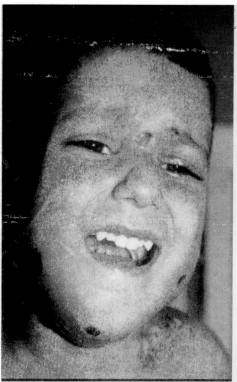

Fig. 23: Immunodeficient child with multiple abscess (chronic granulomatous disease)

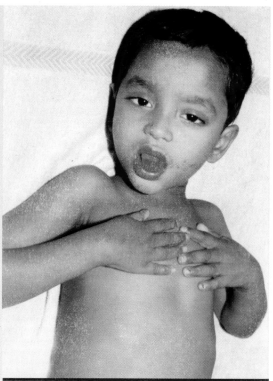

Fig. 24: Strawberry tongue, hand edema and periungual peeling (Kawasaki disease)

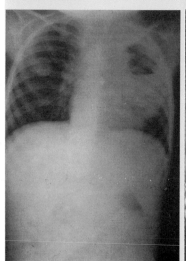

Fig. 25: Lung abscess (Left) and breaking down consolidation (Right) HIV-AIDS

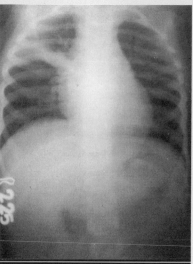

Fig. 26: Spindle shaped minor fissure effusion (Tuberculosis)

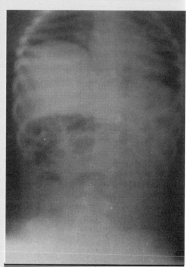

Fig. 27: Eventeration of diaphragm (Right)

Plate 7

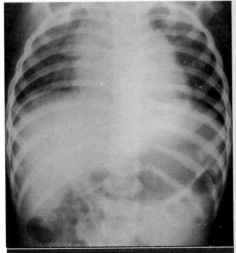

Fig. 28: Sail sign (Thymus)

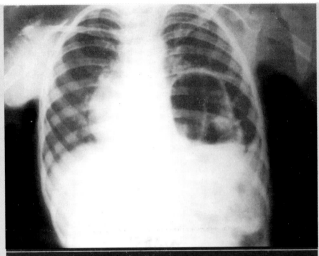

Fig. 29: Diaphragmatic hernia (Lt)

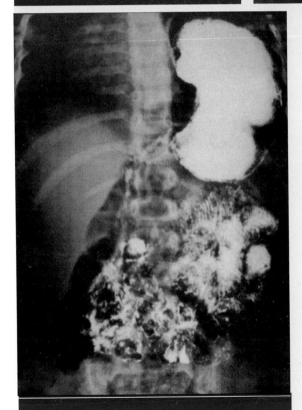

Fig. 30: Barium meal showing diaphragmatic hernia

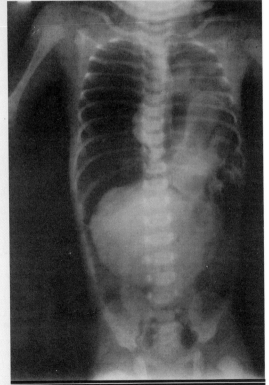

Fig. 31: Newborn with diaphragmatic hernia (Lt) pneumothorax (Rt) and pneumo peritoneum following bag and mask ventilation

Plate 8

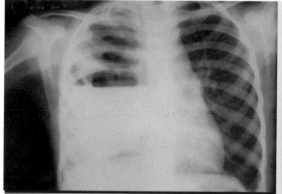

Fig. 32: Pyopneumothorax (Rt) with loculation

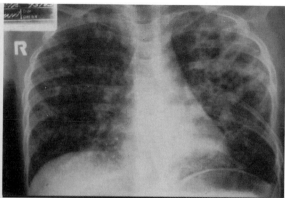

Fig. 33: Bronchiectasis (bilateral) 'Honey Coomb' appearance

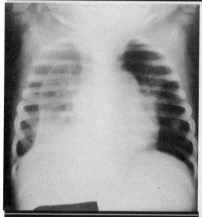

Fig. 34: Pneumothorax (bilateral) with collapsed lung

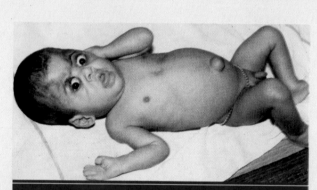

Fig. 35: Cranio-facial dysostosis and syndactyly (Apert syndrome)

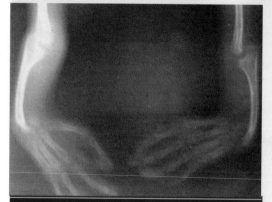

Fig. 36: Absent radius and thumb (Nager type-acrofacial dysostosis)

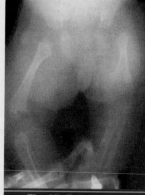

Fig. 37: Focal femoral dysplasia (Left)

Plate 9

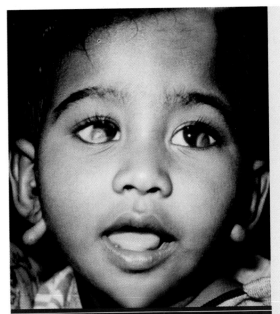

Fig. 38: Bilateral preauricular tags and epibulbar lipoid (Goldenhar syndrome)

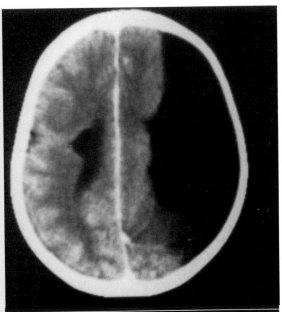

Fig. 39: Schizencephaly (Bilateral) cleft communicating with ventricles

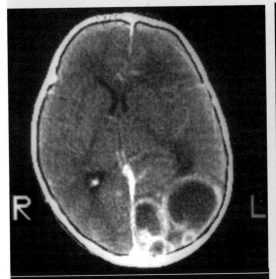

Fig. 40: Multiple brain abscess (congenital cyanotic heart disease)

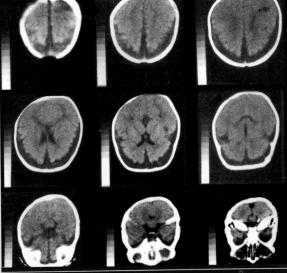

Fig. 41: Frontal atrophy with subarachnoid space widening

Plate 10

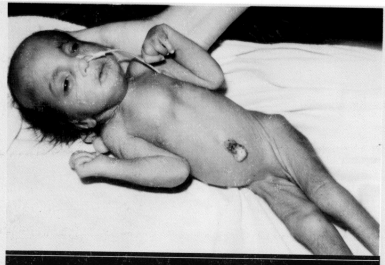

Fig. 42: Arthrogryposis multiplex cogent (congenital muscular dystrophy)

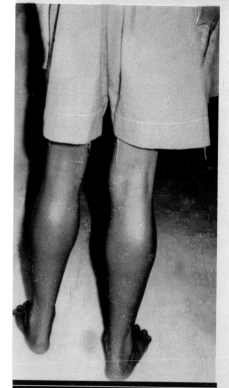

Fig. 43: Pseudohypertropy—Calf muscle (Duschenne muscular dystrophy)

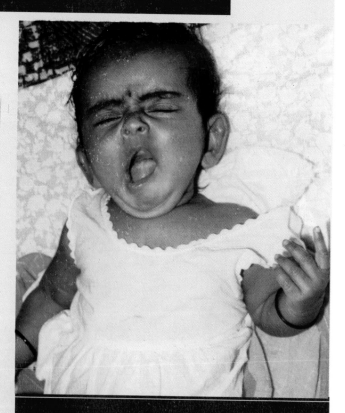

Fig. 44: Hypoplasia of depressor anguli oris (while crying)

Plate   11

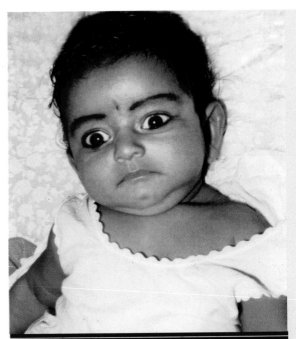

Fig. 45: Hypoplasia of depressor anguli oris
(Normal while not crying)

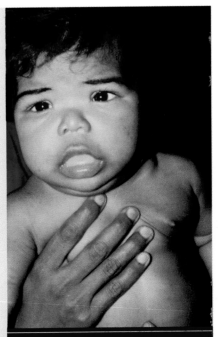

Fig. 46: Congenital hypothyroidism

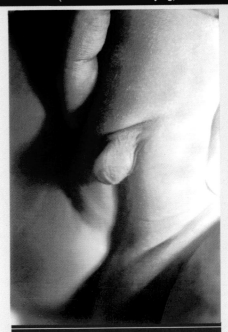

Fig. 47: Clitoromegaly (Congenital adrenal
hyperplasia)

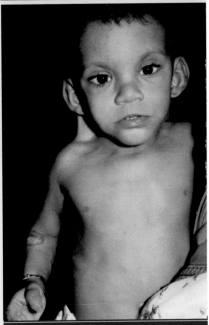

Fig. 48: Webbing of neck and widely
placed nipples (Turner syndrome)

Plate 12

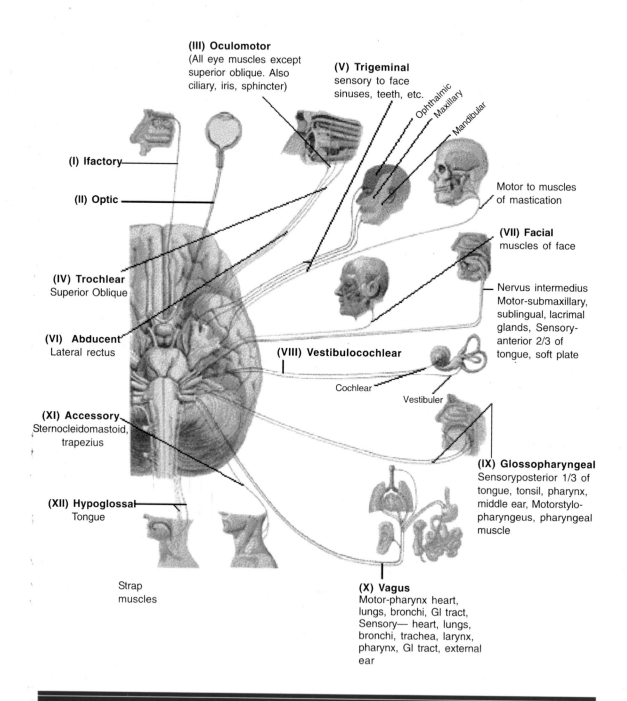

(III) Oculomotor
(All eye muscles except superior oblique. Also ciliary, iris, sphincter)

(V) Trigeminal
sensory to face sinuses, teeth, etc.

Ophthalmic
Maxillary
Mandibular

(I) Ifactory

(II) Optic

Motor to muscles of mastication

(VII) Facial
muscles of face

(IV) Trochlear
Superior Oblique

Nervus intermedius Motor-submaxillary, sublingual, lacrimal glands, Sensory-anterior 2/3 of tongue, soft plate

(VI) Abducent
Lateral rectus

(VIII) Vestibulocochlear

Cochlear

Vestibuler

(XI) Accessory
Sternocleidomastoid, trapezius

(IX) Glossopharyngeal
Sensoryposterior 1/3 of tongue, tonsil, pharynx, middle ear, Motorstylo-pharyngeus, pharyngeal muscle

(XII) Hypoglossal
Tongue

Strap muscles

(X) Vagus
Motor-pharynx heart, lungs, bronchi, GI tract, Sensory— heart, lungs, bronchi, trachea, larynx, pharynx, GI tract, external ear

Fig. 49: The cranial nerves

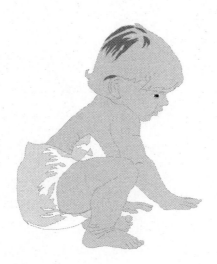

Pediatric Case Recording

SECTION

1.1 HISTORY TAKING

Pediatricians are the custodians of tomorrow as they cater to the future citizens. Some think pediatrics is like veterinary practice as children do not narrate their complaints regarding illness, but it is not so. Older children are good historians like the adults and can contribute to the history of the illness. The smile of the clients and their parents is the greatest reward to the pediatrician. Observation of the child's behavior, feeding vigor and the parental care and attitude can give useful clues to the diagnosis. The consulting room should be attractive with toys appealing to the different age groups. The doctor should greet the child and parents and should make them comfortable before examination.

I. PERSONAL DATA

Name	:
Age	:
Gender	:
Address	:
Informant	: Whether history reliable/not
Date of Admission	:
Date of Examination	:

II. PRESENTING COMPLAINTS: In chronological order.

III. HISTORY OF PRESENT ILLNESS:

Mention if known case of RHD, CCHD, Epilepsy etc.

1. *Fever:* Duration—short (< 2 weeks)
   –prolonged (>2 weeks)
   grade, travel outside to endemic areas
   Continuous–Fluctuation <1° C, never touches baseline
   Remittent—Fluctuation >2° C, never touches baseline
   Intermittent–High fever, touches baseline: Quotidian touches baseline daily. Tertian—alternate day and quartan on 3rd day.
   Eg. Abscess, malaria.

2. *Rigor and chills:* Retroperitoneal/Subdiaphragmatic abscess, UTI–especially in girls associated with hectic intermittent fever, voiding difficulty and pain (chills-symptom/rigor-sign).

3. *Febrile seizure:* Previous history, family history, age group
   - 6 months to 6 years—rarely 3 months to 8 years
   - Not seen in adults
   - Starts as low fever → high grade fever and seizure at peak
   - Rule out intracranial infections–meningitis, metabolic disorders
   - *Simple febrile seizures:* Typical febrile fit
   - Age 6 months to 6 years
   - GTCS < 15 minutes

- Within 24 hours of fever onset
- No neurological sequlae
- No post ictal drowsiness
- *Complex febrile seizures*—Atypical febrile fit
  - Increase in duration > 15 mts, may be partial seizures, family history of afebrile seizures/seizure disorder, abnormal EEG.

4. *Cough:*
   - When it is maximum, day/night (Diurnal variation)
   - URI—Post nasal drip→max. when lying down
   - Asthma→Early morning (2 or 3 o'clock) Spasmodic cough, periodicity, reversibility with bronchodilators, other atopic symptoms, family history.
     - Productive or non productive
     - Colour of sputum (blood stain)
     - Presence of wheeze or stridor, grunt
     - Effect of season→Seasonal variation
     - Response to previous treatment
     - (Lung abscess—foul smelling, copious sputum).

5. *Dyspnoea:*
   - Orthopnea, Paroxysmal Nocturnal Dyspnea—Left ventricular failure. Respiratory Rate—Rise by 6/mt with 1°C fever rise
   - Grade of dyspnea and limitation of activities—mild, moderate, severe
   - Associated edema, decreased urine output (Renal failure)
   - Oxygen saturation.

6. *Palpitation:*
   - Tachycardia
   - Fever—for every 1 degree rise →10 beats rise
   - Rheumatic carditis/myocarditis, arrhythmia
   - Pericardial involvement → pain and rub, effusion.

7. *Vomiting:*
   - Frequency, contents, associated nausea, fever
   - Excessive drowsiness, failure to suck, swallow
   - Headache, convulsions
   - Projectile/non-projectile—Projectile without nausea in increased intracranial pressure
   - Post tussive or not
   - Bilious/non-bilious, blood–Mallory Weiss syndrome following repeated vomiting
   - Associated dehydration/weight loss.

8. *Jaundice:*
   - Family history of jaundice, anaemia
   - Previous babies with jaundice/needing exchange transfusion
   - Family history of neonatal/early infant death due to liver disease
   - Yellow sclera, urine, skin, mucous membrane
   - In carotinemia–skin yellow–not sclera
   - Hemolytic jaundice—Acholuric jaundice
   - Clay coloured stools, itching in obstructive jaundice
   - History of drug intake for fever, viral infections/epidemic fevers
   - Reye's syndrome with drowsiness, convulsion

- History of Anti TB treatment, Cataract in metabolic disorders.

9. *Abdominal pain:*
   - Functional–mostly diffuse/periumbilical
   - Pathologic–localized, away from umbilicus (Appley's law)
   - Drug induced gastritis– blood stained vomiting may occur
   - A/c appendicitis: Pain umbilicus →RIF, fever, vomiting, Abdominal pain, Mc Burney's point tenderness
   - Sick and toxic child, unable to stand erect
   - Rule out surgical causes of A/c abdomen, Abdominal migraine, EEG abnormal in Abd. epilepsy.

10. *Hematemesis:*
    - Drug induced gastritis
    - Viral infections, history of repeated vomiting→fresh blood in vomitus →Mallory Weiss syndrome.

Hematemesis	Hemoptysis
Dark red blood	Fresh blood
Melena	Melena except in swallowed blood
Increased quantity	Decreased quantity
Common in children	Rare in children except Bronchiectasis/Blood stained sputum in pneumonia

11. *Edema:*
    Site–dependent/generalized (anasarca)
    Cardiac disease/renal disease
    Renal–periorbital edema
    Early morning, decrease slightly as day progresses
    Cardiac–dependent, more in the evenings
    Associated Oliguria/not
    Non pitting edema—myxedema.

12. *Hematuria:*
    PSAGN, IGA Nephropathy, Urolithiasis, Loin pain hematuria syndrome, Thin basement membrane disease, tumors, trauma.
    Look for:
    Vomiting, Headache, altered sensorium, abdominal pain
    - Nephrotic syndrome→pervious episodes, no oliguria, hematuria in minimal change lesions
    - AGN → pyoderma/sore throat
    - Oligohydramnios in antenatal period R/o Renal agenesis.

13. *Joint pain:*
    - Which joints–large/small
    - Monoarticular/pauciarticular/polyarticular—5 or more joints
    - Migratory/additive before one subsides
    - Arthritis/arthralgia
    - Difficulty in squatting
    - Abnormal movements, emotional lability→chorea
    - Epistaxis, abdominal pain
    - Previous history of fever, sore throat–similar episodes
    - Continuous fever, multi system involvement
    - Infective endocarditis in heart disease.

14. *Frequency of micturition:*
    - UTI, DM, DI, stones→irritation, pin worm infestation, psychological, neurological disorders.

IV. PAST ILLNESS

- Similar illness in the past
- Previous hospitalisations
- History of allergy, febrile fit, seizure, steroid therapy

- – History of contact with TB patients
- – History of other illness and drug intake
- – CHD, Rheumatic fever prophylaxis.

V. LIFE HISTORY

A. Antenatal/Prenatal History

- Age of mother and father, consanguinity
- Regular ANC
- Para, gravida, abortions
- Whether treatment for infertility
- Antenatal check ups, fetal movements
  - – TT and folifer, calcium intake
  - – History of drug exposure and X-ray exposure, history of fever with rash
  - – History of STORCH intrauterine infections
  - – History of maternal illness
  - – Obstetric–PIH, GDM, PET, Eclampsia
    Nonobstetric–HT, epilepsy, thyroid disorders
  - – History of oligohydramnios, polyhydramnios
  - – USS–normal/anomalies detected (Genetic sonogram).

B. Natal History

- History of APH
- Prolonged rupture of membranes (PROM > 18 hours)
- Maternal fever
- Type of delivery, term, preterm < 37 weeks
- History of prolonged 2nd stage
- Instrumental delivery
- LSCS–Indication–Birth weight.

C. Postnatal/Neonatal History

- First cry/Breath, first feed, cried soon after birth (CSAB)

- Breastfeeding when initiated
- Birth asphyxia—resuscitative measures
- History of seizures
- Meconium-stained liquor
- Neonatal seizure, jaundice, RDS, cyanosis, sepsis
- Days of hospital stay
- Immunization.

VI. DIETARY/NUTRITION HISTORY (Appendix 6)

- Breastfeeding–duration of exclusive breastfeeding, no. of feeds/day
- Sleep duration after feed, urine passed, let down reflex
- Complementary feeds—time and feeds
- Diet prior to onset of illness–calorie and protein content
- 24-hour dietary recall method/food frequency table
- Calorie, protein adequate for age, Vitamins, minerals.

ICMR recommendations (Refer Appendix 6)

Age	Protein	Age	Protein
0-6 m	2.2 g/kg	3-6 years	29 gm
6-12 m	1.8 g/kg	6-10 years	36 gm
1-3 years	22 g	10-12 years	43 gm

Bedside calculation

Age (+100/year)	Energy (Kcal)	Age (+100/year)	Energy (Kcal)
1	1000	7	1600
2	1100	8	1700
3	1200	9	1800
4	1300	10	1900
5	1400	11	2000
6	1500	12	2100

Adolescent Boy – 2400 Kcal			Adolescent Girl – 2200 Kcal		
Food items	Protein	KCalories	Food items	Protein	KCalories
Cow's milk 1 glass/ (200 ml)	6	120	Idli	2	50
Human milk (100 g)	1.1	67	Dosa	2	70
Cooked rice (1 cup)	4	175	Chapathi	2	70
Egg	6	80	Puri	1	35
Fish (30 g)	6	50	Vada/Bonda	1	50
Meat (30 g)	6	50	Uppuma (1 cup)	6	250
Vegetable (30 g)	1	30	Ragiflour (6 tsp)	2	100
Bread (1 slice)	2	70	SAT mix (6 tsp)	2.5	125
Sugar (1 tsp)	–	30	Groundnut (10)	1	20
Jaggery (1 tsp)	–	20	Pappadam	0.5	20
Ghee/Butter (1 tsp)	–	36	Biscuit	0.5	20
Mashed Potato (1 tsp)		40	Coffee (1 cup)	1.5	80
Banana 1	0.5	50	Tea (1 cup)	1.0	60

Holliday and Segar Formula (Energy is calculated for ideal weight and fluid is calculated for present weight)

1st 10 kg.	100/kg.
10-20 kg.	1000 + 50/each kg. > 10
> 20 years	1500 + 20/each kg. > 20

VII. IMMUNISATION HISTORY
(Refer Appendix 9)

• Adequate for age? Fully immunized/ partially immunized/unimmunized–which schedule–UIP/IAP

• If not why? Ignorance/lack of facility/non-availability/illness of child—contraindications/misconceptions

• BCG Scar +/-

• Pulse polio immunization

• Optional vaccines–Hep A, B, HIB, chickenpox, MMR, pneumococcal.

VIII. DEVELOPMENTAL HISTORY
(Refer Appendix 5)

A. Gross Motor

(Control of child over his body—ventral suspension/supine/prone/sitting/standing, walking)—Cephalocaudal progression.

– Head holding–2 m
– Pull to sit no head lag–3 m
– Sits with support–5 m
– Sits without support –8 m
– Rolls over– 6.5 m
– Stand with support –9 m
– Crawls in bed–8 m
– Creeps in bed–10 m
– Cruising around–10 m
– Walk with support and stand without support 1 year

– Walks without support –13 m
– Side step, back step – 15 m
– Tiptoe walking – 2½ years
– Walk backwards and Sideways –15 m
– Runs – 1½ years
– Climbs up stairs (one step at a time) 2 years
– Climb stairs alternate steps–3 years
– Rides tricycle–2-3 years

B. Fine Motor and Adaptive Skills

Hand-eye coordination

– Grasp rattle, reaching for objects, carrying to mouth–4 m
– Transfer of objects hand to hand –5 m
– Hold objects on ulnar side–5 m
– Pincer grasp–index finger + thumb apposition—9 m
– More fine grasp (scooping a pellet)—10 m
– Picks up tiny objects—1 year
– Hold cups in each hand–1 year.

Eye coordination

– Can see red ring or torch in front—1m (4 weeks)
– Can follow objects moved side to side unsteady eyes—2 m
– Can follow objects–side to side steady eyes—2-3 m
– Binocular vision—3-6 m
– Depth perception—6-8 m.

Hand to mouth

– Feeding–spoon to mouth with spilling – 1 year
– Can feed without spoon without spilling – 15 m
– Can feed from cup without spilling – 18 m.

Hand skills

– Turns pages of book (2-3 at a time)—1 year
– Turns pages of book (one at a time)—2 years
– Scribbles on paper with crayon—1-2 years

– Copy horizontal or vertical line—2 years
– Copies a circle—3 years
– Cross or rectangle—4 years
– Tilted cross, triangle—5 years
– Diamond—6 years
– Tower of cubes–2 cubes–15 m, 3 cubes–18 m
– 4-6 cubes—22 m, 9 cubes – 3 years
– Gate out of cubes– 4 years.

Dressing

– Dressing without success, attempts to wear socks —1 year
– Wear shoes and socks—2 years
– Complete dressing—3 years.

C. Language

Turns head to sound of rattle—1 m
Looks around when spoken to—3 m
Cooing—2-3 m
Monosyllable—6 m
Bi-syllables (dada, mama)—9 m
Understands spoken speech—10 m
2 words – with meaning—1 year
4-6 words—15 m
10-15 words—1½ years
2 words sentences and
Pronouns–2 years
250 words–story telling—3 years
Fluent speech—4 years.

D. Social, Personal

– Social smile—2 m
– Recognizes mother—3 m
– Smiles at mirror image—6 m
– Stranger anxiety—7-8 m

- Resist if toy pulled from hand—7 m
- Get toy kept out of reach–9 m
- Bang two cubes—8 m
- Waves bye bye—9 m
- Uncover toys—8 m
- Pretends play—1 year
- Use stick to reach toy—17 m
- Pretend play without doll–17 m
- Knows gender—3 years
- Bladder control—1½ years–dry by day
- 3 years–dry by night (Bowel—1½ years).

IX. FAMILY HISTORY

- Age of father and mother at the time of conception
- Siblings
- History of similar illness in family like TB, DM, RF, CHD
- Neuropsychiatric (Wilson's disease).

X. SOCIO ECONOMIC HISTORY
(Refer Appendix 8)

a. *Income*—per capita income
b. *House*—pucca, concrete, ceiling, brick walls, cement flooring

Kutcha—thatched, mud walls

Floor—impermeable, smooth, concrete, damp proof

Roof—Ht not less than 10 ft.

Rooms—not less than 2 living rooms

Floor area in living room per person not less than 50 sq ft.

Safe water—definition—free from pathogenic agents, free from harmful chemical substances, pleasant to taste, usable for domestic purpose—150 to 200 L/day/head

c. *Source of water*
- Tap/well/boiled water.

Sanitary well
- Not less than 15 m from source of contamination
- At a higher elevation
- Distance between well and house not more than 100 m
- Lining built of bricks and stones upto depth of 6 m
- Lining should be carried 2-3 ft above ground level
- Parapet wall upto height of at least 70 to 75 cm above ground
- Cement concrete platform round the well, 1 m in all directions
- Pucca drain to carry spilled water
- Top of well covered – cement concrete (Uncovered well can't be considered as a sanitary well).

d. *Sanitation*

Does the child wear footwear while walking?

Sanitary latrine

It fulfils following criteria:
- Excreta should not contaminate the ground or surface water
- Excreta should not pollute the soil
- Excreta should not be accessible to flies, rodents, animals and other vehicles of transmission
- Excreta should not create a nuisance due to odor/unsightly appearance

  Eg. Borehole latrine, Dug well latrine, Water seal latrine
- Latrine should not be located within 15 m (50 ft) from source of water supply

- Lower elevation than water supply
- Should have squatting plate, pan, trap
- Water seal–distance between level of water in trap and lowest point in the concave upper surface of trap
- Depth of water seal is 2 cm
- Water seal prevents access by flies and suppresses the nuisance from smell.

e. *Source of pollution*
  - Air pollution, water pollution

- Smokes in house, mosquito/fragrance coils
- Firewood for cooking
- Any pets in house.

XI. PERSONAL HISTORY

For older children/adolescents

Sleep—alteration of daily sleep rhythm

Appetite, Bowel and bladder habits

Addictions.

SECTION 1.2

GENERAL EXAMINATION

I. GENERAL COMMENT—SENSORIUM, GENERAL APPEARANCE, COLOR

A—Alert

V—Verbal Response

P—Pain Response

U—Unresponsive

Ill looking/well looking

Level of consciousness—Glasgow coma scale

Dyspnea

Describe any skin eruption

Halitosis

Abnormal body odour/Smell

Acetone/Fruity   –   Ketosis

Ammonia/fishy.   –   Uremia

Mousy/mercapten   –   Fetor hepaticus

Stale   –   Bronchiotosis

Kerosene   –   Poisoning

II. VITALS

- Temp–in Rt axilla – 37 degree C or 98.4 degree F
- Add 1 degree F for core temp except in NB
- Pulse–rate, rhythm volume, character, no RF delay

All peripheral pulses felt equally on both sides

(bounding pulse, feel dorsalis pedis in PDA)

- RR—regular and abdomino thoracic (count for one minute)

Work of breathing—Lower chest indrawing, suprasternal, subcostal retractions

- BP mm Hg in Right/Left upper limits in supine position
- BP usually between—$70 + (Age \times 2)$ and $90 + (Age \times 2)$
- Cuff size – 3.5 cm, 7 cm or 12.5 cm (standard).

III. HAND—HEAD TO FOOT EXAMINATION SHAKE HAND/OFFER TOY

Start with hands, **"PICCLE"**

Pallor   Clubbing

Icterus   Lymphadenopathy

Cyanosis   Edema

Head: Frontal, parietal and occipital prominence Shape, Scalp, Forehead bulging, Metopic suture, Palpable sutures

Fontannels–depressed/bulging, closed, pulsatile, borders felt/not, size

(AF closes by 9 m–1½ years, PF—3-6 M

If posterior open, R/O hypothyroidism).

Hair: Color, growth, texture, hair lines, hypopigmentation, sparse, seborrheic dermatitis (cradle cap).

Face: Dysmorphism, mooning of face, coarse facies, mid facial hypoplasia, Micrognathia/retrognathia, thick/thin lip, long philtrum, cleft lip palate, Maxilla.

Eyes: Position and slant > 10%—upward (Mongoloid)

Downward—(Antimongoloid)

Pallor, icterus, blue sclera, Vitamin def., Hypertelorism, conjunctival congestion, Microopthalmia, corneal clouding, Coloboma, cataract, Synorphis (eyebrows upto midline), nystagmus, strabismus, muddy conjunctiva.

Ears: Normally set/low set.

Deformities, Preauricular tag/sinuses, Discharge.

Nose: Flat nasal bridge, upturned position, DNS.

Tongue: Glossitis, red/magenta, desquamation, Thrush, Protruded tongue.

Mouth: Oral hygiene, Dental caries, Throat/tonsil, Cleft lip/palate, Vitamin defeciency, Inverted V shaped upper lip, color and no. of teeth, high arched palate.

Neck: Neck length (distance between external occipital protuberance and C_7) Nuchal skinfolds/webbing.

Height divided by neck length (> 13.7 N) Neck—13% of height, Webbing, low hair line, thyroid, lymph nodes, pulsations.

Chest: Pectus excavatum/carinatum).

Absent pectoralis major (Poland syndrome)

Wide spaced nipple, athelia, polythelia (accessory nipples) Sheild chest, precordial bulge, barrel shaped chest.

Abdomen: Umbilical hernia, dilated veins, divarication of recti, distension, ascites.

Genitals: Hernial orifices, ambiguous genitalia, undescended testis, precocious puberty, hydrocoele, scrotal edema, micro penis, macro orchidium.

Upper Limbs: Simian crease, parallel sydney line, poly/syndactyly, arachno dactyly (long finger–Marfan) clinodactyly, camptodactyly, short limbs, broad thumbs, cyanosis, clubbing, palmar erythema, flap, pallor, koilonychia—white nails, dystrophic nails, dermatoglyphics.

Lower limbs: Hypermobility, joint swelling–knee, ankle deformities, weakness, chappal sign (Sandal gap)/Kennedy sulcus, rocker bottom feet (Trisomy 18), pedal edema, arches of foot.

Spine: Dimples, hairy patches, gibbus-swelling, kyphosis, scoliosis, lordosis.

Skin: Neurocutaneous markers, pyoderma scars, S/C emphysema, scabies, skin turgor, phrynoderma, rashes, CFT.

IV. ASSESSMENT OF GROWTH (AUXO-LOGY-ANTHROPOMETRY) (Refer Appendices 1 and 2)

Calculations:

1. Weight for Age (%)

$$\frac{\text{Observed weight}}{\text{Expected weight}} \times 100$$

2. Height for Age (%)

$$\frac{\text{Observed height}}{\text{Expected height}} \times 100$$

3. Weight for Height (%)

$$\frac{\text{Observed weight}}{\text{Expected weight for the height}} \times 100$$

1. *Weight:* Weech's formula (Refer Appendix 1 and 2)

At birth	-	3 kg
3-12 m	-	$\frac{\text{age (m)} + 9}{2}$
1-6 years	-	2 X +8
7-12 years	-	$\frac{7 X - 5}{2}$

IAP Classification (Weight for Age)

71—80%	Gr. I PEM
61—70%	Gr. II
51—60%	Gr. III
< 50%	Gr. IV

Welcome Trust Classification

% of ideal weight	Edema	Interpretation
>80%	–	Normal
60-80%	–	Undernutrition
60-80%	+	Kwashiorkor
<60%	–	Marasmus
<60%	+	Marasmic Kwashiorkor

2. **Height** < 2 y–length

Infantometer Older–stadiometer

Birth	-50 cm
1 years	-75 cm
2 years	-87 cm
4 years	-100 cm (double the birth length)
8 years	-125 cm
12 years	-150 cm (triple the birth length)

(2 × height at 2 years = adult height)

2 – 12 years = 6X + 77 (Weech's formula)

3. **Waterlow Classification for Stunting**

>95%	Normal
90-95%	I degree
85-89	II
<85	III

Waterlow Classification for Wasting

Weight for height	Grade of wasting
>110	Overweight
90-110	Normal
80-90	I degree wasting
70-80	II
<70	III

4. **WHO Grading/Interpetation**

Normal Weight, Normal Height, Normal W for H—Normal nutrition

Decreased W, Normal Height , decreased W for H—A/C malnutrition

Decreased W, decreased H, Normal W for H—C/C malnutrition

Decreased W, decreased H, decreased W for H—A/C on C/C malnutrition

WHO Classification of Undernutrition

Features	Moderate	Severe
a. Edema	No	Yes
b. Weight for Height (Wasting)	70-79%	<70%
c. Height for Age (Stunting)	85-89%	<85%.

5. **Surface Area**

Age	SA
Birth	0.2
3 m	0.3
1 year	0.45
3 years	0.6
6 years	0.75
9 years	0.9
10 years	1.0
Adult	1.73

6. **US:LS Ratio** LS—Symphysis pubis to toes

US (Height—LS)

Age	US/LS	
Birth	1.7:1	US longer→(short
6 m	1.6:1	limbs) achondroplasia
1 year	1.5:1	rickets (bowlegs)
2 years	1.4:1	hypothyroidism
3 years	1.3:1	
4 years	1.2:1	US shorter→(short trunk)
6 years	1.1:1	Spondylo epiphyseal
10 years	1:1	dysplasia, kyphoscolio-sis and MPS

7. **Mid parental height (MPH)—(cm)**

$$\text{MPH (boys)} \quad \frac{\text{paternal H} + \text{maternal height} + 13}{2}$$

MPH (girls) $\dfrac{\text{paternal H + maternal H - 13}}{2}$

6.5 = Mean difference between heights of adult females and males

8. **Head circumferance: Occipitofrontal circumference (OFC)**

Anterior—point above glabella

Posterior—point of occipital protuberance

Birth	35 cm	
3 m	40 cm	
6 m	43 cm	**(2 cm/m – 1st 3 months**
9 m	45 cm	**1 cm/m – next 3 months**
1 years	47 cm	**0.5 cm/m – next 6 months)**
2 years	49 cm	
3 years	50 cm	To say micro/macrocephaly
4 years	50.4cm	a difference of >3 SD should
5 years	50.5 cm	be there i.e., around > 3.75 cm, Compare with **DINE'S**
6 years	51 cm	**formula** (HC in cms) in infants.
9 years	52 cm	
12 years	54 cm	$HC = \dfrac{Length}{2} + 9.5 +/- 2.5$

9. **Chest circumference (CC):** Compare HC and CC (Level of substernal notch in mid inspiration)

Infancy HC >CC, 1 year HC = CC later CC>HC

In PEM CC will remain less than HC > 1 year

CC usually measured upto 2-3 years

Decreased in: Myopathy, Asphyxiating thoracic dystrophy.

10. **Midarm circumference:** (1-5 years)— MAC.

(Lt) triceps, midway between acromion and olecranon.

Arm by side + hanging loose

- 13.5 cms—N
- 12.5-13.5—moderate PEM
- 12.5–severe PEM (< 11—High Risk for Dying is more)
- NB < 9 cm→LBW.

11. **Skinfold thickness:** Over triceps on mid (L) arm (measure from posterior aspect) Harpenden's Calipers—11 mm or more and also subscapularis.

12. **Arm span (AS):**

UL stretched out at right angles to body; Child to stand facing the wall.

Compare with height

AS 2 cms > than height–toddler

AS = height by 7-10 years

AS more than height 2-3 cms—adolescents

AS > height (Marfan Syndrome, Homocysteinuria and spondo epiphyseal dysplasia).

13. **Body mass index (BMI):** Adult

Wt in kg/height in M^2 —18.5–25 N, < 18.5—Chronic energy deficiency.

< 15 moderate PEM

< 13 severe underweight

> 25 overweight (>23 for Indians)

> 30 obesity

Quetlet Index

$\dfrac{w\ (kg)}{Ht\ (cm^2)} \times 100 \to\ > 0.15$ Normal

Ponderal Index

Wt in gm/Ht in cm^3 ×100 — >2.5–Normal

2–2.5 hypoplastic babies (symmetric)

< 2 asymmetric IUGR (malnourished).

14. **SMR** (Tanner's scale)

15. **Teeth development:**

Primary—20 teeth appear between 6 months-2½ years.

(Age in m—6).

Permanent—32 teeth appear between 6 years to adulthood. 3rd Molar (Wisdom Tooth) appear after 18 years.

V. ASSESSMENT OF DEVELOPMENT
(Refer Appendix 5)

- Gross motor
- Fine motor/adaptive
- Language
- Personal social.

$$< 3 \text{ years–DQ} = \frac{\text{Developmental Age}}{\text{Chronological Age}} \times 100$$

$$> 3 \text{ years–IQ} = \frac{\text{Mental Age}}{\text{Chronological Age}} \times 100$$

SECTION 1.3 SYSTEMIC EXAMINATION

I. CARDIOVASCULAR SYSTEM

- Pulse–rate, rhythm, character, volume, Radio-femoral delay
- BP, CFT, JVP
- Peripheral signs of AR, Signs of rheumatic fever.

1. Inspection

- Shape of precordium, dilated veins
- Apex beat, pulsations over precordium, epigastric pulsation
- Suprasternal pulsation, sinuses or scars over chest.

2. Palpation

- Apex–position/site, type, thrill
- Tapping–similar to palpation of a sound
- Forcible–lifts the finger, not sustained
- Heaving–sustained and forceful lifting of fingers
- Palpable P2, thrill, Lt Parasternal Heave →RVH
- Pulsations, rub.

3. Percussion

- Upper border of liver dullness, right border of heart
- Left border of heart.

- PAH→Ribbon sign/dullness in the 2nd left IC space (>2 cm)
- Dullness beyond apex→Pericardial effusion.

4. Auscultation

(Mitral, tricuspid, aortic, pulmonary areas and 2nd AA)

Heart sounds S1,S2, S3 and S4, P2 loud – PAH

Splitting of 2nd sound

— Narrow/wide and fixed, delayed P2, soft P2, single 2nd sound. Single is usually A2 Heart sound

— Muffling in carditis/distant in pericardial effusion

Murmur–Grade

Timing; systolic/diastolic—long/short/pan/ejection/early/late

Intensity–loud/soft or low/high

Pitch–high/low

Conduction/Selective propagation

Change with respiration—Rt sided murmurs better heard in inspiration and Lt sided in expiration

Change with posture—Aortic while leaning forward

Additional sounds–click, opening snap (OS), pericardial rub

Any special characters–Austin Flint (m) Still's murmur, Graham Steel (m).

Grading of Murmur

I. Intense auscultation under ideal conditions/phonocardiogram/intense care needed and may not be audible in all cardiac cycles.

II. Audible in all cardiac cycles.

III. Loud (m) without thrill.

IV. Loud (m) with thrill.

V. Heard with edge of stethoscope.

VI. Heard with chest piece off the chest.

II. RESPIRATORY SYSTEM

1. Inspection

(Remove clothes with permission, whenever indicated)

Upper respiratory tract. Look for adenoid facies, cleft lip palate

- Nose–discharge, bleeding, mucosa and septum, alae nasi flaring → Increased work of breathing
- Nasopharynx or tonsils
- PNS–tenderness
- Throat–mucosa, stridor, hoarseness of voice
- Ear—discharge, mastoid tenderness.

Lower Respiratory Tract (From Larynx to Alveoli)

Inspection

Look for cyanosis and clubbing:

- RR–Rhythm, Abdomino-thoracic/Thoraco Abdominal
- Shape of chest (kyposis/scolosis, Pectus excavatum, carinatum)
- Drooping of shoulders, hollowing of supra/infra clavicular fossa
- Any bulge or recession/indrawing of IC Space
- Retractions—Sub-costal/Inter-costal/Suprasternal
- Respiratory movements—equal on both sides or not
- Trachea–position, Trail's sign in deviation of Trachea
- Dilated veins—flow towards the heart
- Apex beat—visible/not
- Other pulsations.

2. Palpation

- Position of trachea, apex beat
- Respiratory movements equal or not, intercostal tenderness
- Chest expansion, Inspiration, Expiration
- Total (AP: Transverse diameter)
- Vocal fremitus in all areas of lung fields.

3. Percussion

Lung fields:

- Supraclavicular, infraclavicular
- Mammary, inframammary
- Axillary, infra axillary
- Supra scapular, inter scapular, infra scapular
- Upper border of liver dullness, cardiac dullness
- Tidal percussion to eliminate liver dullness, which moves down during inspiration
- Traube's space resonance due to gas in the gastric fundus.

4. Auscultation

Breath sounds:

- Intensity–(n)/decreased/increased
- Type–vesicular/bronchial
- Adventitious sounds–rhonchi, creps (coarse/fine), Pleural rub

– Vocal resonance

Special asucultations–Bronchophony (inc.VR as if near ear piece)

– Whispering pectoriloqy (VR right in ear, while whispering)

– Aegophony/nasal bleat (above the level of effusion)

– Succussion splash in effusion on shaking the patient

– Coin sound.

III. GASTROINTESTINAL SYSTEM

1. Upper GIT

Mouth	Candidiasis, cleft lip/palate
	Lips (colour, eruptions), Gums and teeth
	Dental hygiene, Breath odour→Halitosis
	Tongue–colour, papillations, oral mucosa
	Palate–movement of soft palate, Tonsil., Position of Uvula
Pharynx	Gag reflex, pooling of secretion, congestion
Oesophagus	Tested by asking the patient to swallow water.

2. Inspection–Abdomen

(Examine groin also for completion)

* Shape–(n)/distended/flanks full, scaphoid
* Symmetry
* Movements of all quadrants with resp.
* Umbilicus–(n), everted, hernia
* Dilated venis–direction of flow–away from umbilicus
* Scars and skin over abdomen–striae
* Visible pulsation/peristalsis/lump
* Flanks, hernial orifices, genitalia.

Palpation–Abdomen

* (Warm hand, abdomen relaxed, knees flexed)
* Tenderness–soft/rigid/doughy, temperature
* Feel of abdomen, rebound tenderness
* Palpable pulsations, measure abdominal girth at the level of umbilicus.

Organomegaly

Liver (measure from right costal margin) extend, surface, tenderness, consistency, edge, movement with respiration, pulsatile liver in TR, nodularity.

Gall Bladder—tip of 9th costal cartilage–firm, smooth, globular.

Spleen—extend, swelling with long axis to RIF, consistency moves down with respiration, not bimanually palpable, movement with respiration. Upper border cannot be felt, splenic notch, dull on percussion, lower medial border-notch.

Smooth and firm swelling

Kidneys—bimanual palpation/Ballotable

* Any other mass–fecal mass
* Femorals
* Rectal examination (to be done, when indicated).

4. Percussion

* Upper border of liver dullness
* Any dullness continuous or not with liver/splenic dullness
* Liver span as per age and sex, dullness of renal angles
* Ascites—shifting dullness, fluid thrill, 'Puddle sign' in minimal fluid.

5. Auscultation

* Bowel sound→borborygmi, ileus→ decreased

- Bruit→over liver, epigastrium, spleen, aorta, renal artery
- Rub–hepatic/splenic
- Succussion splash–on shaking abdomen, Seen in–pyloric stenosis, Intestinal obstruction, Paralytic ileus.

IV. CENTRAL AND PERIPHERAL NERVOUS SYSTEM

1. HIGHER FUNCTIONS (ABCDE...)

- Appearance
- Behaviour
- Consciousness
- Delusion
- Emotional status
- Gait
- Hallucination/Handedness
- Intelligence–knowledge, calculations, abstract thinking.
- Memory–recent, remote, past
- Orientation in time, place and person
- Speech–talk, understand spoken speech
- Understand written speech

2. CRANIAL NERVES (Figure 12.1)

I. OLFACTORY NERVE

- Olfactory sensation, olfactory hallucination
- Parosmia, anosmia. In common cold, smell may be temporarily affected.

II. OPTIC NERVE

- Visual acuity–Snellen's chart
- Visual field–confrontation method
- Colour vision–Ishihara chart, 6/6 vision is achieved by around 6 years. Fundus examination.

III. OCCULOMOTOR NERVE
IV. TROCHLEAR NERVE
V. ABDUCENT NERVE

(SO$_4$ (superior oblique) LR 6th Nerve (Lateral Rectus) all others—3rd Nerve) palpebral fissures–equal/not

1. Ptosis, fixed dilated pupil, loss of accommodation
2. Nystagmus and impaired downward movement
3. Strabismus–convergent squint/paralytic squint
   Nystagmus, Diplopia
   — Eye movements in all quadrants—conjugate gaze palsy–Test each eye and both together

Deviation of Eye Ball in Ocular Palsy

Muscle	Nerve	Deviation of eye	Diplopia while looking
Medial Rectus	III	Outward	Towards nose
Superior Rectus	III	Downward and Inward	Upward and Outward
Inferior Rectus	III	Upward and Inward	Downward and Outward
Inferior Oblique	III	Downward and Outward	Upward and Inward
Superior Oblique	IV	Upward and Outward	Downward and Inward
Lateral Rectus	VI	Inward	Towards temple

PUPILS: PEARL—Pupils equal and reacting to light

- Light reflex–direct and consensual (both pupils constricts)
- Accommodation reflex
- Size–compare both pupils
- Shape–circular/irregular/symmetry
- Ciliospinal reflex.

VI. TRIGEMINAL NERVE

Whisp of cotton used to test sensation

Motor–muscles of mastication (Temporalis, masseter)

Open mouth–jaw deviated to paralysed side (due to healthy pterygoids)

Able to chew/not

Sensory–touch, pain, temp, vibration senses (loss of sensation over skin of face, Salivary buccal and lacrimal secretion decreased, corneal ulcers +)

Conjunctival reflex (Corneal reflex is better avoided)—Afferent V and efferent VII

Jaw jerk–Exaggerated in UMN lesions.

VII. FACIAL NERVE

Sensory: Taste sensation anterior 2/3 of tongue.

Motor: Wrinkling of forehead, Tight closure of eyelids, Bell's phenomena (eye ball rolls upward while closing), Blowing, Whistling, Showing of teeth, Nasolabial fold, Deviation of angle of mouth to opposite side, Sprouting lips, Hyperaccusis, Collection of food and saliva in mouth on affected sides, Testing of platysma muscle.

UMN: Lower part of face affected (muscles of upper part of face spared due to bilateral innervation, Taste is not affected.

LMN: Bell's Palsy—one side of face involved completely, Loss of taste, Hyperaccusals (discomfort to loud sound due to

stapedius paralysis), Atrophy of facial muscles.

Secreto-motor: Epiphora, salivation.

VIII. VESTIBULO-COCHLEAR NERVE

Vestibular part—Vertigo, Nystagmus

Cochlear part—Tinnitus

Acuity of hearing—Watch test.

Rinne's test:

Tuning fork in front of ear and then over the mastoid bone.

Air Conduction and Bone Conduction

AC better than BC—normal, BC better than AC in middle ear disease.

Weber's test:

Tuning fork placed on midline of skull

Sound better heard in deaf ears → conduction loss

Sound better heard in better ear→sensory neural.

IX. GLOSSOPHARYNGEAL NERVE

(Supplies middle pharyngeal sphincter and stylopharyngeus)

Sensory: Posterior 1/3 tongue taste, Post pharyngeal wall

Reflex: Gag reflex/pharyngeal reflex.

X. VAGUS

(Motor to soft palate , pharynx and larynx, Sensory and motor for resp. passage and Parasympathetic ganglia—abdomen and viscera)

- Nasal regurgitation, nasal twang
- Position of uvula, palatal movements
- Arch of palate, palatal /gag reflex.

Palatal Palsy

- Affected side flat and immobile (median raphe pulled towards normal side.

- Sternocleido mastoid—weakness on rotation of chin to opposite side.
- Trapezius–upper fibres—shrugging of shoulder against resistance. Lower fibres–bracing of back.

XII. HYPOGLOSSAL NERVE

(Motor to tongue and depressor of hyoid) protrusion of tongue, deviation (tongue pushed to paralysed side)

- Movement of tongue, wasting of tongue
- Fasciculations and fibrillations.

3. MOTOR SYSTEM

(Inspection and Palpation)

1. Bulk of Muscles

Bilateral Midarm circum, Mid forearm circum

Mid thigh circum, Mid calf circum

- Wasting (small, soft, flabby), fibrosis (hard to feel)
- Contractures (due to shortening)
- Pseudo hypertrophy (large but weak muscles in DMD, Hypothyroidism)
- True hypertrophy.

2. Tone of Muscle

- Assess by passive shaking and palpation
- Hypotonia
- Hypertonia—Clasp knife—spasticity
- Cog wheel rigidity

3. Power of Muscle

Grade 0 - No flicker of activity/ contraction

Grade 1 - Flicker of contraction

Grade 2 - Movement if gravity eliminated

Grade 3 - Movement against gravity

Grade 4 - Movement against some resistance

Grade 5 - Normal power

4. Coordination

- Finger nose test with open and closed eyes
- Pick the nose test
- Dysdiadochokinesia—alternate supination and pronation in cerebellar disorders
- Heel Knee test.

5. Gait

Walking in a straight line, walking around a chair.

4. SENSORY SYSTEM

Superficial

Pain, Temperature, Light touch

Deep Sensations

Sense of Pressure, Sense of Position, Sense of Movement.

Cortical Sensation

One point localization, Two point discrimination, Touch localization, Steriognosis–identifying a coin etc. by touch.

Graphesthesia—understanding what is written on palms with closed eyes.

5. REFLEXES

Superficial

Conjunctival	Afferent V and Efferent VII
Abdominal	T6- T12
Cremasteric	L1-L2
Anal	S3-S4
Plantar	S1- S2

Babinski sign—Upgoing Plantars can also be elicited by:

Oppenheim's sign—Firm pressure over tibia from above downwards

Chaddock's sign—Scratch around lateral malleolus

Gordon's sign—Firm squeeze over tendo-achillis/calf muscle

Hoffmann's sign—For upper limb (Babinski equivalent) for lesions above C$_7$. Adduction of thumb and flexion of finger on flicking the nail of middle finger

Wartenberg sign—For upper limb in pyramidal lesions. Adduction and flexion of thumb on pressure after locking the fingers with the patient.

Deep Tendon Reflexes

Jaw Jerk	Pons
Biceps	C5-C6
Triceps	C7-C8
Radial supinator	C5-C6
Knee Jerk	L3-L4
Ankle Jerk	L5-S1

Grading of Tendon Jerks

Grade 0	Absent even with reinforcement
Grade 1	Sluggish +
Grade 2	Normal ++
Grade 3	Brisk +++
Grade 4	Exaggerated ++++

Primitive Reflexes

These get released due to CNS dysfunction/degeneration

Glabellar tap (Diffuse cortical dysfunction)

Palmo – Mental Reflex (Bilateral frontal lobe lesion)

Grasp reflex (Contralateral frontal lobe lesion)

Ciliospinal reflex (Cervical sympathetic paralysis)

Sphincters—Bowel and bladder dysfunction.

6. SKULL AND SPINE

7. CEREBELLAR SIGNS

Ataxia, Nystagmus, Coordination, Dysdiadochokinesia

8. SIGNS OF MENINGEAL IRRITATION
Neck rigidity, Kernig sign and Brudzinskis sign.

9. NEONATAL REFLEXES

Reflex	Age of onset	Age of disappearance
Moro	Birth	12 weeks
Stepping	Birth	6 weeks
Placing	Birth	6 weeks
Sucking	Birth	4-7 months
Rooting	Birth	4-7 months
Palmar grasp	Birth	4-6 months
Plantar grasp	Birth	10 months
Tonic neck	2 months	4-6 months
Landau	3 months	24 months
Parachute	9 months	Persists for life

10. EXAMINATION OF JOINTS

- History—duration, swelling, limitation of movement
- Patellar tap, range of movements
- Deformities, tenderness, measurement of limb length.

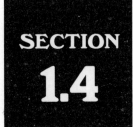

SECTION
1.4 SUMMARY AND DIAGNOSIS

The history and examination findings should be summarised and Diagnosis/Differentials should be written:

1. EXAMPLE OF A SUMMARY AND DIAGNOSIS

A six-year-old child from low socio-economic status and history of sore throat is presenting with fever and migratory polyarthritis. On examination, febrile, polyarthritis+and pallor+, tachycardia, raised JVP, cardiomegaly, pansystolic murmur in mitral area and grade II PEM (IAP).

2. DIAGNOSIS

Example:

Acute rheumatic fever with polyarthritis and carditis—Mitral regurgitation, CCF, anemia and grade II PEM (IAP).

DIFFERENTIAL DIAGNOSIS

Example:

Fever of unknown origin (FUO) with Hepatosplenomegaly.

1. Infections—IMN, Disseminated TB, typhoid fever, HIV (rare).

2. Malignancies—Leukemia, lymphoma.

3. Liver disorders—Chronic active hepatitis, compensated cirrhosis (rare)

4. Collagen vascular disease, systemic onset JRA, SLE (rare).

5. Storage/metabolic disorders with infection.

   MPS, Glycogen storage disease, Osteopetrosis (rare).

6. Others—Macrophage activation syndrome (MAS), Histiocytosis, Amyloidosis (rare).

14

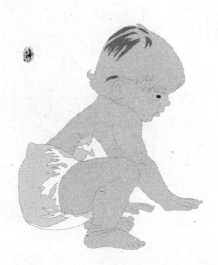

2

Growth and Nutrition

AN ADOLESCENT CHILD WITH SHORT STATURE AND DELAYED PUBERTY

A 15-year-old boy waiting for plus one school admission presented to the adolescent clinic with history of poor growth and delayed puberty. He was good in studies, but appeared depressed due to poor growth and childish voice. He was normal at birth, but was small since childhood.

On examination: Diet intake was adequate. General and systemic examinations were within normal limits except for growth failure, SMR Stage I,

Weight 36 kg, Height 145 cm, OFC 53 cm and upper segment: lower segment ratio 1:1. Bone Age: wrist—7 carpals, epiphysis of lower end of ulna and radius present, elbow—capitulum not fused with shaft. Blood and urine exam normal. Thyroid function test normal.

Parent's height: Father-165 cm, Mother-152 cm.

DIAGNOSIS AND DISCUSSION

Short stature due to Constitutional/Maturational Growth Delay (MGD). DD: Hypopituitarism, hypogonadism. (Also Refer Section 13.1)

The boy is healthy and does not have any systemic diseases, skeletal dysplasia, metabolic errors, chromosomal anomalies etc. to account for growth failure and delayed puberty.

Analysis of present growth shows that weight and height are below 3rd centile (NCHS) and OFC is between 3rd and 50th centile. The 3rd centile values are weight - 40.9 kg, Height 153.8 cm and

OFC 52 cm and the 50th centile values are weight 56.7 kg, Height 169 cm and OFC 54.8 cm, Height age=11.5 years, weight for height age= 37 kg., Bone age reduced (Appendix 3).

Auxology (Refer Appendix and Section I)

Weight for Age %=36/56.7 × 100= 63.5%

(61-70.9% grade II PEM- IAP Classification as applied to underfives).

Height for Age % = 145/169 × 100 = 85.7% (85-90% - 2° stunting—Waterlow).

Weight for Height % = 36/37 × 100 = 97.3 i.e., >95 %

(No wasting—Waterlow).

US:LS ratio reveals, he has proportionate short stature, corresponding to his age. This will practically rule out disproportionate dwarfism like, skeletal dysplasias and also hypothyroidism with infantile proportions. Even though, his weight for age is low and he is stunted, his weight for height is normal. So, it is clear that he is not a case of acute malnutrition.

The three possibilities here are: (i) he is not having acute malnutrition, but chronic malnutrition, (ii) he is a treated case of acute malnutrition and (iii) he is a case of short stature. There is no history of chronic malnutrition resulting in nutritional dwarfing in this child. **So the differential diagnosis includes constitutional delay of growth/Maturational growth delay (MGD) and hypopituitarism/hypogonadism.**

Analysis according to family history: Constitutional/maturational delay is the most likely diagnosis, which is due to a slow running clock leading to late blooming. These children are **'late bloomers'** and usually there will be a family history of similar delayed growth especially in one of the parents, especially the father. This boy's father also gave history of similar delayed growth on subsequent interrogation.

Analysis according to bone age: His bone age was less than his chronological age. In malnutrition and constitutional delay, bone age will be less than chronological age, but equal to height age. This is a positive sign, denoting further potential for growth. In genetic/familial short stature, the bone age will be equal to chronological age and the potential for further growth is less as the bones will fuse earlier. In hypopituitarism and hypothyroidism, bone age will be more retarded than both chronological age and height age. Bone age is assessed using the **Greulich-Pyle bone age atlas or Tanner-Whitehouse scoring system.** The former consists of representative hand radiographs for both gender at all ages and the best match for the child should be selected to get the bone age of the child. The latter scoring system is precise, but time consuming. The **Bayley Pinneau charts** can be used to assess the extent of growth already occurred and the growth potential left in the child. Thus with the bone age, the predicted adult height can be assessed (Refer Appendix 3).

Analysis according to Mid Parental Height (MPH): MPH is the **'target height'** for the child, i.e., the predicted adult height with a variability of plus or minus 5 cm.

MPH = (165+ 152+13 *) /2 = 165 cm (*-13 is taken for girls).

The child's growth potential is 165 cm as per MPH. Now find out the percentile of 165 cm corresponding to 18 years as per the gender of the child. Comparison is made to that of 18 years, the time when maturity is attained. This target height is above 3rd centile, approximately 5th centile. Thus the child's growth potential is in the

5th centile, but he is now at 3rd centile. Hence, there is reason for concern. Otherwise reassurance is all that is needed. It is important to plot the height on a growth chart and mark MPH on it. Even when it is < 3rd centile, a line can be drawn below 3rd centile curve parallel to the 3rd centile curve.

Puberty is said to be delayed if secondary sexual characters do not appear in boys by 14 years and in girls by 13 years of age.

In constitutional delay, reassurance works in majority of cases. But, if psychological stress is more and if the child is 14-15 years old, testosterone monthly injections may be given for 3 months to kick off puberty in boys. In girls, low dose cyclical pills may be given.

If there is no family history of constitutional delay and if signs of puberty are not appearing after a period of observation for 3-6 months, growth hormone assay may be done to rule out hypopituitarism using clonidine stimulation test. Basal level of GH is done early morning. Then 2 samples are taken 30 minutes and 1 hour after giving 5 mcg/kg/dose of clonidine. It may also be done after 20 minutes of exercise. Insulin stimulation test is not done as it is dangerous especially in a case of hypopituitarism with associated hypoglycemia. The other agents used are glucagon, arginine, L dopa. Three days of estrogen priming is also said to be beneficial. GH value < 7 mcg/L is diagnostic of hypopituitarism and GH >10 mcg/L rules out hypopituitarism. GH hormone therapy is discussed in Chapter 13.

In central hypogonadism, FSH and LH will be low and in peripheral cause, S. testosterone or estradiol will be low. LH is a better indicator than FSH.

The causes and types of short stature are given in Tables 2.1 and 2.2.

The term 'maturational growth delay (MGD)' is preferred to the conventional 'constitutional growth delay (CGD), Constitutional refers to inherent and largely unmodifiable compared to the term maturational.

SECTION 2.2 AN INFANT WITH FAILURE TO THRIVE (FTT)

A four-month-old female baby was admitted with loose stool, poor feeding and fever. Baby was born full term with a birth weight of 2.6 kg. Baby was on breast milk, but was stopped abruptly due to mother's employment in a local factory. Baby was on dilute cow's milk 1:1 dilution, 2 glass per day since last 2 weeks and baby was started on 3 tsp cooked ragi powder in a feeding bottle.

On examination: Febrile, AFT normal, respiratory rate 40/mt, pulse rate 120/mt, thirst not increa-sed, skin turgor normal, hair sparse. Socioe-conomic status—poor.

Auxology: Weight 3.0 kg, length 55 cm and OFC 39 cm.

Loose skinfold noted in axilla, groin, chest and abdomen. Baby had social smile, partial head control, voluntary grasp and cooing sounds+.

Liver enlarged 2.5 cm below costal margin. Other systems within normal limits. Hb 9 g/dl, TC 13500/cum. P75%, L24 % and E 1%. CRP 8 mg/dl.

DIAGNOSIS AND DISCUSSION

Severe malnutrition clinically presenting as marasmus (non-edematous malnutrition) with acute diarrheal disease, no dehydration and probable sepsis/meningitis.

Sepsis is probable due to positive CRP, leukocytosis and associated fever and poor feeding. LP is indicated before starting antibiotics.

AF may not be full in partially treated meningitis and in cases with dehydration. Antibiotics like ampicillin and gentamicin or 3rd generation cephalosporin and amikacin may be started after doing blood culture and LP, as per the hospital protocol.

Baby is severely malnourished. Nutritional intake is inadequate. Four-month-old baby should be ideally on exclusive breastfeeding. Abrupt stoppage of breast milk, early introduction of dilute cow's milk and dilute and unhygienic comple-mentary food has led to diarrheal disease. Poor socio-economic status and poor health aware-ness of the family adds to the present illness.

Auxology

Weight for Age = 3/6 × 100 = 50% (Grade IV PEM-IAP)

Height for Age = 55 /62 × 100 = 88.7% (2° stunting - Waterlow)

Weight for height = 3/4 × 100 = 75% (2° wasting-Waterlow)

OFC 39 cm-expected 41cm (2 cm below normal).

Baby has acute on chronic malnutrition due to presence of both wasting and stunting. With respect to development, there is slight gross motor delay which is attributable to malnutrition.

Another question to be answered is that: Is the baby eligible for any allowance with respect to growth and development?

The baby was full term with a birth weight of 2.6 kg and does not have any congenital anomalies to suggest a hypoplastic baby. Only preterm babies and hypoplastic babies with reduced growth potential are eligible for such allowance like growth and development on par with corrected age instead of chronological age or unique growth as in case of syndromes. This baby is not eligible for any such allowances as the baby is not preterm and not hypoplastic.

What Nutritional Advice should be given to the Mother? (Refer Appendix 6 and 7)

Even though breastfeeding is stopped, she should try relactation by restarting suckling. This will promote orofacial growth of the baby (non-nutritive sucking), mother-infant bonding and relactaction and optimum growth especially brain development. Meanwhile, she should give 150-165 ml/kg undiluted cow's milk/formula milk, whichever is affordable.

Fluid Requirement:

Milk/Fluid=3 x 150=450 ml and 3 × 165= 595 ml, i.e. 500-600 ml/day. Maximum upto 200 ml/kg may be given in hyperalimentation.

As the baby is marasmic, the requirement is 200 kcal/kg and 4 g/kg/day protein. At present the baby is getting 400 ml dilute milk amounting to 200 ml undiluted milk. That provides roughly 130 kcals. 3 tsp ragi flour gives 50 kcals making a total of 180 kcals and the protein intake is 7 g/day.

Energy required = 3 × 200 = 600 kcal/day.

Protein requirement = 3 × 4 = 12 g/day.

500 ml of dilute cow's milk can be converted to high energy milk to give 500 kcals by adding 1 tsp sugar and ½ tsp coconut oil to each 100 ml milk. Visible fat intake may be restricted to 10-15% of the total energy intake. In this case, upto 10 ml of oil can be added to give 80 kcals, which is <15% of the total energy intake. In the usual diet, the fat intake is 25% of the energy from invisible fat. It can be pulled to 35-40% by adding visible oil. Further oil will lead to a ketogenic diet.

The rest 100 kcals can be made up by breast milk if relactation is feasible. If not, 3 tsp cereal flour and 2 tsp sugar with 100 ml cow's milk may be given to make up the energy. The baby should also be prescribed calcium, phosphorus, iron, zinc and other micronutrients including vitamins (Refer Appendix 6).

The normal requirements in health are roughly as follows:

Protein→2-2.5 gm/kg/24 hours.

Carbohydrate→5 gm/kg/24 hours.

Fat→0.5-1 gm/kg/24 hours.

Dehydration should be prevented by giving approximately 10 ml/kg/dose ORS per each purge till diarrhea stops. Hypo-osmolar ORS is preferable in young infants. Fresh fruit juice also may be started after control of diarrhea to supply vitamin C and potassium.

Failure to thrive (FTT) is diagnosed when a baby is persistently below 5th centile or is showing down crossing of two major centiles over a period of given time, say 3-6 months or so. The major centiles are 3rd, 5th, 10th, 25th, 50th, 75th, 90th, 95th and 97th.

This is a case of low intake FTT, unlike in hyperthyroidism or malabsorption, which may be a high intake FTT. As no organic cause is detected for the FTT and as the low intake is due to poverty, ignorance etc, this is a case of Non-Organic/Environmental FTT.

Nutrition recovery syndrome: It represents apparent deterioration in the 3rd week of treatment, resolving by the 6th week. The clinical features include abdominal distension, increasing hepatomegaly, hypertrichosis and tremors (Kwashi shake). The causes may be increased protein/solute load, nutritent imbalance between supply and demand, dyselectrolytemia, rapid recovery of endocrine organs, dysmyelination and neurotransmitter imbalance.

The different causes of FTT are given in Table 2.3. 80% of the cases are due to non-organic causes and only 20% are due to organic causes.

SECTION 2.3 — AN EXTREMELY PRETERM BABY WITH FAILURE TO THRIVE

A preterm baby, 6-week-old male, born at 28 weeks gestation was brought with feeding difficulty and poor weight gain. Birth weight was 1 kg, length 37 cm and OFC 25 cm.

Mother had a precipitate labor, no history of APH. Baby was on breastfeeding and dilute formula feeds and multivitamins.

On examination: Baby alert, sucking at breast. Weight 1.4 kg, length 42 cm and OFC 29 cm. Social smile not attained. Vitals stable and systemic examination and baseline investigations were within normal limits.

DIAGNOSIS AND DISCUSSION

FTT with severe malnutrition, probably due to non-organic cause and faulty feeding:

Obviously, the baby has growth faltering. The first attempt is to analyse the growth at birth with the help of intrauterine curves (Refer Appendix 2). Accordingly a 28 weeker is expected to have an ideal weight of 1.2 kg, length 38 cm and OFC 26 cm (50th centile values). This baby's growth at 28 weeks was around the 10th centile, the corresponding 10th centile values are: weight–1 kg, length 36.5 cm and OFC 24.5 cm.

And on analysing the present situation, the baby born at 28 weeks gestation is now 6 weeks old and the corrected age is that of a 34 weeker. As the baby has not crossed the expected date of childbirth (EDC), his present growth should be equated to intrauterine growth curves of a 34 weeker. **He cannot be compared to that of a 1½ month (6 weeks) old normal baby born at term.**

For a 34 weeker, as per intrauterine growth curves, the 50th centile values are: weight 2.2 kg, length 45.5 cm and OFC 31.5 cm and the 10th centile values are: weight 1.8 kg, length 43 cm and OFC 29.5 cm. This baby's measurements are below the 10th centile. Considering the fact that the baby's growth was around the 10th centile at birth, and now it is below the 10th centile, there is definite growth retardation. The cause for the failure to thrive is probably faulty feeding. There is no obvious organic cause for the FTT. In a preterm extremely low birth weight (ELBW) baby, the nutrition should support growth on par with the baby's potential, and in this case, it is the 10th centile and it should also promote catch up growth in order to catch up with the peer group by 1- 2 years of age. This baby is not a hypoplastic baby with reduced growth potential. So, feeding should be optimized. The baby should be given a fair trial of exclusive breastfeeding, prolonged suckling and also expressed breast milk (EBM) after finishing sucking. EBM will promote growth in the baby with minimal effort and energy expenditure and will lead to complete emptying of breast, which will promote more milk production. Proper nutrition and micronutrient supplements should be ensured to the mother with adequate intake of fluids (10-12 glasses/day). She should also be advised galactogogues like LACTIN power available in the market.

Indigenous home remedies may also be tried. Metaclopromide 10 mg 1-1-1 × 5 days is also useful.

If weight gain is not adequate or EBM is practically nil, infant milk substitutes (IMS) may be prescribed as it is now medically indicated. This can be done with due respect to the 6th clause in the ten steps and ten policies of Baby Friendly Hospital Initiative (BFHI) i.e; no food or drink should be given unless medically indicated. IMS can be prescribed in a dose of 150-165 ml/kg/day. In hyperalimentation, upto 200 ml/kg may be given. The formula feed should be reconstituted as 1:1 formula (1 level scoop powder in 30 ml). Cow milk is not desirable, but if it is the only solution due to poverty, it is advisable not to dilute it, as dilution will lead to lesser calories and less nitrogen content. The total calories and net nitrogen content are the same in breast milk and cow milk. But in view of the high osmolarity and high solute load and chance for constipation, boiled and cooled water may be offered in between if necessary. It is also very important not to use feeding bottle that leads to contamination, acute diarrhea and also nipple confusion. Gokarnam (Palada) feeding or cup and spoon feeding is recommended.

The next question to be answered is this: **Has the baby got adequate growth potential for normal growth and catch up growth?** The answer is yes, because this LBW baby was normal at birth except for prematurity. He was not having congenital anomalies suggestive of a hypoplastic baby with reduced growth potential. Such hypoplastic babies present as symmetric IUGR, with very low weight, length and OFC.

The ponderal index (PI) of this baby at birth was 1.97 indicating a LBW baby who is malnourished and not hypoplastic. (Normal PI >2.5, malnourished <2 and hypoplastic 2-2.5). Hence, this baby has adequate growth potential for normal growth and catch up growth if proper nutrition is provided. However, as this is a case of FTT, all attempts should be made to rule out organic or biological causes of FTT like systemic malformations or dysfunctions including inborn errors of metabolism. He has not attained social smile, but is eligible for some more time to achieve it. The baby may take at least 8 weeks post term to attain it. Here the corrected age is only 34 weeks gestation.

The baby should be given minerals like calcium, phosphorus, zinc and iron along with multivitamins. Iron is started only later. Vitamin E is important to prevent hemolytic anemia of prematurity and Vitamin D is important to prevent osteopenia of prematurity. This may become evident when rapid growth and catch up occurs. Rickets will not manifest when there is no growth, but will manifest when growth spurt starts especially during nutritional rehabilitation. It can occur as early as 8 weeks of age with wide metaphysis and double maleoli.

$$\text{Ponderal Index} = \frac{\text{Weight (g)}}{\text{Height (cm)}^3}$$

Postnatal growth velocity is given in Table 2.8. complete catch up in weight may take upto 24 m, length upto 40 m and OFC upto 18 m.

<table>
<tr><td>SECTION
2.4</td><td># A TERM BABY WITH CONGENITAL ANOMALIES AND FTT</td></tr>
</table>

A 2-month-old male baby with facial dysmorphism and Congenital Heart Disease, large VSD was brought with recurrent respiratory infection and congestive cardiac failure. He was born term with 1.4 kg at birth, length 40 cm and OFC 29 cm.

At present, he is 2 kg, length 47 cm and OFC 32.5 cm. He is on breast milk and 4 oz of 1:1 dilute cow milk. Social smile attained.

DIAGNOSIS AND DISCUSSION

FTT—Hypoplastic Baby with Acyanotic Congenital Heart Disease, Large VSD, CCF and severe malnutrition (Grade IV PEM-IAP) and 3° stunting.

He is a term very low birth weight (VLBW) baby with IUGR. Ponderal index at birth was 2.2. He is a hypoplastic baby with congenital anomalies and reduced growth potential. It is a case of symmetric IUGR with low weight, length and OFC. All measurements were below the 3rd centile. The expected measurements of a normal 2-month-old baby are: weight 5 kg, length 58 cm and OFC 40 cm.

Now, let us analyze his growth as per his chronological age. In comparison to a 2-month-old baby with normal growth potential.

His weight is only 40% (2/5 × 100)—Grade IV protein energy malnutrition according to IAP classification.

Length is 81% (47/58 × 100) 3° stunting according to Waterlow classification and

OFC is 32.5 as against 40 cm (3 standard deviations below the normal).

All these parameters are unacceptably low.

Next query to be answered is that: Is he eligible for any allowance than a normal child and Is he going to follow a unique growth pattern? The answer is Yes. Being a hypoplastic baby with reduced growth potential, he is unable to catch up with peer group. Such babies may follow unique growth pattern and may need disease specific or syndrome specific growth charts for comparison (Appendix 4).

After giving allowances, let us see where he stands when he has completed 8 weeks post term. Considering the fact that his potential for both normal growth and catch up growth is reduced, let us analyze his present growth. He is 2 months or 8 weeks old. As there is practically no weight gain in the first 10 days of life, except regaining birth weight after initial loss. So, his weight gain may be approximated for 7 weeks instead of 8 weeks. This exercise is necessary only in very young babies less than 3 months old. Assuming a weight of gain of 200 g/week, he is expected to gain 1.4 kg (7 × 200 = 14000 g).

Thus the expected weight is at least 2.8 kg and expected length is 46 cm (3 cm/month—40+6 =46 cm) and expected OFC is 29 + 4 = 33 cm (2 cm/month).

But, it should be remembered that this rate of growth will not allow any catch up growth. To attain catch up growth, LBW babies should grow faster than this usual growth (Table 2.8).

Anthropometry after giving allowance for being hypoplastic

Weight for age (%) - $\underline{2/2.8 \times 100} = 71\%$ (Grade I PEM- IAP).

Length for age (%) - 47/46 ×100 =100% (No stunting).

Weight for height % - 2/2.9 × 100 = 69% 3° wasting—Waterlow (This is according to intrauterine curve, Refer Appendix 2).

OFC—32.5 cm as against an expected of 33 cm.

Now we can see that if feeding is optimized, he can grow at a unique curve acceptable for the child's condition. It is the weight which has to improve more than the length and the OFC.

His medical conditions like LRI, CCF and electrolyte imbalance should be corrected. Breastfeeding and EBM is the best food for the baby as it is lowest in salt content. EBM will avoid exhaustion and energy expenditure on sucking. Emptying will promote more milk production also. If EBM is less, IMS can be prescribed at a dose of 2/3 the fluid requirement in view of CCF. The baby should also be on multivitamins, iron, zinc, calcium and potassium. Developmentally, attainment of social smile is a good sign in this baby and the development is acceptable for a 2-month-old baby. The baby is likely to benefit more from optimum nutrition and early stimulation.

Disease specific growth charts are included in Appendix 4.

SECTION 2.5 AN INFANT WITH SEVERE MALNUTRITION

An eight-month-old female baby was admitted with poor feeding, cough and oral thrush. She was born to a mother with RHD, who died in the immediate postnatal period. She was under the care of the mother's sister. Baby had only BCG and OPV. Dietary intake was 1:1 dilute cow milk x 2 glasses, 1 cup tea, 3 biscuits and 3 teaspoon ragi+2 tsp sugar in dilute form given in a feeding bottle. Baby could roll over and had head control and voluntary grasp and social smile.

On examination: She was lethargic, irritable, hypotonic, hypothermic with loose skinfolds in axilla, groin, chest and back. Buccal pad of fat was present. Scaling and erythema of skin creases were present. Nails were grown with dirt inside. Liver was palpable 2.5 cm below costal margin. Oral thrush, cheilosis and glossitis + Dryness of skin and conjunctiva +. Bilateral pitting edema + Respiratory rate 42/mt, pulse 90/mt, temp 36.5°C. Bilateral crepitation present. Birth weight was not known.

Present weight 4 kg, length 62 cm, OFC 42 cm. Hb 8.5 g/dl, TC 8500/cumm, P 60, L30, E10, peripheral smear: hypochromic microcytic anemia with increased red cell distribution width (RDW). ESR 40 mm/1st hour, CRP 10 mg/dl. X-ray chest showed increased bronchovascular markings and patchy opacities. Urine albumin trace, pus cells 4-5/HPF, sugar nil.

DIAGNOSIS AND DISCUSSION

Non Organic FTT due to faulty feeding and multi deprivation, Grade IV PEM-IAP clinically presenting as marasmic kwashiorkor, multiple micronutrient deficiency disorders (MDDs) and 2nd degree stunting, Sepsis and Bronchopneumonia. This is a case of edematous malnutrition.

This female baby is an example of multi deprivation; deprived of nutrition and maternal tender loving care (TLC), breastfeeding and proper complementary feeding, immunization, growth monitoring, medical care, personal hygiene and environmental health.

On analyzing growth, we see that all anthropometric parameters are below the expected range.

Weight for Age %—4/8.2 × 100 = 49%—Grade IV PEM-IAP.

Length for Age %—62/69 × 100 = 89.8%—2nd degree stunting – Waterlow.

Weight for Height (height age = 4 months)—4/6 × 100 =66.6 %—3rd degree wasting waterlow.

OFC—42/44 cm, 2 cm less than normal.

Baby has clinical features of marasmus like loose skinfolds in the axilla, groin, thigh, buttocks, chest and back. As buccal pad of fat is preserved, it is 3rd degree marasmus. As edema is there, it is a case of Marasmic kwashiorkor. Baby has other features of kwashiorkor like skin changes, apathy, hepatomegaly and mucus membrane changes.

Investigations point to iron deficiency anemia. Other MDDs are vitamin A deficiency and B complex deficiency. EFA deficiency, protein deficiency and zinc deficiency lead to skin changes. Hypomagnesemia, cerebral edema and electrolyte imbalance may be the cause for apathy.

Fever, tachypnea and tachycardia are absent in spite of pneumonia and sepsis due to severe malnutrition and low BMR. Relatively faster respiratory rate >40/mt, cough, chest signs denote pneumonia.

Hypothermia and positive CRP point to sepsis.

Analysis of present nutritional intake:

2 glasses of 1:1 Dilute cow milk = l glass milk = 67 Kcals + 6 g protein

1 cup tea = 60 Kcals + 1g protein

3 biscuits = 60 Kcals + 1.5 g protein

3 tsp Ragi = 50 Kcals + 1 g protein

1tsp sugar = 20 Kcals

Total 257 Kcals + 9.5 g protein

The current energy intake is only 31% of the expected. This is in comparison to the expected RDA for a reference child of this age with an ideal weight of 8 kg.

As per RDA for age (ideal weight) = 8 × 110 = 880 Kcals (Refer Appendix 6).

Energy requirement as per therapeutic calculation for malnutrition

150-200 Kcal/kg and protein 3-4 g/kg. In this child with marasmus/severe PEM, the calculation is = 4 × 200 = 800 Kcals.

Protein requirement (Marasmus) 4 × 4 =16 g

Fluid requirement (infant) (150-165 ml/kg) 4 × 165 = 660 ml. In hyperalimentation, upto 200 ml/kg fluid may be given orally. In heart disease and conditions with syndrome of inappropriate ADH secretion (SIADH), it is restricted to 2/3rd of the requirement. **The energy administered should never be more than 150% of the RDA for age in any therapeutic calculation.** Total calories are given in 8 feeds, 6 feeds during day time on a 2 hourly basis and a late night and an early

morning feed to prevent hypoglycemia at night, ensuring adequate sleep.

Baby can be given 2 glasses of undiluted cow milk instead of the diluted milk made into high energy milk leading to 400 Kcals/400 ml. High energy milk is prepared by adding 1 tsp sugar and ½ tsp coconut oil to 100 ml milk. Preparations that give 100 Kcals/100 ml are called isodense preparations (Refer Appendix 6). Coconut oil is preferred as it provides medium chain triglycerides (MCT), that can be absorbed straight into portal vein, even when there is fat malabsorption. The amount of visible oil that can be given is as much to provide around 10% of the total calories, i.e.; 80 kcals. This is obtained from 2 tsp oil and it is acceptable in this child. Baby also can be given 6 tsp of ragi, 3 tsp sugar in 100 ml milk to supply 100 + 60 + 60 = 220 Kcals and isodense fruit juice (100 ml =100 kcals). The rest of the calories can be made up by idli, rice or cereal pulse combinations liké SAT mix (Refer Appendix 6).

Oral thrush should be treated vigorously with clotrimazole mouth paint. Blood should be drawn for RBS, RFT, LFT, Blood culture. She should be started on broad spectrum antibiotics like ampicillin and gentamicin in view of LRI and septicemia. The baby should be given tube feeds if oral intake is inadequate. Initially, in view of lethargy, 4 ml/kg 10% dextrose push may be given followed by 6 hours of maintenance fluid containing potassium in view of hypokalemia, if oral intake is very poor. The other supplements needed are calcium, phosphorus, multivitamins and minerals including zinc. As the anemia is not severe, 'top up' packed cell transfusion is not needed. Oral iron can be started after stabilization of the patient and control of infections. Early iron therapy may be poorly tolerated initially with an increased infectious morbidity. Bacteria like E. coli may thrive on unbound iron in the gut due to low levels of carrier proteins. Vitamin A deficiency is treated by giving 2 doses of vitamin A concentrate on two consecutive days followed by 6 monthly doses 0.5 lakh unit is given below 6 months, 1 lakh unit is given below 1 year of age and 2 lakh units after 1 year of age. Refer Tables 2.6 and 2.7. The various age independent anthropometric parameters are given in Table 2.5.

Clearance of edema and apathy marks improvement. Return of social smile is a good prognostic sign. The immediate goal of therapy in the intensive phase of therapy (initial 2-3 months) is weight for height, i.e., 6 kg and not weight for age (8 kg). The expected weight gain is 500 g/week or 70 g/kg/week. This is usually achieved in 8-12 weeks.

Developmental delay needs detailed evaluation and early stimulation after control of infection. Gross motor delay is the rule in PEM, whereas global delay occurs in brain damage. Personal social and language delay may occur due to poor stimulation and lack of proper human interaction with the baby. Immunization should be given soon after stabilization (Refer Appendix 10).

CHAPTER 2

GROWTH AND NUTRITION

SECTION 2.6

A TODDLER WITH NUTRITIONAL EDEMA

1½-year-old female child is brought with generalized edema, anemia, apathy, cough and recurrent bouts of diarrhea of 1 month duration with perianal excoriation and reduced urine output. She was refusing feeds. Mother had stopped giving breast milk at 10 months of age and she was on rice kanji, dilute milk 1:1 dilution x 2 glasses and 4 biscuits/day. BCG, OPV and DPT given. Measles vaccine and 1st boosters were not given. She had exanthematous fever 2 weeks back, treated with homeopathic medicines.

On examination: Hypothermic, capillary filling time 2 seconds, skin pinch 2 seconds, RR 30/mt, pulse 100 /mt, BP 80 systolic.

Weight 8 kg, length 72 cm and OFC 45 cm. Erythematous and blackish scaling in creases and groin were present. Peeling of skin in the lower limbs and brownish pigmentation and desquamation of skin noted. Hair sparse and straight. Mooning of face and pitting edema of feet and paraspinal area +. Skin and eyes were dry. Oral thrush, erythema of mouth and angular stomatitis +. Pallor +. CVS ejection systolic murmur +. Apex beat 5th space in the MCL. Liver felt 5 cm below costal margin with a span of 11 cm, no ascites. Generalised hypotonia + and plantar B/L up going. DTR just elicited. X-ray—B/L mottled opacities. Hb 6.5 g/dl TC 4000 /cu mm, P 50, L 30, E 10, PS: Dimorphic anemia with eosinophilia. B. Urea 20 mg/dl. S.Na 130 and K 3 mEq /L. RBS 40 mg/dl. Motion sugar 1%.

DIAGNOSIS AND DISCUSSION

Severe malnutrition clinically presenting as kwashiorkor (edematous malnutrition) with 2nd degree stunting, persistent diarrhea and lactose intolerance, nutritional anemia and bronchopneumonia with probably miliary TB.

With abrupt stoppage of breast milk, she had recurrent infections and diarrhea adding to malnutrition. 2 weeks back, she had probably measles (unimmunised against measles) that worsened her nutritional status and led to pneumonia and recurrence of diarrhea and probably flaring up of TB. Absence of tachypnea, tachycardia and fever does not rule out infection and pneumonia, but is attributable to low BMR in malnutrition. She is also having helminthiasis, eosinophilia and nutritional anemia. Present dietary intake is unacceptably low. Baby has malnutrition, nutritional edema, nutritional dermatosis and multiple MDDs namely iron, folic acid and B_{12} deficiency (Dimorphic anemia), vitamin B Complex, vitamin A, essential fatty acids (EFA) and potassium deficiency. Mild hyponatre-mia denotes dilutional hyponatremia/hyponatre-mic dehydration.

Assessment of Growth

Weight for Age %—8/11 x 100 = 72.7%—Grade I PEM-IAP with edema. This is represented as Grade I K to denote kwashiorkor. With edema feet, mooning of face and paraspinal edema without ascites, it is grade III kwashiorkor (Table 2.4).

Length for Age %—72/81 × 100 =88.8 %—2nd degree stunting.

Weight for Height)—8/9 × 100 =88 %—1st degree wasting—Waterlow.

OFC—45/47 cm, 2 cm less than normal.

It is interesting to note that child has demonstrable wasting in spite of edema. Practically, no kwashiorkor is found to be >90% of the expected weight, even with edema. Child has medical emergencies like hypothermia, hypoglycemia, fluid electrolyte imbalance, that are to be corrected immediately by providing warmth, broad spectrum antibiotics like ampicillin and gentamicin, 10% dextrose 4 ml/kg push followed by potassium and dextrose containing IVF. Fluid intake is restricted to 2/3 of the requirement, i.e., 70 ml/kg/day due to edema. Rapid ration may be omitted in view of edema and poor cardiac reserve. 50% of this may be given as 10% glucose and 50% as normal saline due to increased total body sodium with 1-2 ml of 7.5% kcl/100 ml IV fluid to correct hypokalemia. One ml/100 ml is added if SK is normal and 2ml/100ml if SK is low. Oral fluids, ORS, rice kanji water, cereal, pulse and semi solids, should be started as the child improves. It is better to avoid cow milk as there is evidence of secondary lactose intolerance, which may last for 1-2 weeks, following which cow milk can be started. Soya milk/ground nut is an initial option if the child does not accept semi solids and solids.

The child should be investigated for tuberculosis using gastric aspirate, Mantoux test and repeated X-ray chest especially looking for clearance after antibiotics. If there is a close contact with TB, it is better to start Anti TB treatment initially itself. It is desirable to start ATT after checking LFT. In sick children and those with severe types of TB like miliary, TB meningitis, progressive pulmonary TB, pleural, pericardial/peritoneal effusions and AFB positive cases, CAT I ATT is given.

Nutritional Requirement—Therapeutic Calculation

Energy = 8 x 200 = 1600 Kcal.

RDA for age/expected weight = 1200 kcal (11 × 110=1210) ICMR RAD is 1240 in 1-3 years old child.

This therapeutic calculation of 1600 Kcal is 133% above RDA (upto 150% is acceptable).

Protein–8 × 4 = 32 g (as against RDA of 22 g) upto 7 g/kg may be given or as much to supply 15% of the total calories.

Fluid Requirement= 8 × 100 = 800 ml (Excess fluid is not advisable and initially 2/3rd fluid may be started in view of edema, fluid retention and poor cardiac reserve).

Visible oil – 1600 x 10% = 160 Kcals/day = 4 tsp/day.

50% Mg SO_4 -0.2 ml/kg/dose Q 12 H may be given deep IM x 2 days (This is found to revert mental changes quickly).

Clearance of edema and return of social smile mark signs of recovery. Child should be on potassium, Mg, multivitamin and mineral supplements including zinc, iron and vitamin A x 2 doses on 2 consecutive days.

As the anemia is severe (<7 g/dl) with hemodynamic impact and cardiomegaly, packed cell transfusion 10 ml/kg may be given sandwiched with frusemide 2 mg/kg. In mild to moderate anemia (7-11 g/dl), deworming and oral iron can be started after stabilization, preferably in the 2nd week when synthesis of carrier proteins starts (Dose 3-6 mg/kg element iron/day × 3 months).

The treatment is divided into 3 phases: **Resuscitation** (tackling the medical emergencies), **Restoration** (restoring weight for height and micronutrients) and **Rehabilitation** (long-term treatment to achieve further growth and to prevent further malnutrition). Initially frequent tube feed may be needed in very sick children and those with severe apathy and anorexia (Table 2.7).

Tube feed may be given as bolus feeds that mimic physiologic feeds, but this may evoke nausea and reverse peristalsis and vomiting. Another way to give enteral feeding is to give as continuous infusions in 3-4 rations. This will avoid reverse peristalsis. Aspiration of feed is an important cause of death in children with malnutrition. Lactose free commercial feed are available for tube feed, e.g., isomilk, soyal, nusobee etc. Lactose and sucrose free formula are also available, e.g., prosoyal.

SECTION 2.7

AN INFANT WITH CHRONIC DIARRHEA AND SKIN CHANGES

Eight-month-old female baby is admitted with chronic diarrhea of 3 months duration. Baby looks puffy with sparse depigmented hair, with a reddish discoloration and alopecia noted in some areas of scalp. There is peri-orificial and perianal excoriation and peeling of skin. Abdomen is distended. No pitting oedema. Baby is irritable. Baby was born to consanguineous parents. Both parents healthy. Weight 6 kg, length 66 cm OFC 44 cm.

Auxology

Weight for age—$6.0/8.2 \times 100 = 68\%$ grade II PEM – IAP.

Length for age—$66/71 \times 100 = 93\%$ I degree stunting—Waterlow.

Weight for Height – $6.6/7 \times 100 = 86\%$ $1°$ wasting—Waterlow.

OFC 44 cm, Expected 45 cm.

DIAGNOSIS AND DISCUSSION

Chronic Diarrhea with PEM—Acrodermatitis Enteropathica

Differential diagnosis gluten enteropathy, cystic fibrosis, congenital/acquired immunodeficiency. Prekwashiorkor is an alternate diagnosis as there is no edema.

Consanguinity in the parents, chronic diarrhea, peri-orifical excoriation and peeling of skin, alopecia and reddish discolorisation of hair point to the diagnosis of acrodermatitis enteropathica.

There will be dramatic improvement with 100-150 mg. of Zinc sulphate to supply 2 mg/kg elemental zinc. This will have to be continued indefinitely. Supportive care and broad spectrum antibiotics are also indicated. Topical application of antibiotics and zinc sulphate creams are also useful for excoriation.

Acrodermatitis enteropathica is a genetic condition with autosomal recessive inheritance leading to defective absorption of zinc. Lymphocyte function and free radical scavenging may be defective in this condition. The baby also needs nutritional rehabilitation and developmental stimulation.

Food Groups, Major Nutrients and Micronutrients

The major food groups are cereals, legumes (pulses), roots and tubers, vegetables, fruits, milk and milk products, meat group (meat, fish and egg), oil, fats and oil seeds, sugars, condiments and spices etc. These food groups yield the major nutrients namely carbohydrate, lipids and proteins and the protective foods like vitamins, minerals and antioxidants. Lipids are divided into saturated, monounsaturated and polyunsaturated fatty acids (PUFA). The essential fatty acids (EFA) are unsaturated fatty acids that cannot be synthesized like linoleic acid (LA) (Omega 6) and alpha linolenic acid (ALA)-Omega-3. The long chain polyunsaturated (LCP) fats derived from LA are arachidonic aid and adrenic acid and that from ALA are eicosa pentaenoic acid (EPA) and docosa hexaneoic acids (DHA). EPA is heart-friendly and DHA is brain-friendly.

Micronutrients are vitamins and minerals needed in small quantities e.g. milligram or microgram. Antioxidants are betacarotene, vitamin E and C, selenium, lycopene etc.

Smart Nutrients and Super Nutrients

Smart nutrients are the brain-friendly nutrients like folic acid, vitamin B_1, B_6, B_{12}, iron, iodine, vitamin A, EFA, LCPs like DHA (omega 3 fats) etc. Four out of the above are called super nutrients namely vitamin A, iron, folic acid and omega 3 fats.

Theories Regarding Development of Kwashiorkor

1. Viteri's time bound theory—More time to adapt leads to marasmus and less time leads to kwashiorkor route.

2. Dietary hypothesis—Marasmus is energy deficiency and kwashiorkor is protein deficiency.

3. Jelliffe's catastrophy hypothesis—Kwashiorkor is event related like infection, maternal deprivation, death in the family etc.

4. Gopalan's theory of adaptation—Marasmus is due to extreme biochemical adaptation and kwashiorkor is due to dysadaptation.

5. Golden's free radical theory—Kwashiorkor is due to overproduction of free radicals and reduced antioxidants.

6. Toxin mediated—Aflatoxin is a cause for kwashiorkor.

Fig. Nos. 1-10 (Plates 1 to 3) show various nutritional deficiencies and conditions with short stature.

Table 2.1: Causes of short stature
1. Racial/Genetic/Familial e.g. Pygmies—Proportionate
2. Primordial—IUGR/Hypoplastic babies, Syndromic/Non syndromic e.g. Russel Silver, Seckel—Proportionate
3. Constitutional/Maturational growth delay (MGD), Late bloomer—Proportionate
4. Nutritional—chronic PEM—Proportionate
5. Emotional Deprivation—Psychosocial—Proportionate
6. Chromosomal/Single gene disorders—Proportionate/Disproportionate
7. Skeletal dysplasias—Usually disproportionate
8. Metabolic disorders—Proportionate/Disproportionate
9. Endocrine disorders, e.g. Hypopituitarism—Proportionate, Hypothyroidism—Infantile proportions

Table 2.2: Types of short stature	
Proportionate	*Disporportionate*
1. Normal variants	1. With short limbs
Familial short stature	
Maturational growth delay	
2. Prenatal onset IUGR/Primordial	2. With short trunk
Intrauterine infection, genetic disorder	
3. Postnatal causes	
PEM, anaemia	
due to systemic illness	
Psychosocial short stature	
4. Endocrine	
• Hypopituitarism	
• Hypothyroidism (Infantile proportions)	
• Hypogonadism	

Table 2.3: Causes of failure to thrive (FTT)

I. Non Organic/Environmental/Socio-Economic–80%

II. Organic/Biological–20%

1. GIT Causes—Cleft tip, palate, GERD. Pyloric stenosis, food intolerance, hepatobiliary/pancreatic disorders, intestinal atresias. aganglionic megacolon, inflammatory bowel diseases, malabsorption
2. Renal—CRF, UTI, RTA
3. Neurologic—CP, MR
4. CVS—CHF, CCHD, PAH
5. Respiratory—TE Fistulas, Chronic Bronchitis, Chronic asthma, Bronchiolitis obliterans, pulmonary fibrosis
6. Endocrine—Hypopitutarism, Hypothyroidism, adrenal insufficiency
7. Metabolic—In born errors of Metabolism
8. Infections and infestations—Intrauterine infections, TB, HIV, giardiasis, whip worm colitis
9. Immunodeficiency/Immune related Disorders
10. Miscellaneous—IUGR, Hypoplastic baby, heavy metal poisoning, syndromic and non-syndrome anomalies.

Table 2.4: Grading of marasmus and kwashiorkor

Grade	Marasmus		Kwashiorkor
1	Loose skinfolds in axilla and groin	1.	Pedal edema
2	Loose skinfolds in thigh and buttocks	2.	Facial edema/puffiness
3	Loose skinfolds in chest and back	3.	Edema over body and paraspinal region
4	Loss of buccal pad of fat	4.	Ascites/serous effusions

Table 2.5: Age independent anthropometric parameters

1. Mid Arm Circumference (MAC) 1-5 years (N>13.5 cm)
2. Bangle Test (Internal Diameter of 4 cm)
3. Shakir tape (Coloured tape for MAC)
4. MAC/HC Ratio—Normal > 0.32-0.33
5. Chest circumference/HC Ratio (> 1 year > 1)
6. QUAC Stick (Relates Height and MAC)
7. Nabarrow's Thinness Chart (Relates Height and Weight)
8. Skinfold thickness
9. Ponderal/BMI/Quetlet Index.

Table 2.6: WHO grading of Vitamin A deficiency (VAD)

1.	X_1A	–	Xerosis conjunctiva
2.	X_1B	–	Bitot's spots—conjunctiva
3.	X_2	–	Xerosis cornea
4.	X_3A	–	Corneal ulceration
5.	X_3B	–	Keratomalacia
6.	XN	–	Night blindness
7.	XF	–	Fundoscopic changes
8.	XS	–	Corneal scarring

Treatment of Keratomalacia: 5000 IU/kg IM × 5 days followed by 25,000 IU/day till recovery.

(Nelson Textbook, 15th ed)

VAD (WHO/UNICEF, 1988) 1-2 lakh units Vitamin A orally on 2 consecutive days, followed by 1 dose after 1 month.

CHAPTER 2

GROWTH AND NUTRITION

Table 2.7: Various steps in the management of PEM

Hospitalisation
Ensure health and nutrition education, social interview, counselling, TLC

↓

Resuscitation
(Goal: Treatment of medical emergencies)

↓

Restoration
(Goal: Weight for height)

↓

Rehabilitation
(Goal: Weight for age)

↓

Prevention

Investigations
Blood counts, smear, urine and motion—RE and cultures, RBS, blood urea, electrolytes, LFT, Mx, X-ray chest, malarial parasite

Hypoglycaemia, hypothermia, infections, dehydration, CCF, severe anaemia, convulsion, tremor, tetany, electrolyte, mineral and vitamin deficiencies

Nutritional therapy, deworming, mineral and vitamin supplementation

Food supplementation

NIMFES

* Exclude causes of FTT like genetic, metabolic, endocrine disorders and causes of oedema.
TLC—Tender Loving Care.

NIMFES—Nutrition, Immunization, Medical care, Family health, Education and Stimulation. FTT—Failure to thrive.

Table 2.8: Growth velocity and RDA (Bedside calculation)

Age group (month)	Weight (g/wk)	Height (cm/mo)	OFC (cm/mo)	Energy (Kcal/kg)	Protein (g/kg)
1-3	200	3.0	2.0	120	2.0
4-6	150	2.0	1.5	120	2.0
7-9	100	1.5	0.5	110	1.7
10-12	50	1.0	0.5	110	1.7
(Year)	(kg/year)	(cm/year)	(cm/year)	(Kcal/kg)	(g/kg)
1-2	2.0	12.5	0.5	100	1.6
2-3	2.0	7.0	0.5	100	1.6
4-6	2.0	6.0	—	90	1.5
7-9	3.0	6.0	—	80	1.4
Adolescent	Variable	Variable	—	60	1.4
Adult	—	—	—	40	1.0

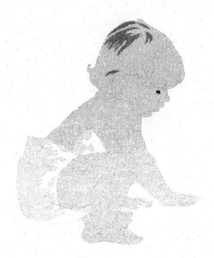

3

Developmental and Behavioral Medicine

A PRETERM BABY WITH DEVELOPMENTAL DELAY

Five-month-old baby, born 2 months preterm was brought with excessive crying, feeding difficulty and lack of social smile. Baby had multiple episodes of seizures since newborn period.

On examination: A stiff baby with hypertonia and brisk DTR, plantar bilaterally up going. Neonatal reflex: Moro partial, stepping and placing +, sucking and rooting +, palmar and plantar grasp +, Adductor spread of knee jerk +, Tonic neck reflex +, Landau and parachute reflex absent. Primitive reflexes: Palmo-mental reflex and glabellar tap +ve. Head control absent. Pulling to sitting—head in plane with body and stiff back. Vertical suspension—tendency for scissoring. Hand always kept closed with thumb adducted leading to 'Ape thumb'. No cooing sounds, no social smile, does not turn head to rattle, follows object to 90 degrees. Amiel Tison angles—all reduced (Refer Appendix 5). Adductor angle thigh—30, popliteal angle 60, dorsiflexion foot—45, jaw jerk exaggerated. Auditory blink and startle +. Other systems within normal limits.

Weight 3.5 kg, Length 54 cm, OFC—35 cm (Expected weight—6 kg, length—61.0 cm, OFC—40.6 cm) Chronological age – 5 months, Corrected age = 3 months. Developmental age = 1 month.

DIAGNOSIS AND DISCUSSION

Spastic Cerebral palsy—Quadriparesis with global developmental delay, malnutrition and seizure disorder.

Developmental age is only one month.

DQ = 1/5 × 100 =20, leading to severe retardation (Tables 3.1 and 3.2).

Neonatal reflexes preserved. Abnormal persistence of neonatal reflex is noted in brain damage. Decreased Amiel Tison angles and tendency for scissoring, adductor spread of knee jerk and brisk reflexes denote spasticity. Hypertonia is also there indicating spasticity. This is a case of Spastic CP with global developmental delay and seizure disorder.

Vision and hearing appear normal. But it needs objective assessment. Sequelae of birth asphyxia or neonatal seizure is the most likely etiology. OFC is very low 35 cm, i.e., 5 cm below that of corrected age and 8 cm below that for chronological age. Excessive crying and lack of Mother Infant Bonding is noted in infants with cerebral palsy. Difficulty in feeding is often due to pseudobulbar palsy as evidenced by exaggerated jaw reflex or due to gastroesophageal reflux disease (GERD).

As the baby is preterm and growth is much below that of chronological age, analysis should be done as per corrected age.

Growth as per Corrected Age

Weight for age—3.5/6 × 100 = 58% (grade III PEM IAP).

Height/length for age—54/61 × 100 = 88% (II degree stunting—Waterlow).

Height age–1 month.

Weight for height—3.5/4.3 x 100 81% (I degree wasting—Waterlow).

OFC—35 is 5 cm below that of corrected age.

This baby needs nutritional therapy, micronutrient supplements, neuro- developmental patterning (NDT) and early stimulation. As the retardation is severe, baby needs custodian care, preferably with mother as the caretaker and therapist. **Community based rehabilitation (CBR) and Home based Rehabilitation (HBR) are most relevant in these cases** (Refer Chapter 16—Disabled child).

The baby should also get regular physical therapies to reduce spasticity and also muscle relaxants like diazepam and baclofen. Baclofen may worsen uncontrolled seizures. Seizure control with pheno, phenytoin or valparin should be achieved. Botulinum toxin (Botox) is useful in severe spasticity.

Neurodevelopmental Patterning

It aims at establishing milestones as per chronology in a cephalocaudal pattern. For e.g., first aim for head control, then sitting followed by standing. The Child Development Centre, Trivandrum follows a systematic schedule like this. The Bobath approach is another one in this field.

SECTION 3.2 A CASE OF DYSLEXIA

A 5½-year-old girl was brought with poor school performance. She was a loner in class. She could climb up and down stairs, could skip and copy a diamond. She was noted to repeat spoken words several times.

Examination was within normal limits including anthropometry. Vision and hearing were normal. She used to develop temper tantrums when her mother cleaned up her room or arranged her clothes and books. Thyroid function test normal.

DIAGNOSIS AND DISCUSSION

Autism/Pervasive Developmental Disorder (PDD)

Growth, development, vision and hearing appear normal, but child is having poor school performance. Hence, autism is considered. Autism is also called **Kanner's syndrome** and it means aloof/alone. The child has impaired capacity for communication and human relationship and severely restricted range of activities and interests. Symptoms always occur before 3 years of age and may be evident very early as lack of social smile or bonding (Table 3.3). The related conditions are non autistic PDD, **Asperger's syndrome, Rett syndrome, Heller's syndrome** etc. ADHD is another differential diagnosis when child is very hyperactive and has attention deficit.

In Asperger's syndrome, speech is well developed. But there is impaired social interaction, clumsiness and unusual interests that impair adaptive function. Rett syndrome is deceleration of head growth, loss of hand skills, social, cognitive and speech skills after a period of normal growth seen exclusively in girls and associated with typical hand washing stereotypy, ataxia/seizure. Heller's syndrome is a similar condition seen in boys.

Childhood Disintegrative Disorder (CDD) is a condition characterized by normal period of growth before 10 years of age followed by loss of acquired skills at least in two areas namely language, personal social, motor skills, play or bowel/bladder control. Usually children with ADHD have dyslexia, but are very hyperactive and usually destructive. This child is a loner with impaired verbal and non-verbal communication. Echolalia is present, i.e., repetition of spoken words. This child should have a formal IQ assessment and evaluation by a clinical psychologist. EEG and MRI brain may be done to rule out organic lesion/seizure activity.

Attention Deficit Hyperactivity Disorder (ADHD) is diagnosed when duration of symptoms is more than 6 months and onset before 7 years of age. Secondary ADHD occurs in certain drugs, toxins, infections, degenerative conditions, epilepsy etc (Table 3.4). **Tourette syndrome** is a genetic subtype with ADHD and tics.

Pediatric Autoimmune Neuropsychiatric Disorders Associated with Streptococcal Infection (PANDAS) describe a group of neuropsychiatric disorders, obsessive compulsive disorders and tic disorders that occur following group A streptococcal infections and may recur with repeated infections. These are similar to Tourette syndrome. It is more common in boys and in the age group 6-7 years. MRI has shown enlargement of basal ganglia, probably due to inflammation. Antibodies that cross react with basal ganglia suggest local autoimmune reactions due to a molecular mimicry. The comorbidities are emotional lability and separation anxiety and Sydenhams chorea.

The diagnostic criteria of PANDAS are the following:

1. Presence of obsessive compulsive disorder and or tic disorder.
2. Pediatric onset with peak at prepubertal age.
3. Episodic course of symptom severity— relapsing remitting course.
4. Temporal association with group A Beta Streptococcal Infection and exacerbation with repeated infection as evidenced by positive ASO titre or throat swab.
5. Association with neurological abnormalities during exacerbation. Treatment includes antibiotic therapy, plasma exchange and IV immunoglobulins in severe cases along with symptomatic management.

Counselling and behavioral modifications are useful in PDDs.

Autism is highly resistant to treatment. Drug therapy using opiate antagonists, haloperidol, trifluoperazine may be tried. A team work between psychologist, child psychiatrist and neurologist and special educators may show some success. Autism is said to have a link with in utero exposure to high testosterone. It is almost 4 times more common in boys (Refer Table 3.4). Dyslexia is a specific reading disability, but it is often used to denote scholastic backwardness.

SECTION 3.3

A CHILD WITH DEVELOPMENTAL DELAY AND SMALL HEAD

A 2-year-old boy was brought with developmental delay. Growth was adequate, but head circumference was only 43 cm. General examination was normal except for large bat ears. He could walk sideways holding to furniture, had pincer grasp, could babble mama, dada, amma and acha and he enjoyed repetitive play. He had temper trantrums and breath holding spells. He had no spasticity.

DIAGNOSIS AND DISCUSSION

Microcephaly with Developmental Retardation:

Chronological age–24 months.

Developmental age—11 months.

DQ 11/24 × 100–45.8 (Moderate Retardation).

OFC very low 43 as against 48-49 cm.

The baby does not have any demonstrable motor defect and hence a diagnosis of cerebral palsy cannot be made. The diagnosis is microcephaly with developmental/mental retardation. The bat ear points to primary microcephaly or fragile X syndrome (FRAX). Family history and consanguinity should be elicited. CNS imaging will help to look for developmental malformations. Macro orchidism in FRAX may become evident only at puberty. Neuronal migration defects are unlikely in this child due to absence of seizures. This child will need special schooling. Iron supplementation is said to improve breath holding spell (Refer Tables 3.1 and 3.2).

The developmental assessment tools are:

1. Denver Developmental Screening Test (DDST)
2. Gessel Developmental Schedule
3. Bayley Scale of Infant Development (BSID)
4. Baroda Developmental Screening Test
5. Trivandrum Developmental Screening Chart (TDSC)
6. Brazelton Neonatal Behavioral Assessment Scale
7. Developmental Assessment Scale for Indian Infants (DAASI).

The IQ assessment tools are:

1. Stanford Binet Intelligence Scale
2. Binet Kamat Test
3. Wechsler Intelligence Scale for Children (WISC)
4. Malin Intelligence Scale for Indian Children (MISC)
5. Good enough's Draw a man test
6. Seguain Form Board.

The usual psychosocial problems noted in children are the following:

1. Resistance to feed/sleep
2. Three-month Colic
3. Breath holding spell
4. Head banging
5. Thumb sucking

6. Nail biting
7. Teeth grinding (Bruxism)
8. Stuttering
9. Pica
10. Nocturnal enuresis, encopresis
11. Temper tantrums
12. Stealing
13. Tics
14. Masturbation (Boys)
15. Gratification (Girls)
16. Dyslexia
17. Juvenile delinquency
18. ADHD

19. Psychosomatic disorder
20. Rumination
21. Anorexia nervosa, Bulimia nervosa.

Categorisation of Hearing Loss	
Slight	(16-25 dB)
Mild	(26 - 40 dB)
Moderate	(41-65 dB)
Severe	(66-95 dB)
Profound	(>96 dB)

Hearing tests are Oto-Acuostic Emission (OAE), Brainstem Evoked Response Auditory (BERA), Free field audiometry and formal audiogram (> 3 years).

Table 3.1: Grading according to IQ score

IQ Score	Grade
>90	A
>80	B
>70	C
>60	D
>50	E
<50	F

Table 3.2: IQ score (American Association on Mental Retardation—AAMR) and guidelines for rehabilitation as per IQ

Level of retardation	IQ	Remarks
Genius/Very superior	>130	Genius
Superior	120-129	Extraordinary
Very Intelligent	110-119	Very good in studies
Intelligent	90-109	Good in studies
Dull/normal	80-89	Normal/average
Borderline retardation	70-79	Vulnerable to educational problems
Mild/educable	50-70	Often need special classes
Moderate/trainable	35-50	Trainable in workshop setting
Severe	20-35	Trainable for selfcare skills
Profound	<20	Need custodian care

CHAPTER 3

Table 3.3: Clinical criteria for identification of autism (Adopted from Sabina Ahmed, Guwahati)

1. Difficulty in mixing and playing with other children.
2. Inappropriate laughing or giggling.
3. Avoids eye contact.
4. Lack of pretend play or unusual and repetitive pretend play.
5. Doesn't respond when called, sometimes appears to be deaf.
6. Not responsive to normal teaching methods.
7. No understanding or fear of real dangers.
8. Can do something very well, but not tasks involving social understanding.
9. Unusual behaviour or body movements such as flapping hands or rocking and jumping.
10. Standoffish in manner.
11. Indicates needs by gestures or leading adults by the hand.
12. Echoes words or phrases.
13. Enjoys spinning or rotating objects.
14. Likes sameness in everyday routine, does not enjoy change.
15. Apparent insensitivity to pain.
16. Inappropriate attachments to objects.
17. Sometimes does not like to be hugged or touched.
18. Crying tantrums, extreme distress for no apparent reason.
19. Extreme restlessness, hyperactivity or extreme passivity.

Table 3.4: Barkley's ADHD rating scale

ADHD–DSM IV (American Psychiatric Association 1994/ ICD 10 (WHO, 1992))
1. Fails to give close attention to details or makes careless mistakes in work.
2. Fidgets with hands or feet or squirms in seat.
3. Difficultly sustaining attention to task or fun activities.
4. Leaves seat in classroom or in other situations in which remaining seated is expected.
5. Doesn't appear to listen when spoken to directly.
6. Feels restless.
7. Doesn't follow through on instructions/fails to finish work.
8. Difficulty engaging in leisure/fun activities quietly.
9. Has difficulty in organizing tasks and activities.
10. Feels "on the go" or acts as if "driven by a motor".
11. Avoids, dislikes or is reluctant to engage in work that requires sustained mental effort.
12. Talks excessively.
13. Loses things necessary for tasks or activities.
14. Blurts out answers before questions have been completed.
15. Easily distracted.
16. Has difficulty awaiting return.
17. Forgetful in daily activities.
18. Interrupts or intrudes on others.
    Score 2-3 is positive, a positive score of at least 12 items is diagnostic
    0–Never
    1–Sometimes
    2–Often
    3–Very often

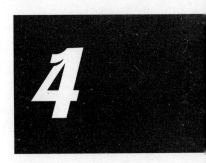

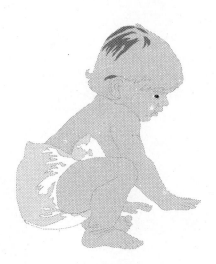

Neonatology

Neonatology

SECTION 4.1

A NEWBORN WITH BIRTH ASPHYXIA AND MECONIUM ASPIRATION

A term newborn with history of birth asphyxia and thick meconium stained liquor, delivered by LSCS for fetal distress, was admitted to NICU. Baby received bag and mask ventilation in the local hospital. Baby developed one episode of convulsion after admission.

On examination: Weight 2.8 kg, RR 70/mt, HR 100/mt, Apex beat 4th Lt. ICS outside MCL, Heart sounds—Normal, Air entry reduced on right side, percussion note tympanic on right side, crepitions on left side. Baby drowsy, poor suck, hypotonic, DTR brisk, pupils contracted, periodic breathing noticed.

DIAGNOSIS AND DISCUSSION

Neonatal Encephalopathy/Hypoxic Ischemic Encephalopathy–Stage II, Meconium Aspiration Syndrome (MAS) and Pneumothorax Rt.

Baby has 2 major medical problems, namely respiratory and CNS. The respiratory problem is secondary to meconium aspiration and vigorous resuscitation.

Bag and mask ventilation is contraindicated in meconium aspiration.

The clinical features are suggestive of pneumothorax on the right side.

The CNS problem is typical of neonatal encephalopathy/Hypoxemic Ischaemic Encephalopathy—Stage II (Refer Table 4.1). Vasopressin level will be elevated in asphyxia and prolactin in seizures. This may help in confirmation.

Baby needs immediate X-ray chest, under water seal, needle aspiration and intercostal drainage. EEG may be done to look for low voltage delta waves or periodic discharges (Table 4.1). USS Head and CT head will delineate the CNS injury and haemorrhage if any.

Treatment consists of supportive care, vitamin K, calcium, O_2 inhalation, broad spectrum antibiotics, anticonvulsant (especially phenobarbitone due to its cerebroprotective effects) and anti oedema measures. Artificial ventilation may be needed in case of impending respiratory failure, apnoea or bradycardia. Steroids are better avoided in MAS, but may be given in this case as part of antiedema treatment. In case of meconium aspiration/meconium stained liquor, suction may be done at delivery, first mouth and then nose followed by intubation and suction. As in case of diaphragmatic hernia, bag and mask ventilation is contraindicated in MAS. Stomach wash should also be done in MAS. Meconium passage in utero occurs in fetal distress and postmaturity. In preterms, it is less likely and fetal diarrhea in preterm leading to meconium staining can occur in 'listeriosis'.

In case of HIE, some may develop intraventricular or intracerebral hemorrhage (IVH/ICH) in 24-48 hours. HIE may be due to birth asphyxia. Asphyxia may be due to cord round the neck, difficult and prolonged delivery or CNS malformations. The sequelae include neurodevelopmental abnormalities, cerebral palsy, seizures, mental retardation, special sense organ defects like vision, speech and hearing, dyslexia and hyperactivity. Persistently low APGAR score at 5, 10 or 20 minutes and early neurological findings suggest sequelae.

Preterm babies can tolerate hypoxia for longer periods (5-7 minutes) without sequel. Preterms have more superficial vascularity of the cortex through communicating cortical and meningeal vessels and suffer more periventricular hypoxia due to less deep penetrating vessels. Preterms suffer periventricular leukomalacia and cerebral diplegia or monoplegia, usually without seizures and mental retardation.

Term babies suffer more of superficial and cortical ischemia due to non-communicating vessels than periventricular insults. They develop more extensive focal or multifocal/extensive insults/necrosis and porencephalic cysts and hydranencephaly. They develop hemiplegia, double hemiplegia with more affected upper limbs or quadriplegia with equal upper and lower limb involvement and also MR, seizure and sense organ defects. Basal ganglia involvement leads to 'status marmoratus' and is often seen following bilirubin encephalopathy.

The initial response to hypoxia is the 'diving reflex' and redistribution of cardiac output to the brain. But this hyperperfusion may result in damage of 'cerebro vascular autoregulation' and cerebral edema. Initially there is glucose influx followed by neuronal glucose and glycogen depletion, potassium leakage, failure of sodium potassium pump, lactic acidosis and failure of ATP dependent energy metabolism. These changes and seizures will aggravate cerebral edema. There will also be multi organ dysfunction syndrome (MODS) involving kidney, heart, liver, coagulation and hematological profile, acute respiratory distress syndrome (ARDS), hemorrhagic gastroenteropathy etc. There may also be DIC, adrenal hemorrhage, shock and syndrome of inappropriate ADH secretion (SIADH).

ICH should be suspected when there is bulging fontanel, apneic attacks and fits. There may be increasing or sudden pallor and jaundice. Imaging should be done for confirmation. CSF study will help to diagnose or exclude meningitis and subarachnoid haemorrhage. Intraventricular hemorrhage (IVH) occurs in preterms and may follow rapid boluses of hyperosmolar solutions like 25% glucose/soda bicarb. The sequelae of ICH and IVH include brain damage and hydrocephalus.

The level of vasopressin will be elevated in cord blood in fetal distress. Another simple way to screen for asphyxia is an elevated urine lactate to creatinine ratio > 0.62.

Enhancement of the posterior limb of the internal capsule (PLIC) in MRI may be an early indicator of HIE.

SECTION 4.2

A PRETERM NEWBORN WITH POOR FEEDING AND POOR ACTIVITY

A 36-hour-old newborn with poor feeding and poor activity was admitted to NICU. Baby was delivered at 35 weeks gestation following maternal febrile illness and leaking membranes for 30 hours. Birth weight 2 kg.

On examination: Baby pale, cry and activity poor, abdominal distension +, hypothermic (Temp—36 ºC), icterus upto thigh, AFT normal.

Hb 14 g/dl, RDT +, CRP 10 mg/dl, ANC 1500/cumm, micro ESR 18 mm/1st hour.

DIAGNOSIS AND DISCUSSION

Early onset neonatal sepsis and LBW due to Prematurity

Baby has 3 risk factors leading to neonatal sepsis (1) Prematurity and low birth weight (LBW); (2) Maternal febrile illness; and (3) Prolonged rupture of membranes (PROM) > 24 hours. The Bhakoo sepsis score is given in Table 4.2. This baby has a score of at least 6.

All the C/F are suggestive of neonatal sepsis and investigations highly favour probable sepsis. Rapid diagnosis test (RDT) is considered positive when 2 out of the 3 parameters are positive and is considered equivalent to getting culture positivity. It is positive when CRP is > 6 mg/dl, Absolute Neutrophil Count (ANC) is > 5000/cumm or < 1750/ cumm and micro ESR > 15 mm/1st hour or > 5 + No of postnatal days. (For e.g., this baby is 2nd postnatal day and so 5+2 = 7 may be considered positive).

Neonatal sepsis is considered possible, probable or confirmed. Confirmation is by positive culture. Other sepsis screen items include increased band forms >20% of neutrophils, shift to the left in peripheral smear, Immature to Total neutrophil ratio (IT ratio > 0.2). Other acute phase reactants are alpha1 antitrypsin, acid glycoprotein, haptoglobin, platelets and fibrinogen. Prealbumin and transferrin reduce during acute infections and increase during recovery. These are called **'negative reactants'**.

Newborn sepsis is divided into early onset (<72 hours) and late onset (>72 hours). Early onset neonatal sepsis (EONS) is usually due to organisms from the mother or maternal genitourinary tract like Group B strept (GBS), E Coli, listeria etc. Hypothermia is more common in EONS and fever in LONS. Treatment consists of supportive care, IVF, EBM/breastfeeding and broad spectrum antibiotics to give gram positive and gram negative cover like CP and Genta or Ampi and Genta, as per hospital protocol. The drug of choice for listeria is ampicillin. Twice daily injections are enough upto 7 days of age except in meningitis. The second line drugs are 3rd generation cephalosporin cefotaxim/ceftazidime and amikacin. The 3rd line drugs are vancomycin and aztreonam. Meningitis is not usual in EONS compared to late onset neonatal sepsis (LONS), but it is better to do LP and rule out meningitis if baby is RDT positive. Neonatal sepsis is the 3rd major cause of neonatal death next to LBW and birth asphyxia.

LONS is usually due to hospital acquired strains like MRSA, klebsiella, pseudomonas etc., and meningitis is more common in LONS.

Intrauterine infections may also present as neonatal sepsis and they usually may have hepatosplenomegaly, icterus and thrombocytopenia in addition to specific findings like chorio retinitis, cataract, CHD etc.

Gastric aspirate can also give valuable clue in neonatal sepsis. > 5 neutrophils/HPF is a predictor. Hospital outbreaks of neonatal sepsis is usually due to ceftazidime resistant klebsiella. Umbilical and ear swab culture of newborns should be done prior to NICU admission periodically to contain such infections.

Thorough cleaning, periodic disinfection and proper housekeeping practices are valuable in controlling sepsis. Isolation and barrier nursing are helpful while handling highly infected babies.

SECTION 4.3 A FEBRILE NEWBORN

A 5-day-old newborn who had cord round the neck, fetal distress and history of neonatal resuscitation was admitted to NICU with fever and poor feeding. BW 3.3 kg.

On examination: Febrile, AF flushed non pulsatile. Baby was hypertonic with abdominal distension RDT +ve, Hb 14 g/dl.

DIAGNOSIS AND DISCUSSION

Late Onset Neonatal Sepsis (LONS) with meningitis

Baby had fever and features of neonatal sepsis. As the manifestation is after 72 hours, Late onset neonatal sepsis (LONS) is the diagnosis. History of neonatal resuscitation is a risk factor for sepsis. It may be a nosocomial infection from labour room or 'lying in ward'.

LONS usually leads to meningitis. Positive RDT and flushed non pulsatile AF warrants LP. LP showed purulent CSF with high protein and low sugar. CSF hypoglycorrhachia is diagnosed when CSF sugar is below 50% of blood sugar or < 40 mg/dl. Normally CSF sugar is 2/3rd of blood sugar, usually > 50 mg/dl. It may be as high as 75% of RBS in preterm.

The baby should be treated with broad spectrum antibiotics in antimeningitic dose for 14-21 days so as to cover nosocomial infections as well. The usual organisms are pseudomonas, klebsiella, MRSA, acinetobacter etc. The drugs needed are 3rd generation cephalosporin (cefotaxime/ceftazidine) and amikacin with or without vancomycin. In multi drug resistant (MDR) bacteria, aztreonam, meropenem and ciprofloxacin may be needed as 2nd line drugs. LP should be done at the end of the course to document that meningitis has cleared. Supportive care includes feeding, control of cerebral edema and anticonvulsants.

If gram negative organisms are cultured from blood or CSF, 21 days of treatment is necessary. The sequelae of neonatal meningitis are extensive including ventriculitis, hydrocephalus, brain infarct , brain damage, seizure disorder, brain abscess, subdural effusion/empyemia, paralysis and special sense organ defects. Hypoglycorrhachia may rarely occur in IVH. The normal CSF findings are given in Table 4.3.

Rarely, viral meningitis or meningoencephalitis can occur with herpes simplex, enteroviruses etc. It may be part of intrauterine infection.

CHAPTER 4

NEONATOLOGY

SECTION 4.4

A NEWBORN BABY WITH INDIRECT HYPER-BILIRUBINEMIA

A four-day-old newborn was referred from local hospital with jaundice. Jaundice was noticed within 24 hours of birth and was increasing in spite of sun exposure. Birth weight 3 kg. Mother's blood group was O +ve and baby's group was not known. Baby had a difficult delivery and had a large cephal haematoma. Baby was born to a short primi mother.

On examination: Yellow staining of palms and soles present. Baby had poor suck, lethargy, shrill cry, hypertonia and an episode of convulsion. Baby had persistent downward gaze. Liver and spleen palpable 2 cm below the costal margin. S bilirubin 25 mg/dl, Direct 0.6 mg/dl, SGOT/ SGPT 45/50, SAP 300 IU/L Blood group A +ve. Hb 10 g/dl, Peripheral Smear: Evidence of hemolysis with numerous spherocytes. RBS 60 mg/dl, Thyroid function test normal, Direct Coomb's test positive.

DIAGNOSIS AND DISCUSSION
(Also Refer Table 7.6)

Hemolytic Disease of the Newborn (HyDN) due to AO incompatibility and Bilirubin encephalopathy (Kernicterus), cephal hematoma and possible neonatal sepsis

AO incompatibility manifests in the first baby itself unlike in Rh incompatibility, which affects subsequent pregnancies. It should have been anticipated and diagnosed by doing umbilical cord blood grouping, cord blood bilirubin and Hb in O group mothers. Cord blood bilirubin > 5 mg/dl and

Hb < 10 g/dl warrant immediate and efficient phototherapy. Exchange transfusion is needed when S. bilirubin is in exchange zone or if S. Br. rise is > 0.5 mg/hour. Hypoglycemia, sepsis hypoxia and acidosis aggravate hyperbilirubine-mia. Cephal hematoma, intestinal obstruction and hypothyroidism are other risk factors. Clinical severity of jaundice is assessed by skin colour (Table 4.4).

AO incompatibility is the most likely diagnosis as the jaundice appeared within 24 hours of birth and the mother O +ve and Baby is A +ve. Spherocytes can occur in AO incompatibility. However, hereditary spherocytosis is yet another possibility. In direct hyperbilirubinemia, direct S. Br. is > 20% of the total. Direct bilirubin increase is noted in associated sepsis. Difficult delivery, poor suck and increase in direct bilirubin point to possible sepsis. Elevated liver enzymes also may occur in sepsis. The lifespan of RBCs in newborn is about 90 days compared to 120 days in others. The liver is immature in them and hence most newborns develop physiological jaundice, that occur after 24-48 hours of birth and clear off in 1-2 weeks (Table 4.5).

Baby has typical features of Kernicterus/ Bilirubin Encephalopathy including sun setting sign. This baby is the victim of 'missed opportu-nities' in neonatal care.

The treatment options are immediate efficient phototherapy using green, blue or white light or halogen lamp and biliblanket. Adequate hydration, with N saline, 10- 20 ml/kg bolus, single donor plasma or albumin infusion, are also beneficial. Broad spectrum antibiotics and double blood volume exchange transfusion using 160-180 ml/kg O +ve blood compatible to both mother and baby are warranted. The sequelae are brain damage, status marmoratus, choreo-athetoid cerebral palsy, high tone deafness, developmental retardation, permanent staining of teeth and upward gaze palsy.

The different diagnosis for hemolysis is hereditary spherocytosis. In this condition Coomb's test will be negative and osmotic fragility will be increased. TFT may be repeated later as TSH may take time to rise.

Short mother may have difficult delivery. UNICEF has put up a goal for prospective mothers to achieve at least 40-45 kg and 140-145 cm height to reduce LBW and other complications.

In Rh incompatibility, mother is Rh negative and baby is Rh positive. Previous Rh +ve pregnancy, abortion or transfusion will sensitize the mother to produce antibodies, which get transferred during subsequent pregnancy. Anti D antibody (300 mcg) injection within 72 hours of delivery or abortion is recommended for prophylaxis.

In ABO, mother is O +ve and baby may be A or B +ve. It is a universal preformed antibody and hence can occur even in the first pregnancy. Phenobarbitone may help to induce liver enzymes and hence may be beneficial. IV immunoglobulin will decrease hemolysis and competitively block antibodies. Phototherapy leads to photo-oxidation and photo isomerization of bilirubin (lumirubin) and help in excretion. Direct bilirubinemia will result in 'bronze baby' with pigmentation following phototherapy.

In Rh -ve mothers, 2 doses of Anti D globulin (300 mcg = 1 ml Rhogam) may be administered at 28-32 weeks and then at birth to prevent sensitization. This dose is sufficient to eliminate 10 ml of antigenic fetal cells.

SECTION 4.5

A NEWBORN BABY WITH DIRECT HYPERBILIRUBINE-MIA AND MICROCEPHALY

A 25-day-old term newborn was brought with poor feeding, poor activity, jaundice and reddish blue lesions over the body. Mother had several episodes of febrile illness and urinary tract infection from 1st trimester onwards and was on medications. Birth weight was 2.2 kg.

On examination: Sick baby, cry and activity poor, eyes, body, palms and soles show icterus, pallor, purpura and blue berry muffins +. Hepatosplenomegaly +, microphthalmia and microcephaly (OFC 30 cm), CVS and RS within normal limits. Hypertonia +, S Br 15 mg/dl. Direct 4 mg/dl. SGOT/SGPT 90/102 IU/L, SAP 250 IU/L, TFT N, RDT +ve, platelet count 80,000/cumm. Babygram—Whole body X-ray—epiphyseal hypoplastic centres in the knee and talus, calcaneum and cuboid in the ankles +. CT head—Ventriculomegaly with calcification around the ventricle.

DIAGNOSIS AND DISCUSSION (Table 4.5)

Intrauterine infection probably CMV with conjugated hyperbilirubinemia, thrombocytopenia and microcephaly

Maternal febrile illness during pregnancy, low birth weight, microcephaly ventriculomegaly, periventricular calcification, thrombocytopenia, conjugated hyperbilirubinemia, anaemia and hepatosplenomegaly favour the diagnosis of intrauterine infection, most probably cytomegalovirus. Baby has to be investigated for chorio retinitis and deafness. 'Blue berry muffins' are secondary to

cutaneous extramedullary erythropoiesis. Microcephaly with ventriculomegaly is unique for CMV.

Among the other infections, rubella usually present with CHD-PDA or pulmonary branch stenosis, corneal opacity, cataract and 'celery stalk/broom stick appearance' of long bones with alternate dense and lucent longitudinal bands.

Toxoplasmosis present with large head, hydrocephalus, and diffuse brain calcification apart from jaundice, hepatosplenomegaly, anemia, purpura and meningoencephalitis.

Herpes simplex present with vesicles, cicatricial scars, keratitis, conjunctivitis, apart from jaundice, hepatosplenomegaly and anaemia.

Congenital syphilis usually has normal birth weight, snuffles, anemia, meningoencephalitis and osteochondritis. Congenital rubella babies are called 'cloudy babies' as they shed the virus for 1-2 years and are potential risk to women in the child bearing age. They may retain the virus in the eye for a decade and pose threat of infection to ophthalmologists who do cataract surgery.

CROTCHES is a new acronym similar to TORCH and STORCH that includes Coxsakie, Rubella, others like HIV, HBV, TB etc., Toxoplasma, CMV, Herpes, Enteroviruses and Syphilis.

The differential diagnosis is other intrauterine infections and teratogenic effect of antenatal medications. Medications usually produce congenital heart and skeletal defects. Septicemia is another differential diagnosis which can explain poor feeding, poor activity, pallor, hepatospleno-megaly thrombocytopenia and positive RDT. But, microcephaly, microphthalmia and periventricular calcification point to intrauterine infection rather than post natal infection.

CMV inclusion bodies can be detected in urine in CMV. Positive CMV IgG and IgM in the baby and IgG in the mother are diagnostic. After 3-4 months of age, rising titre of IgG, more than that in the mother is diagnostic as IgM start waning off after 3 months of age. Treatment includes gancyclovir for 6 weeks especially if chorioretinitis is present. Other treatment option is cytosine/adenine arabinoside. Acyclovir is not effective in CMV that belongs to the Herpes group of virus.

Hypothyroidism usually produces indirect hyperbilirubinemia due to reduced enzyme function. Breast milk jaundice is due to transfer of conjugation inhibitor like 3 Alpha 20 Beta pregnanediol. Driscoll Lucy syndrome is due to transplacental transfer of inhibitor like ortho-aminophenol.

CHAPTER 4

NEONATOLOGY

SECTION
4.6   A BLEEDING NEONATE

A 3-week-old term female newborn was admitted with crops of purpuric spots, hematuria and melena. Birth weight 3 kg. Hb 16 g/dl, WBC normal, Coomb's test–ve, platelet count 28,000/cumm. Peripheral smear no evidence of hemolysis or abnormal cells. LFT, PT and APTT–Normal. RDT and TORCH IgM–ve. Mother's blood count, ESR, ANA, DsDNA, APLA and Coomb's test–ve. Mother gave no history of any drug intake.

DIAGNOSIS AND DISCUSSION

Thrombocytopenic Purpura most probably Alloimmune Thrombocytopenia Purpura (AITP)

The most common cause of thrombocytopenia and bleeding in the newborn is sepsis with DIC, in which RDT will be +ve and PT, APTT prolonged with thrombocytopenia in a sick looking baby. The 2nd possibility is intrauterine infection with thrombocytopenia in which baby will be LBW with other stigma of infection and TORCH IgM will be positive. The 3rd possibility is immune thrombocytopenic purpura due to transfer of antiplatelet antibodies in which mother will have thrombocytopenia (ITP) or autoimmune disease with +ve markers of SLE/ ITP/ Evan's syndrome. Evan's syndrome is antibody mediated destruction of platelet and RBCs. In the case, Coomb's test will be positive and there will be evidence of hemolysis and thrombocytopenia. The duration of such thrombocytopenia due to transferred antibodies is 2-3 months. Corticosteroids avd IVIG given to

the mother 1 week prior to delivery is found beneficial. Antiplatelet antibodies will be positive in the baby and mother. Rarely aplastic anemia or leukemias may be the cause of thrombocytopenia in the newborn. Other differential diagnosis includes Amegakaryoctic thrombocytopenia/ Thrombocytopenia absent radius (TAR) syndrome, Kasabach Merritt syndrome with cavernous hemangioma etc. In newborn, thrombocytopenia is <1,50000 unlike <1 lakh in others.

With normal platelet count in the mother and –ve markers of auto immune disease and no other obvious cause of thrombocytopenia in the baby, a diagnosis of AITP can be made in the baby. It is due to the presence of platelet antigens, especially PLA1 in the fetus that the mother does not have. The mother may produce high titres of anti platelet antibodies that cause thrombocytopenia in the baby. The first born as well as subsequent pregnancies may be affected. Treatment includes platelet transfusion and corticosteroids/IVIG to the baby. This is similar to ABO incompatibility and alloimmune neonatal neutropenia. Washed platelets from the mother are usually preferred for transfusion to the baby.

In platelet function defect like thrombasthenias, platelet count will be normal or only mildly reduced. In Wiskott Aldrich syndrome, only boys will be affected. There will be eczema, immunodeficiency and draining ears. These conditions usually manifest later in life. There was no evidence of thrombosis or gangrene to account for thrombotic thrombocytopenic purpura (TTP).

In ITP and AITP, Bone marrow will show proliferation of megakaryocytes with increased budding as against markedly reduced megakaryocytes in pancytopenia, Amegakaryocytic thrombocytopenia and leukaemias.

Late onset hemorrhagic disease of the newborn (HgDN) is not considered because thrombocytopenia is the cause of bleeding and not coagulation defect. Early HgDN occurs within 1 week and late occurs after 1 week. In this condition, factors II, VII, IX and X are reduced. PT, APTT will be prolonged without thrombocytopenia in HgDN. In 'May Hegglin anomaly', there may be reduced neutrophils and platelets with irregular blue cytoplasm and are usually asymptomatic.Hemophilia with coagulation defect manifest with umbilical stump bleeding, APTT will be prolonged.

CHAPTER 4

NEONATOLOGY

SECTION
4.7   A CONVULSING NEWBORN

Three-day-old neonate was admitted to NICU with repeated episodes of convulsions. It was a term baby with BW 3.8 kg and no history of birth asphyxia. Baby had glucose push in the postnatal ward, but convulsion recurred and the RBS came as 55 mg/dl before push. Mother was not on any medications, but one value of FBS was recorded as 120 mg/dl. There was no family history of seizures or any neurocutaneous markers in the parents or baby. Baby had no birth asphyxia.

On examination baby conscious, AF normal, all systems including CNS were within normal limits in between convulsions.

DIAGNOSIS AND DISCUSSION

Infant of Gestational Diabetes Mellitus (IGDM) Baby with Neonatal Seizure probably due to hypocalcemia or hypo magnesemia

Relatively larger birth weight and one FBS value > 120 mg/dl in the mother points to Gestational Diabetes Mellitus (GDM). Mother should have had a GTT and proper control of blood sugar, which was overlooked in this case.

GDM infants are prone to seizures due to hypoglycemia, hypocalcemia and hypomagnese-mia. Here hypoglycemia is ruled out. So, hypocalcemia (NB–9-11.5 mg/dl) and hypom-agnesmia (NB–1.2-2.6 mg/dl) are the most possible clinical situations to be considered. Other possibilities are HIE stage II and Intracranial hemorrhage (ICH), which are unlikely in this baby due to non-contributory history and normal CNS examination. Pyridoxine deficiency/dependency is possible if the mother had been on pyridoxine for hyperemesis or oxaluria. Drug/alcohol withdrawal is possible if the mother was on any such medications/alcohol.

Hypocalcemia and hypomagnesemia usually do not lead to sequelae unlike hypoglycemia, HIE and ICH. LGA babies especially > 4 kg may preferably be on IV glucose or under close monitoring with early frequent feeds to prevent hypoglycemia. This baby responded to 10% calcium gluconate 2 ml/kg IV and 0.2 ml/kg 50% Mg sulphate diluted and given as slow infusion.

In newborns, the anticonvulsants given are phenobarbitone, 15-20 mg/kg loading dose followed by 5 mg/kg/day and phenytoin 15 mg/kg loading dose followed by 5-8 mg/kg/day. Diazepam is avoided as it will displace bilirubin from binding site.

In adults 75 g glucose is given for GTT. Interpretation of GTT is given in Table 4.6. 1.75 g/kg/glucose is given for GTT in a child.

SECTION 4.8 A NEWBORN WITH RESPIRATORY DISTRESS

A 2 kg 34 weeker was rushed from labor room to NICU with respiratory distress with RR 80/mt, chest retractions and audible grunt. Baby was cyanosed. Apex beat was not palpable. Heart sounds were better heard on the right side and heart rate was 90/mt and percussion note was tympanic on the left side. Abdomen was not distended. Baby was intubated due to bradycardia and on giving 100% oxygen colour improved. There was no history of gestational diabetes.

DIAGNOSIS AND DISCUSSION

Respiratory Distress Syndrome most probably Congenital Diaphragmatic Hernia (CDH)

Differential Diagnosis: RDS – HMD with pneumothorax Lt

Tachypnoea, RR> 60/mt, chest retraction and grunt lead to the diagnosis of RDS. Scoring is done as per the Downey Scoring system (Table 4.7). Oxygen saturation/Colour improving on giving after 100% Oxygen confirms respiratory cause for cyanosis (Hyperoxia test) Tympanic percussion note on left, mediastinal shift/ dextroposition of heart and non distended abdomen (scaphoid abdomen) point to CDH. Tympanic note on the right side also may be noted due to compensative emphysema or pneumothorax. A Ryles tube should be put to decompensate the stomach and erect X-ray chest should be taken with ryle tube in situ. For confirmation, barium study may also be done. Bag and mask ventilation is contraindicated in this condition. The

baby should be stabilized and if needed ventilator care should be given and then taken up for early surgery. Fetal surgery is also useful. Bag and mask ventilation is contraindicated and may lead to pneumothorax, pneumomediastinum and pneumoperitoneum. Pulmonary hypoplasia in CDH usually results in poor prognosis.

Hyaline Membrane Disease (HMD) occurs in preterms below 32 weeks and manifestation usually start a few hours after birth. There will be ground glass/whitewashed appearance in X-ray. It can occur in near term or term IDM babies due to immaturity of lung, even when gestational age is more than 32 weeks. Surfactant therapy and nasal or bubble CPAP are beneficial in babies with HMD.

Congenital pneumonia occurs with early onset neonatal sepsis (EONS), maternal pyrexia, PROM etc. Gastric aspirate will be positive for polymorphs (> 5 HPF). In this case, RDT will be positive.

Meconium Aspiration Syndrome (MAS) is diagnosed with history of meconium aspiration or meconium stained amniotic fluid (MSAF) and X-ray findings.

Transient Tachypnea of the Newborn (TTN) is usually seen in C section babies due to fluid filled lung which improves in 2-3 days with or without oxygen administration. It is usually seen in term babies. The causes of RDS are given in Table 4.8

Congenital lobar emphysema (CLE) is more common on the left side with overdistension of lung. Lung markings will be present unlike pneumothorax.

Cystadenomatoid malformation of lung (CAM) is more common on the right side. It may be microcystic, macrocystic or solid. Microcytic variety has better prognosis.

Wilson Mikity syndrome is due to lung dysmaturity in VLBW babies occurring around 2-3 weeks after birth.

Bronchopulmonary dysplasia (BPD) is due to high oxygen concentration in premature babies coupled with ventilator barotrauma and PDA shunt.

Pulmonary lymphangiectasia is a rare, but fatal disease with RDS and cyanosis from birth.

LBW is < 2.5 kg, VLBW is < 1.5 kg and extremely LBW (ELBW) is < 1 kg.

A SICK NEWBORN—ONE AMONG TWINS

Term 2.2 kg newborn, one among twins was admitted 24 hours after delivery to NICU with lethargy, poor feeding and distress. Baby was hypotonic, irritable and jaundiced. There was tachycardia, tachypnoea, cyanosis, cardiomegaly, abdominal distension and enlarged palpable kidneys. Hb 24 g/dl, PCV 70%, RDT – ve, B urea 25 mg/dl, S Br. 15 mg/dl. The other twin was with the mother (weight 1.8 kg) and the Hb was 12.5 g/dl and PCV 30%. S Br 4 mg/dl.

DIAGNOSIS AND DISCUSSION

Polycythemia of the Newborn due to Twin to Twin Transfusion:

The history and C/F are suggestive of twin to twin transfusion, one developing anaemia and the other one developing polycythemia. Lethargy, poor feeding, irritability, seizure, hyperbilirubine-mia, cardiomegaly, tachypnoea, cyanosis, tachycardia and renal vein thrombosis are the features of polycythemia. PCV >55% is diagnostic. Hb in newborn is usually around 17 and < 13 indicates anemia.

Early recognition and prompt treatment is rewarding. Partial plasma or N saline exchange transfusion is the treatment of choice.

Volume to be taken out/transfused

Observed PCV–Desired PCV (55) x Blood volume/Observed PCV.

Blood volume is 85 ml/kg in normal babies and 100 ml/kg in LBW babies.

The other baby may benefit from a 'top up' transfusion of packed cells 10 ml/kg. in the newborn, Hb < 8g/dl needs intervention like transfusion.

Feto-maternal hemorrhage may be the cause for anemia in some babies. This can be diagnosed by Kleihauer-Betke test in maternal blood. Fetal RBCs are resistant to acid elution and will remain darkly stained, while adult RBCs will appear like

CHAPTER 4

NEONATOLOGY

A PRETERM BABY WITH DIARRHEA

ghost cells.

A newborn 1 kg, 35 weeker was born with pallor, poor cry, poor activity, meconium stained liquor and the baby was found to have diarrhea. RDT was positive.

DIAGNOSIS AND DISCUSSION

Listeriosis

Preterm babies are prone for early onset neonatal sepsis (EONS), but meconium passage in utero does not usually occur in preterm babies. Usually, fetal distress in term babies and postmaturity lead to passage of meconium in utero. +ve sepsis screen, C/F and fetal diarrhea is diagnostic of listeriosis. The drug of choice is Ampicillin.

A NEWBORN WITH CYANOSIS

A term newborn baby 3.5 kg was admitted with cyanosis and tachypnea.

On examination: Tachycardia +, hepatomegaly +; Grade 2/6 systolic murmur +, mild edema+.

DIAGNOSIS AND DISCUSSION

Cyanotic congenital heart disease.

Differential Diagnosis: Cyanosis due to Respiratory cause, CNS cause or Methemoglobinemia.

Marked cyanosis without severe RDS is suggestive of cardiac cause. Severe RDS, chest retractions and mild cyanosis that improve with oxygen is suggestive of respiratory cause. CNS depression of respiratory failure/apnea may also cause cyanosis. In methemoglobinemia, cyanosis is present, but oxygen saturation will be normal. In cyanotic heart disease, clubbing appears in 3-6 weeks.

Cardiac causes for cyanosis are transposition of great arteries (TGA). Pulmonary atresia tricuspid atresia, anomalous pulmonary veins and Ebstein anomaly. In right to left shunt, cyanosis increases on crying. Administration of 100% oxygen will not relieve cyanosis nor increase arterial PO_2.

Hyperoxia test is done by administering 100% oxygen for 10 minutes followed by ABG. PaO_2 <70 will confirm CCHD and > 150 mm will favour respiratory condition.

Features of cardiac failure like edema, hepatomegaly point to cardiac cause. Cyanosis usually manifest when arterial PO_2 is <40 torr and when oxygen saturation is <85%. Polycythemic babies manifest cyanosis more rapidly as reduced Hb > 5 g/dl is achieved faster in them than anemic babies.

Fig. Nos. 11-22 (Plates 4 to 5) show various disorders and anomalies in the newborn.

Table 4.1: Clinical staging of HIE (Sarnat and Sarnat)

No	Parameter	I	II	III
1	Consciousness	Alert	Drowsy	Comatose
2	Sucking	Active	Poor	Absent
3	Muscle tone	Normal	Hypotonic	Flaccid
4	Tendon reflex	Brisk	Exaggerated	Absent
5	Moro reflex	Exaggerated	Incomplete	Absent
6	Doll's eye	Normal	Exaggerated	Reduced
7	Pupils	Reacting	Constricted	Dilated, fixed
8	Respiration	Normal	Periodic	Apneic attacks
9	Heart rate	Normal	Bradycardia	Bradycardia
10	Seizure	Absent	Common	Absent
11	EEG	Normal	Periodic discharges/ low voltage/ delta waves	Isoelectric/ periodic discharges

Table 4.2: Neonatal sepsis score (Bhakoo, *et al*)

No	Risk item	Score
1	LBW/<37 weeks	3
2	Maternal pyrexia	2
3	Foul smelling liquor	2
4	Unclean vaginal examination	2
5	Birth asphyxia	2
6	PROM >24 hours	1
7	Duration of labor >24 hours	1

Interpretation

Score 0 - 3—Observe

Score 4 - 5—Investigate

Score 6 and above—Full sepsis work up and antibiotics pending culture report.

Table 4.3: Normal CSF findings in various age groups

Age	Cells/ cumm	Protein mg/dl	Sugar mg/dl
Term	7 (0-32) 60% neurophils	90 (20-170)	52 (34-119) > 50% of RBS
Preterm	8 (0-29) 60% neutrophils	115 (65-150)	50 (24-63) > 75% of RBS
<2 mo	< 5 75 % lymphocytes	20-45	> 50 mg/ > 50% of RBS

Table 4.4: Clinical correlation of jaundice with skin color (Cramer's)

Clinical Jaundice	S.Bilirubin
Face	5 mg/dl
Upto Nipple	7 mg/dl
Face + Trunk	10 mg/dl
Face + Trunk + Thigh	12 mg/dl
Face + Trunk + Legs	15 mg/dl
Whole body + Palms and soles	> 20 mg/dl

Table 4.5: Causes of neonatal jaundice as per time of onset

< 24 Hrs	24-72 Hrs	>72 Hrs
Blood group incompatibility (Rh, ABO and minor groups)	Physiological jaundice Exaggerated physiol.	Neo. sepsis
Intrauterine infections	jaundice	Neo. hepatitis
Maternal drugs—	Prematurity, acidosis,	Neo. cholestasis
Vitamin K,salicylates,	hypoxia, polycythemia,	Biliary atresia
sulfisoxazole	cephal hematoma	Breast milk jaundice
Hemolytic anemias	Hypothyroidism and	Intestinal obstruction,
Crigler-Najjar syndrome	All causes <24 hrs	Pyloric stenosis
Lucy Driscoll syndrome		Metabolic causes—
		Galactosemia, tyrosinemia
		Hypothyroidism
		Inspissated bile syndrome
		Intrauterine infections
		Gilbert's syndrome, Dubin -Johnson syndrome

Table 4.6: Interpretation of GTT and blood sugar values (mg/dl)

Time	Abnormal GTT (GDM)	Impaired glucose tolerance	Diabetes mellitus
Fasting	> 105	> 126	>126
1 hour	> 90	–	
2 hours	> 165	140-200	>200
3 hours	> 145		

No	Item	0	1	2
	Table 4.7: Clinical scoring of respiratory distress in the newborn (Downey score)			
1	RR	<60	60-80	>80
2	Cyanosis	No	No cyanosis with 40% oxygen	Requiring >40% oxygen
3	Retractions	None	Mild	Moderate–Severe
4	Grunt	None	Audible with steth	audible without steth
5	Air entry	Good	Decreased	Barely audible

Table 4.8: Causes of RDS

No	Condition	Age of onset	Remarks
A	**Respiratory Causes**		
1	Aspiration/MAS	At birth	LBW, prematurity/postmaturity Fetal distress, meconium stained liquor
2	Congenital pneumonia	1-2 days	Maternal pyrexia, foul smelling liquor, PROM, Birth asphyxia
3	Postnatal aspiration/ pneumonia	1-3 weeks	LBW, cleft palate, untrained nurse. GERD, neonatal sepsis
4	HMD	1-6 hours	Prematurity, GDM
5	TTN	1st day	Term CS baby, materno-fetal Transfusion
6	Congenital malformations, CDH, atresias, Congenital lobaremphysema, CAM	At birth/Variable	Other anomalies, specific features
B	**CVS Causes**		
1	CCF	Variable	CHD, anemia
2	Pulmonary hypertension/ Anomalous pulmonary venous connections	Variable	PPHN, TAPVC
C	**CNS Causes**		
1	CNS immaturity, malformation, trauma, asphyxia	Variable	Prematurity, difficult delivery
2	Respiratory muscle paralysis, diaphragm, intercostals	Variable	Breech/traumatic delivery, myasthenia gravis, congenital polio, SMA, myopathy
D	**Metabolic Disorders**		
1	Organic acidemias, hypoglycemia, hyperammonemia	Variable	Inborn errors of metabolism, positive family history
E	**Others**		
1	Sepsis, shock	Variable	GBS infections

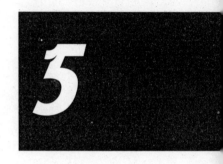

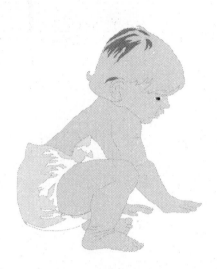

Infection and Infestations

SECTION 5.1

A CHILD WITH PROLONGED FEVER WITHOUT A FOCUS

A 10-year-old girl with history of recurrent oral ulcers for the last 6 months developed fever, that was persisting for more than 3 weeks and hence was admitted. She was on levamisole for the last 2 months for immuno modulation for oral ulcer from a local hospital.

On examination: Temp 102°F. RR 30/mt, HR 100/mt BP 100/60. Capillary filing time 2 seconds, oral ulcer +, Throat congested, whitish patches +, multiple cervical lymph nodes palpable. Liver palpable 3 cm, spleen not palpable. Other systems within normal limits. Hb 9 gm/dl, TC 3000/cumm, P15, L 85, platelet count 1.1 lakh/cumm, ESR 95 mm/1st hr, CRP 12 mg/dl, X-ray chest–Increased bronchovascular markings.

DIAGNOSIS AND DISCUSSION

FUO/PUO- Febrile Neutropenia probably Agranulocytosis secondary to Levamisole

History of prolonged fever, documented fever >1 week duration on several occasions and failure to reach diagnosis despite 1 week of investigations is diagnostic of fever/pyrexia of unknown origin (FUO/PUO). The child's absolute neutrophil count (ANC) is < 500/cumm, which clinches the diagnosis of febrile neutropenia. Levamisole is well-known to cause agranulocytosis. Blood culture may be rewarding. But empirical antibiotic therapy should include ceftazidime or 4th generation cephalosporin + Vancomycin + CP or Metrogyl for anaerobic cover. Crystalline penicillin (CP) is usually started for infection above the diaphragm and Metrogyl for those below the diaphragm. In penicillin/beta lactam antibiotic hypersensitivity, meropenem is an alternate drug for febrile neutropenia. Absent eosinophils/Eosinopenia is indicative of a stressful condition to the body with outpouring of corticosteroids.

Durack and Street-Fever of Unknown Origin (FUO) Classification

1. Classic FUO
2. Nosocomial FUO
3. Neutropenic FUO
4. FUO Associated with HIV infection.

Control of fever should be achieved by tepid sponging and paracetamol 10-15 mg/kg/dose. Other antipyretics used are ibuprofen, mefenamic acid, aspirin nimesulide etc. These are better avoided due to toxicity and interactions with drugs and viruses.

CHAPTER 5

INFECTION AND INFESTATIONS

SECTION 5.2 AN INFANT WITH FEVER, RASH, DIARRHEA AND SHOCK

A 5-month-old baby with acute onset of fever, rash and diarrhea was admitted with circulatory collapse.

On examination: Febrile, Temp 103° F, Generalized erythematous rash +, Mouth and Pharynx congested, BP 60 mm Systolic, CFT 3 seconds, profuse watery Diarrhea +, Skin turgor 3 seconds. Hb 9 g/dl, TC 15000, P72, L28, ESR 42/mm 1st Hr, Platelet count 90,000/cumm, B Urea 45 mg/dl, S creatinine 1.8 mg/dl, S Na 135 mEq/L, S K 3.5, S Br. 2 mg/dl, SGOT/SGPT 82/102 IU/L, ASO 100 U, Urine Alb trace, Pus cells 5-10/HPF. PT and APTT within normal limits. Blood and stool cultures were also taken. Baby also gave a history of immunization 2 days back in a peripheral camp.

DIAGNOSIS AND DISCUSSION

Toxic Shock Syndrome (TSS) Probably Staphylococcal

The diagnosis of TSS is based on fever, rash, hypotension and at least 3 organ involvement (Table 5.1). This baby was having GIT, hematological and renal involvement. The history of an immunization in a peripheral camp is a predisposing factor for the same.

Differential Diagnosis: Dengue fever, Kawasaki disease, septicemia with DIC, Rickettsial fever, Leptospirosis and measles. GIT symptoms are rare in these conditions.

Blood culture yielded methicillin sensitive staph. aureus (MSSA) in this case confirming the diagnosis. Absent eosinophils noted is a grave sign indicating a stressful state with outpouring of corticosteroids.

Cloxacillin 200 mg/kg/day Q 6 H and supportive care were given to the baby. The baby recovered, but developed desquamation of palms and soles in the 2nd week.

Streptococcal TSS can also occur, but rare. In adults, TSS may be associated with menstruation and is usually staphylococcal. The diagnosis is based on major and minor criteria (Table 5.1).

Diagnosis of other exanthematous fever and positive blood culture will exclude TSS. Staph. aureus produces abscess, boils and carbuncles (ABC), empyema, TSS and scalded skin syndrome (SSS). The different toxins elaborated by Staph. aureus are the following:

Hemolysins (Alpha→tissue necrosis, Beta→hemolysis and gamma→disruption of cell membrane), Leukocidin→neutrophil and macrophage leakage, exfoliative toxin→bullous impetigo and SSSS, enterotoxin→food poisoning and TSS (non menstrual—enterotoxin A and B) and TSS toxin I (menstrual TSS). The enzymes are coagulase, catalase, penicillinase, hyaluronidase, lipase, phosphodiesterases. Penicillinase/Beta lactamase inactivate→Betalactum antibiotics (Cephalosporins, Penicillins) and extended Spectrum. Betalactam inhibitors (ESBL) inactivate—3rd generation cephalosporins.

A CHILD WITH FEVER AND SHOCK

A 4-year-old child with history of fever, sore throat seen in local PHC in the morning was admitted to PICU the same night with extensive rash all over the body. Child also had purpuric lesions and blackish discoloration of 2nd toe (left).

On examination: Febrile, RR 35/mt, pulse 130/mt, rapid and thready, BP systolic 70 mm of Hg, CFT – 3 seconds. Ashen grey face with lethargy and drowsiness.

Hb 9 g/dl, TC 10,000/cumm , P74, L 24, E 2, platelet count 1 lakh/cumm.

DIAGNOSIS AND DISCUSSION

Meningococcemia with Shock probably adrenal hemorrhage – Waterhouse Friderichsen syndrome

Differential Diagnosis: Septicemia with DIC.

Febrile illness with rash, purpura, gangrene and rapidly progressive shock are diagnostic of meningococcemia/Sepsis and DIC. Associated shock and rapid progression is usually due to adrenal haemorrhage leading to shock. There may also be meningitis.

Swab from the skin lesion may yield meningococci (gram negative diplococci). Blood culture and gram stain may confirm the diagnosis. Treatment includes supportive care including steroid and empiric antibiotic therapy. CP 3 lakh/kg/day, Q4 H or cefotaxime 200 mg/kg/day Q 6 H/ceftriaxone 100 mg/kg Q12 H or Chloramphenicol 100 mg/kg/day Q 6 H for 7-10 days. The diagnosis of meningococcemia is important as it warrants Rifampicin prophylaxis to household contacts. H. Influenza (HIB) also warrants prophylaxis. The dose of rifampicin is 20 mg/kg/day Q 12 H for 2 days in meningococcemia. Ceftriaxone 125-250 mg IM single dose and ciprofloxcin 500 mg PO single dose also are useful in prophylaxis.

DIC can occur in any case of septicemia including meningococcemia. The features are prolonged PT, APTT, thrombocytopenia and increased FDP or D Dimers. Septicemia usually produces a warm shock with narrow pulse pressure initially. There is capillary leak and multi organ dysfunction (MODS). Supportive care includes organ by organ support namely CNS (Ventilation and oxygen), Resp system (Acute respiratory distress syndrome—Ventilation and O_2) CVS (fluid management and ionotropes) GIT (Hemorrhagic Gastroenteropathy-H2 receptor blockers, proton pump inhibitors, renal (fluid management and ionotropes) etc. Protein C replacement therapy is also tried.

Meningococcal vaccine (Meningovax) is not completely protective as it is immunogenic against A/C/Y/W – 135 only, but not against B subunit.

SECTION
5.4   A CHILD WITH BULL NECK

A 3-year-old child with history of fever and sore throat was admitted with extensive cervical adenopathy amounting to 'Bull neck'. He was only partially immunized and had missed many of his injections. He was having drooling and difficulty in swallowing, ENT consultation was done to rule out peritonsilar abscess. The swelling in the right side of the submandibular region increased and an I&D was done which resulted in a fistula through which swallowed fluids were coming out. He was on CP, Ceftriaxone and Cloxacillin for 2 weeks. In the second week, he developed palatal paralysis and nasal regurgitation. MRI brain did not reveal any CNS or cranial nerve involvement. Repeat ENT examination revealed a pharyngeal membrane which was negative for diphtheria, but positive for fungus. He did not develop any evidence of myocarditis, ophthalmoplegia or symmetric spinal nerve paralysis (Table 5.2). He was given Anti Diphtheritic Serum (ADS) 1 lakh unit and flucanazole orally.

He was on supportive care including partial parenteral nutrition. Subsequently, general condition, neck swelling and paralysis improved and the cutaneous fistula healed.

DIAGNOSIS AND DISCUSSION

Diphtheria with Palatal Paralysis

Bull neck is due to massive lymphadenopathy.

This partially immunised child's pharyngeal membrane was not visualised initially due to drooling and oedema which prevented proper examination. The I & D from outside could have been avoided, if ADS was administered early leading to resolution of nodes. In the 2nd week, ADS was given after developing local paralysis and on seeing the membrane. As fungal growth was noticed Flucanazole was given. The child received 1 lakh units, Anti Diphtheretic Serum (ADS) IV. Diptheria Immunoglobulin (Dipglob) can also be given, 0.3 ml/kg IM for prophylaxis and 0.6 ml kg/IM for treatment. Schick test positive sensitive contacts need prophylactic antibiotics, oral penicillin or erythromycin. Benzathine penicillin single dose IM may also be given. Ventilator care and tracheostomy may be needed in some cases.

It is due to corynebacterium diphtheriae and the toxin production is bacteriophage mediated. The various manifestations and the onset timings are given in Table 5.2.

Prevention is by administering 3 primary doses of DPT at one month interval, starting at 6 weeks of age and Boosters at around 18 months of age (DPT) and 5 years (DT). In children older than 7 years of age, Td is preferred to DPT/DT with lesser dose of diphtheria toxoid.

SECTION 5.5

A CHILD WITH PROLONGED FEVER AND HEPATO-SPLENOMEGALY

A 12-year-old boy was admitted with fever of 10 days duration. He had anorexia, headache, myalgia, abdominal pain, loose stool for 3 days and occasional cough. There was history of travel to an outstation temple 3 weeks ago. He gave a history of bathing in the temple pond. No history of contact with pets.

On examination: Pallor +, Temp 103°C, RR-30/mt/HR 88/mt, abdomen distended with diffuse tenderness, Liver and spleen palpable 3 cm below costal margin, discrete small lymph nodes in the cervical area, other systems within normal limits. He had Grade II PEM and mild first degree stunting.

Hb 9 g/dl, TC 4000/cumm, P 50, L40, E 10, ESR 58, platelet 1 lakh, Peripheral smear—no malarial parasite, S Br. 1.8, SGOT/SGPT 84/104.

DIAGNOSIS AND DISCUSSION

1. Enteric fever/Typhoid fever
2. Leptospirosis/Weil's disease
3. Disseminated TB
4. Dengue/IMN/other viral infection
5. Malaria/Other protozoa infection
6. Collagen vascular disease
7. Hematological malignancies.

History of travel to outstation temple, prolonged fever, GIT symptoms, hepatosplenomegaly, relative bradycardia and leucopenia favour the diagnosis of enteric fever, which can be confirmed by Widal test and culture of salmonella typhi. Widal is positive in the 2nd week of illness. Absence of relative bradycardia and presence of hepatomegaly/hepatosplenomegaly, rather than splenomegaly alone, are unique for children as against the manifestations in the adult. 'Rose spots' also may be seen in the second week. Encephalopathy and perforation of gut are dreaded complications of this condition. Widal O titre > 160 is diagnostic of acute infection, H titre indicates convalescent case. In titre > 100, rising titre may be looked for (Table 5.3).

Leptospirosis is also likely in view of history of bathing in pond, myalgia and deranged liver enzymes. CPK may be elevated and Weil's antibody IgM will confirm recent infection. Conjunctival congestion and icterus may also be seen. It is due to leptospira ictero-hemorrhagica (spirochete). It responds to CP/Doxycycline.

Disseminated TB (Table 5.4) is a common condition in India, which present with lymphadeno-pathy and hepatosplenomegaly. History of contact with TB, Positive Mantoux test, X-ray chest and USS abdomen showing lymph nodes/ascites may confirm the diagnosis. Sputum AFB/ascitic fluid AFB may also be looked for. Evidence of acute and chronic malnutrition is contributory to the diagnosis. 'BACTEC' is special culture that will yield TB bacilli in 2 weeks unlike 8 weeks in ordinary culture. A negative Mantoux test will not rule out TB.

Dengue fever (DENV), Chickungunya (CHIKV) and other endemic/reemerging viral infections should also be considered in the DD. These are transmitted through mosquito bite (Aedes Agyptiae). Headache, Rash, Leukopenia, thrombocytopenia and hemoconcentration and positive touurniquet test are noted in DENV. Dengue IgM will confirm recent primary infection. Positive IgM and low titers of IgG will be seen in reinfection. Reinfection and primary infection in infants with maternal antibodies are prone for Dengue Hemorrhagic Fever (DHF) (Table 5.5). This is due to Antibody dependent enhancement (ADE) of immune responses and also cell mediated immune responses. DF may show a Biphasic fever. The afebrile phase may mark the hemorrhagic manifestations. The 3 phases are the febrile phase, the leaky phase and the congestive phase. The critical stage may last for 3-10 days. Appropriate fluid management is life saving. DENV is flavi virus belonging to Togaviridae.

CHIKV present with myalgia and arthralgia or arthritis lasting for several weeks or months. It is an alpha virus. Chloroquine 250 mg/day (5 mg/kg/day) for several weeks may be needed to suppress the symptoms. Chloroquine has anti inflammatory, anti protozoal and anti viral effects.

IMN due to EB virus presents with prolonged fever, lymphadenopathy especially epitrochlear nodes and rash usually following ampicillin. Leukopenia, pancytopenia etc., may also occur.

It is an oncogenic virus and X-linked lympho-proliferation (XLP), Burkitt's lymphoma etc. may occur later. 'Alice in Wonderland syndrome' with perceptual problems may also occur in IMN. The other names of IMN are 'glandular fever' and 'kissing disease' due to increased incidence among adolescents following close contact.

Malaria is possible in case of travel to endemic area. Malaria may also be a co-infection with any of the above fevers. Usually paroxysms of fever, mild jaundice, pallor and splenomegaly with a positive smear during peak of pyrexia confirms the diagnosis.

Malaria is treated with chloroquin and primaquin. In presumptive treatment, chloroquin is given 10 mg base/kg orally followed by 5 mg/kg after 6 hours and 5 mg/kg/day for 2 days more. In radical treatment, primaquin is given 0.3 mg/kg/day for 5-14 days in falciparum infection. In vivax, a single dose of primaquin is given as gametocidal. In drug resistance, quinine is given 25 mg/kg/d for 10-14 days. Other drugs are sulfadoxine-pyrimethamine and artesunate.

Drug resistant malaria is treated with artesunate, quinine, pyrimethamine—sulphadoxine combination etc. Table 5.6 shows the levels of malarial parasites in peripheral smear in different types of drug resistance.

High ESR, pancytopenia or Leukocytosis with blast cells if present will point to leukemia. High ESR, positive ANA and anti ds DNA will point to collagen vascular disease in cases of PUO.

SECTION 5.6

AN INFANT WITH RECURRENT INFECTIONS AND DIARRHEA

A 5-month-old male baby was readmitted with diarrhea and cough. Baby was getting treatment from local hospital for 1 month for pneumonia. Then baby was admitted in a tertiary care hospital and discharged one week back after treatment with cefotaxime and Amikacin for 2 weeks for diarrhea and sepsis. Baby also had delayed milestones and head control was only partial. Thirst was increased and baby was irritable. Skin turgor 2 seconds, RR 56/mt. HR 112/mt, BP 60 systolic, pallor +, extensive oral thrush +, cervical and axillary nodes +, hepatosplenomegaly +, weight was < 60% of expected and there was mild pedal edema. (Weight 3.5 kg. previous admission 4 kg), Hb 8 g/dl, TC 3500, P 76, L20, E 4, platelet 1 lakh, CRP 8 mg/dl, X-ray chest RUL collapse consolidation, Lt Lower zone haziness. Elder sibling was 6 years old normal, parents appeared healthy.

DIAGNOSIS AND DISCUSSION

HIV–AIDS with Opportunist Infection (OI) and Marasmic Kwashiorkor

Baby had a prolonged illness starting around 3 months of age. Fever, recurrent pneumonia, recurrent/persistent diarrhea, oral thrush and weight loss point to immunodeficiency syndrome. Leukopenia and lymphopenia are contributory to the diagnosis. HIV ELISA was positive in the baby and both parents, but elder sibling was negative. Father was reported to have high risk behaviour. P24 Antigen study was also positive in the baby.

Upto 18 months of age, transplacental antibodies are detectable and hence retesting is mandatory at 18 months. But, P24 antigen positivity and clinical features are suggestive of HIV infection. P24 antigen testing may give false positive result in newborn babies. The other test is PCR. PCR RNA is qualitative and PCR DNA is quantitative.

The opportunistic infections are bacterial, fungal and probably parasitic-cryptosporidium. Treatment approach includes control of opportunistic infections, nutritional support and Highly Active Anti Retroviral Therapy (HAART). The diagnostic criteria are given in Table 5.7.

C section and avoidance of breastfeeding are advisable if HIV status is known antenatally. If formula feeding is not affordable/feasible, it is better to give exclusive breastfeeding for 3-4 months to reduce colonization by opportunists and then abruptly stop breastfeeding and go for complementary feeding. Breastfeeding raises the transmission rate of HIV from 30% to 45%.

Absolute lymphocyte count (ALC) equal to 1200 is said to be adequate in adults, corresponding to a CD_4 count of 200/cumm. In infants $CD_4 < 750$ is an indication for HAART (Table 5.8). CD_4 count is usually done after stabilization and treatment of opportunistic infection.

Pneumocystis (carini) pneumonia (PCP) pro-phylaxis is beneficial, starting early. The human strain of pneumocystis is now identified to be Pneumocystis jerovecci. PCP treatment includes trimethoprim sulpha in a dose of 20 mg/

kg/day in 4 divided doses IV initially followed by oral therapy for 21 days. PCP prophylaxis includes 5 mg/kg/day as a single dose. The WHO staging is given in Table 5.9 and treatment is given in Table 5.10.

The centres that undertake counselling and testing for Prevention of Parent to Child Transmission (PPTCT) are called SNEHA Centres attached to major maternity hospitals. Voluntary Counselling and Testing Centres (VCTC) are now called—JYOTHIS. HAART Centre are called USHAS and STD clinics are called PULARI.

These are the names of such centres in Kerala. Live viral vaccines are contraindicated in symptomatic patients.

Post Exposure Prophylaxis (PEP) is given is Table 5.11.

Patients with HIV, HBV and other blood borne infections pose biohazard threat and it may be necessary to take universal standard precautions to prevent spread. The label and logo of 'Biohazard' may be used to indicate this need (Table 5.12).

A CHILD WITH FEEDING DIFFICULTY AND MUSCLE SPASM

SECTION 5.7

A 10-year-old girl with history of chronic ear discharge was admitted with inability to eat/drink and stiffness of muscles. She was unimmunized and was belonging to the coastal area. She had generalized convulsions several times.

On examination: Conscious, inability to open mouth completely. Hypertonia +, Plantar down going. RR 28/mt, HR 100/mt, BP 128/80 mm of Hg.

DIAGNOSIS AND DISCUSSION

Otogenic tetanus

She is unimmunized and has a focus of infection for spore bearing bacteria like CSOM, trismus, muscles spasm and convulsion point to tetanus. Spatula test or Spoon test will be positive in tetanus. There will be clinching on to the spatula while trying to take it out from the mouth. Normally when spatula is pulled out, child will open the mouth and it can be taken out easily.

Differential Diagnosis: Brainstem encephalitis and strychnine poisoning. Due to primary immunization and prompt treatment of wounds, tetanus is rare, but otogenic tetanus do occur, especially among partially/unimmunized.

Complete primary immunizations and booster immunization including TT at 10 years and 15 years are essential for continued immunity. Those with ear discharge should have proper cleaning and prompt treatment in collaboration with an ENT surgeon. 3000-5000 units tetanus immuno-globulin (TIG) is usually given IM for treatment. TIG 500 units may be given for prophylaxis in ear infections. 500-2000 units are given in tetanus prone injuries for prophylaxis. Crystalline penicillin for 10-14 days is the antibiotic of choice.

Neonatal tetanus is now very rare. It manifests between 3-15 days and it usually presents with lock jaw (trismus), inability to feed, spasm of muscles and opisthotonos. Treatment includes 250 mg Tetanus Immunoglobulin, CP for 14 days and diazepam 0.3–1 mg/kg dose IV 3–4 hourly. Other useful drugs are chlorpromazine 1 mg/kg/dose, and mephenesin 3.0 mg/kg/dose and methacarbonol 25 mg/kg dose to control seizures and spasm. Some centres also give 250 units TIG intrathecally in tetanus.

The poor prognostic features are injury on the face (cephalic tetanus), short time of onset of seizures from trismus and respiratory compromise.

SECTION 5.8 AN INFANT WITH EXANTHEMATOUS FEVER

A 10-month-old baby was admitted with fever of 4 days duration.

On examination: Eyes red, flushed face, maculopapular rash over face and mouth +, loose stool and vomiting +, cough +, runny nose +, Immunization—Complete except measles vaccine.

DIAGNOSIS AND DISCUSSION

Exanthematous Fever—Measles

Exanthematous fever are common in children. Measles caused by Morbili RNA virus is the most common. It is called Rubeola/5 days measles as the rashes appear on 4th or 5th day of fever starting on the face and hair line. The prodromal stage has the 3Cs, cough, coryza and conjunctivitis plus the exanthem and the enanthem, Koplik spots. Lower eye lid congestion is called 'Stimson's line'. The complications include bacterial/viral/giant cell pneumonia, ear discharge, flaring up of TB, malnutrition, diarrhoea, protein losing entero-pathy, encephalitis etc. Slow virus infection (SSPE) subacute sclerosing pan encephalitis is a rare long-term complication.

Other Exanthematous Fevers

1. *Rubella/Three-day Measles:* It is caused by Rubi virus. Fever is mild with mild rash and posterior cervical/posterior auricular lymphadenopathy. It is a teratogenic virus leading to congenital rubella syndrome.

2. *Roseola/Exanthem subitum:* It is caused by HHV-6 and here rash occurs after control of fever, especially in an infant.

3. *Erythema Infectiosum/Fifth Disease:* It is caused by parvovirus B_{19}. It causes slapped cheek appearance and rash. The virus also causes aplastic crisis in hemolytic anemias.

4. *IMN:* It is caused by EB virus and causes prolonged fever, lymphadenopathy, hepatosplenomegaly and rash following ampicillin.

5. *Others:* Typhoid fever/enteric fever, scarlet fever, Rickettsial fevers, CHIKV, DENV infections (Table 5.5).

6. *Hand-Foot-Mouth Disease:* It is caused by coxsackie A_{16}. Various other enteroviruses and coxsackie B also may produce this Vesicular lesions appear in mouth, palms, soles, buttocks and genitalia. Usually self limited, encephalitis may rarely occur with enteroviruses. It spreads by fecal-oral route.

7. *Kawasaki Disease* (Refer Chapter 7).

Treatment of exanthematous fevers is symptomatic with antibiotics for secondary infections. Measles and Rubella can be prevented by vaccination. The day of onset of rash/vesicle can be remembered by this acronym.

'Very sick person must not take exercise'.

V—Varicella (chickenpox)—Day 1

S—Scarlet fever–Day 2

P—Pox (smallpox)—Day 3

M—Measles—Day 4 and 5

N—Nil other than measles

T—Typhus—Day 6

E—Enteric fever—Day 7.

SECTION 5.9	# A CHILD WITH PULMONARY TB

A 3-year-old unimmunized child was brought with fever—1 month, cough and weight loss. His grandfather was on irregular treatment for TB.

On examination: Weight < 60% of expected, loose skinfold in axilla and thigh, Tachypnoeic, reduced air entry (Rt) with bilateral crepitations.

DIAGNOSIS AND DISCUSSION

Pulmonary TB with Marasmus

1. Epidemiological data—Intrafamilial contact with TB +, unimmunized.

2. Clinically—Weight loss, marasmic, fever, cough and respiratory findings.

3. Investigation—Mantoux test strongly +ve (> 20 mm). X-ray chest hilar node with minor fissure opacity, right lung infiltrates, gastric aspirate for AFB—negative.

4. Response to treatment—Child promptly responded to CAT-I treatment.

Primary focus (Ghon's focus) may remain quiscent or may lead to progressive primary TB and also disseminated TB (Table 5.4). Simon's focus in RUL usually caseates in Reactivation TB. Primary complex may be asymptomatic. Other primary sites are eye, ear, skin, tonsil, GIT etc. AFB in sputum/gastric aspirate are scanty and hence may be difficult to demonstrate. BACTEC culture yield AFB in 2 weeks compared to conventional 8 weeks duration. Endobronchial TB may lead to bronchiectasis. Pleural effusion, serous meningitis, Phlycten, Poncet's arthritis etc. may mark hypersensitivity reactions. Progressive disease will lead to pleural effusion, bone and joint destruction and genitourinary TB. Miliary TB, TB Meningitis (TBM) and tuberculoma are serious forms of TB. Tuberculoma indicates immuno-logical competence to localize the infection.

Mantoux test is positive only in one third pulm TB cases and some with disseminated/lymph node TB. An induration more than 10 mm in a child and 14 mm in an adult indicate disease. BCG, atypical mycobacteria. Sarcoidosis etc. produce some induration with Mantoux test (ITU = 0.00002 mg purified protein derivative—PPD). 0.1 ml of 1 TU with Tween 18 is used for the test and the induration is read at 48-72 hours. Mantoux positivity may remain even after treatment. False negative Mantoux test occurs in malnutrition, immunosuppression due to viral infections, drugs, and in severe forms of TB like TBM and miliary TB. BCG test is not standardized and is better avoided.

Revised National TB Control Programme (RNTCP) has unified case categorisation and management (Table 5.13). Anti TB treatment is given 3 days/week as directly observed therapy short course (DOTS).

Table 5.1: Criteria to diagnose TSS

No	Criteria
I. Major:	
1	Fever >38.9° C
2	Rash, diffuse erythroderma with desquamation of palms and soles, 1-2 weeks later
3	Hypotension/orthostatic syncope
4	Involvement of 3 or more of the following organs
II. Minor:	
1	GIT upset
2	Muscular—myalgia/CPK > twice the normal
3	Renal—abnormal RFT/>5 pus cell/HPF
4	Hepatic—abnormal LFT
5	Hematologic—platelet < 1 lakh
6	CNS—disorientation/drowsiness without focal deficits
7	Negative tests for leptospira, dengue, measles etc.

Table 5.2: Time table of diphtheria progression

Incubation period: 1 -7 days

1st week	Conjunctival, nasal, pharyngeal, laryngeal membrane and bull neck
2-3 weeks	Local paralysis of soft palate, pharyngeal and laryngeal muscles and toxic myocarditis
5th week	Focal paralysis— Ophthalmoplegia
2-3 months	Symmetric Post Diphtheretic Paralysis (PDP)

Table 5.3: Time table for salmonella diagnosis

1st week	Blood culture/Bone marrow
2nd week	Widal test 1 in 160 titre O is diagnostic of acute infection. In titres 1 in 100, rising titre may be looked for. H titre suggests old infection and A or B suggests paratyphi infection
3rd week	Stool culture
4th week	Urine culture

Table 5.4: Time table of TB infections — Welgren's Calendar

1.	TB Meningitis and Miliary TB	6 months to 1 year
2.	Bone and joint TB	3 to 5 years
3.	Genitourinary	5 to 10 years

Reactivation TB – Simon's focus in RUL

Primary focus – Ghons focus usually subpleural

Table 5.5: Manifestations of dengue fever– Flavivirus (DF virus 1–4 serotypes)

Types	Symptoms	Lab
DF	Fever with 2 or more symptoms Headache, Retroorbital pain Myalgia, arthralgia	Leukopenia
DHF I	Above + Positive Tourniquet Test	Thrombocytope-nia < 1 lakh/ cumm and PCV rise > 20%
DHF II	Above + Spontaneous bleed	
DHF III/ DDS	Above + Spontaneous bleeding Circulatory failure	
DHF IV/ DSS	Above + Profound shock	

Table 5.6 Diagnosis of malaria drug resistance

	PS on day 7	PS on ay 14	PS on day 28
R1 Resistance	Disappear	Reappear	Persist
R2 Resistance	75% Reduction	Reappear	Persist
R3 Resistance	75% Persist	Persist	Persist

Table 5.7: WHO criteria for diagnosis of AIDS

Major	Minor
1. Weight loss/FTT/Wasting syndrome	1. Oropharyngeal candidiasis
2. Fever > 1 month	2. Lymphadenopathy
3. Diarrhea > 1 month	3. Pruritic dermatitis
4. Severe/repeated pneumonia	4. Repeated infections
	5. HIV +ve mother

Table 5.8: Interpretation of CD_4 counts

CD_4 count	Normal	Abnormal
% of total lymphocytes	> 25%	< 15%
Adult	> 500	< 200
Underfives	> 1000	< 500
Infants	> 1500	< 750

Table 5.9: WHO staging of HIV infections

Stage 0	Asymptomatic/Acute primary infection/seroconversion/Acute retroviral syndrome (upto 6 weeks)
Stage I	Early Asymptomatic HIV infection: persistent generalized lymphadenopathy (CD_4 >500)
Stage II	Intermediate HIV infection/organomegaly, lymphadenopthy, wart, molluscum, herpes zoster, papular urticaria, recurrent/chronic respiratory infection, fungal nail infection (CD_4: 200 - 500)
Stage III	Symptomatic HIV Disease: unexplained moderate malnutrition, persistent fever, diarrhea, oral candidiasis, oral lesions, lymphoid interstitial pneumonia (LIP), severe persistent pneumonia, pulmonary TB, bronchiectasis, unexplained pancytopenia
Stage IV	Late HIV Disease: severe malnutrition, extensive pneumonia, chronic diarrhea, severe extrapulmonary TB, Mycobacterium avium complex (MAC) infection, HIV encephalopathy, esophageal candidiasis, opportunistic CNS infections, progressive multifocal leukoencephalopathy (PMN), Kaposi sarcoma, lymphomas, (CD_4: 50–200).

Table 5.10: HIV treatment

3 Drugs Therapy—2 NRTI + 1 PI or 2 NRTI + 1 NNRTI

(NRTI —Nucleoside Analogue Reverse Transcriptase inhibitor and Non NNRTI)

PI – Protease Inhibitor—small doses added to 2 NRTI + 1 NNRTI regimen will result in PI boosting effect.

Drugs available

NRTI	NNRTI	PI
Zidovudine	Nevirapine	Indinavir
Lamivudine	Efavirenz	Ritonavir
Stavudine	Delaviridine	Saquinavir
Zalcitabine		

PPTCT Schedule

Early Pregnancy : Since 14 weeks: oral ZDV, intrapartum IV ZDV + Baby ZDV x 6 weeks

Late Pregnancy : > 36 weeks: oral ZDV, intrapartum IV ZDV Baby ZDV x 6 weeks

In Labour : Nevirapine to mother and baby (Single dose)

Table 5.11: PEP – Post exposure prophylaxis (Within 2- 72 hours)

Basic regimen	– ZDV 300 mg BD and Lamivudine 150 mg BD
Expanded regimen	– Basic + One Protease inhibitor
Duration	Minimum 4 weeks
HIV testing	6 weeks, 12 weeks, 6 months

CHAPTER 5

INFECTION AND INFESTATIONS

\	Table 5.12: Directions for biohazard waste disposal		
No	Item	Color	Disposal
1.	General Waste—Food Item	Green	Municipal waste
2.	Blood stained/Body parts	Yellow	Disinfection and Incineration/Deep burial
3.	Plastics/Disposables	Blue	Disinfection/Recycling
4.	Sharps	White/ Black	Hub cutting and Sharp pit disposal

Table 5.13: Anti TB treatment—categorywise		
Category	Types of cases	Treatment
I	AFB +ve cases, seriously ill cases, Neuro TB	2 (HRZE)3 (2 months) + 4 (HR)3 (4 months)
II	Defaulter, Retreatment	2 (HRZES) 3+ (2 months) 1 (HRZE) 3+ (one month) 5 (HRE)3 (5 months)
III	AFB -ve cases, Extrapulmonary TB, TB adenitis	2 (HRZ)3 + (2 months) 4 (HR)3 (4 months)

* Prednisolone 1 mg/kg/day × 6-8 weeks in Neuro TB, pleural effusion.
* INH chemoprophylaxis in contacts.
* 6 HR for asymptomatic Mx + ve, < 3 years, Mx +ve with PEM < 5 years.
* BCG adenitis—Excision/6 HR if size > 2 cm.

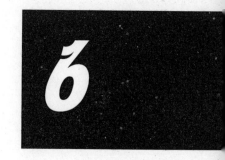

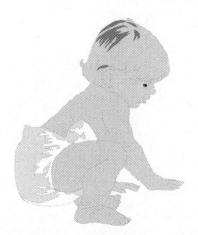

Immunity and Allergy

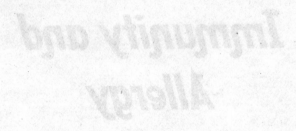

Immunity and Allergy

SECTION 6.1

A 3-YEAR-OLD BOY WITH MULTIPLE ABSCESSES

A 3-year-old boy attended OP with multiple abscesses. He had similar illness since 6 months of age and had I & Ds done several times in the neck, groin and submandibular region. He had eczematoid dermatitis, lymphadenopathy and hepatosplenomegaly. No history of sinopulmonary infections, diarrhea or candidiasis. Other systems within normal limits. Hb 9.5 g/dl, TC 6500/P 44, L 55, E1, ESR 80/1st Hr, LFT, RFT normal. Growth–Grade II PEM, 2nd degree stunting.

DIAGNOSIS AND DISCUSSION

Chronic Granulomatous Disease (CGD)

Multiple crops of draining abscesses favour the diagnosis of CGD. Sinopulmonary infections and meningo encephalitis occur in B Cell deficiency and viral and fungal infections in T Cell deficiency. Thymus, Tonsils and lymph nodes will be atrophic in T cell defects whereas these will be enlarged in B cell defect and combined immunodeficiencies.

Differential Diagnosis: Congenital neutropenia and neutrophil function defects. HIV infection should be ruled out by serology.

Neutrophil function and number of defects are the following: **Pelger Huet anomaly** with hyposegmented neutrophils, **Alder Reily anomaly** with large lavender blue granules in neutrophils and **May Hegglin anomaly** with irregular blue cytoplasmic inclusion in neutrophils and platelets. These conditions are usually asymptomatic.

Cyclical Neutropenia and Neutropenia associated with Shwachmann Diamond syndrome, Cartilage hair hypoplasia (CHH), Dyskeratosis congentia (DC) and Chediak Higashi syndrome (CHS) also came in the DD. CHS present with neutropenia with azurophil granules, partial albinism, photophobia, blond hair and platelet aggregation defects. Under the microscope, hair looks non- pigmented with black dots in between. 'Accelerated phase of lymphohistiocyte proliferation' may prove fatal in the above condition.

In CGD, Nitro Blue Tetrazolium (NBT) test is diagnostic, NBT reduction occurs only with adequate levels of superoxide anion. Due to reduction in NADPH oxidase complex, there is defective killing of catalase positive microbes in phagocytes leading to increased infection. In Wiskott Aldrich syndrome, there is T cell deficiency, skin involvement, draining ears and thrombocytopenia occurring in boys.

Treatment includes antibiotics and I & D whenever indicated. Cotrimoxazole prophylaxis (5 mg kg/day single dose) and Vitamin C and Copper supplements are also useful.

The various immunodeficiency states are summarised in Table 6.1.

Fig. No. 23 (Plate 6)

CHAPTER 6

IMMUNITY AND ALLERGY

A BOY WITH PROLONGED FEVER, ARTHRITIS AND RASH

A 10-year-old boy presented with fever of 6 weeks duration. He had several crops of evanescent rash and joint pain and swelling involving major and minor joints.

On examination: Febrile, hepatosplenomegaly and lymphadenopathy +. Sepsis screen –ve, Hb 8 g/dl, TC 15,000, P 74. L 22, E 3, ESR 110 mm/1st Hr, ANA -ve, DsDNA -ve, RA factor -ve, Mantoux test -ve, X-ray chest—Increased. Bronchovascular markings. Eyes—No iridocyclitis.

DIAGNOSIS AND DISCUSSION

Systemic Onset Juvenile Rheumatoid Arthritis (JRA)/Juvenile Idiopathic Arthritis

Differential Diagnosis: Systemic Lupus Erythematosus, Leukemia, atypical presentation of infections like Typhoid, TB, Brucella, IMN, HIV etc.

PUO like presentation with fever, rash, arthritis/arthralgia, negative ANA and RA factor point to systemic onset disease. The other types are Pauciarticular, Type I and II and Polyarticular sero positive and sero negative types. Bone marrow test may be done to rule out leukemia if clinical/hematologic parameters are suggestive. It is also wise to do HIV ELISA before starting long-term steroids/NSAIDs as HIV may induce various autoimmune antibodies.

Pauciarticular Type I JRA is more common in girls and affect upto 4 major joints. ANA is +ve. Iridocyclitis is seen in 30%. **Pauciarticular Type II JRA** is more common in boys and affects upto 4 major joints, especially sacroiliac joints ANA – ve, but HLA B 27 is positive. **Polyarticular sero-negative–JRA** occurs in girls and affects 5 or more joints. ANA + ve in 25%, Iridocyclitis rare. **Polyarticular seropositive JRA** is also more common in girls. ANA +, RA +ve. **Systemic Onset JRA** is more common in boys. Iridocyclitis, ANA and RA –ve.

SLE is diagnosed when 4 or more of the 11 criteria are satisfied (Table 6.2).

Treatment of JRA includes Aspirin/NSAIDs like Naproxen in a dose of 10 mg/kg/day Q 12 H. Steroids are warranted in non responders/those with organ dysfunctions. Iridocyclitis needs topical steroids.

Keeping the patient ambulant is of prime importance in view of crippling arthritis. In SLE, cyclophosphamide in a dose of 15-25 mg/kg as monthly pulses or 2-3 mg/kg OD and azathioprine in a dose of 1mg/kg/day are also beneficial. Steroids remain the first line drug in SLE also. Anti histone antibodies are pathognomonic of drug induced SLE.

SECTION 6.3

A BOY WITH FEVER, IRRITABILITY AND RED EYES AND MOUTH

A 4-year-old child with history of fever for 7 days was admitted with redness of eyes with non purulent discharge and redness of lips and mouth. He was highly irritable and the restlessness appeared after 5 days of fever.

On examination: He had generalised erythematous rash, oedema of feet, joint swelling and multiple unilateral cervical lymph nodes, extreme irritability +, HR 120/mt, RR 34/mt. Temp 102 °F, Hb 10.5 g/dl. TC 15,000/cumm, P 75 L 24, E1, ESR 110/mm, CRP 32 mg/dl. Platelet count 5.5 lakh/cumm. S Br 0.5 mg/dl, SGOT/SGPT 88/96.

DIAGNOSIS AND DISCUSSION

1. Kawasaki Disease (KD)/Mucocutaneous lymph node syndrome
2. Viral Exanthematous fever/Measles/Chikungunya/Rickettsia/Den V
3. Collagen Vascular Disease
4. Scarlet Fever/Staph. septicemia/Toxic shock syndrome
5. Drug reaction/Erythema multiforme/Stevens-Johnson syndrome
6. Acrodynia—Mercury poisoning.

KD is diagnosed based on the clinical criteria, usually in children below 5 years of age (Table 6.3). Juvenile KD is also reported in older children. Staphylococcal superantigen in the young and streptococcal superantigen in older children have been postulated in the etiology of KD.

With fewer than 4 positive criteria, incomplete KD is diagnosed. Those with complications are also referred to as atypical KD. Other manifestations are arthritis. GI upset, hepatosplenomegaly, extreme irritability, aseptic meningitis, seizures, renal involvement, sterile pyuria, and CVS involvement like coronary vasculitis, artery dilatation, aneurysm, pancarditis, CCF and arrhythmia. Pleural effusion and hemorrhagic serous effusions have been rarely reported.

The boy had B/L proximal coronary artery lesion (CAL) in the form of dilatation. He responded to IVIG 1g/kg/dose × 2 days. It may also be given as 2 g/kg single dose or 400 mg/kg/day × 5 days. IVIG is most effective within 10 days of onset. Non responders or relapses may need repeat course or pulse doses of methyl prednisolone.

Aspirin is given in a dose of 75-100 mg/kg/day (Anti inflammatory dose) × 2 weeks or till defervescence followed by 5 mg/kg/day for 6 weeks (Anti-platelet dose).

Coronary Artery Lesion (CAL) may resolve with treatment. Long-term follow up is needed. Antiplatelet low dose aspirin may be given for 6-8 weeks or more depending on the cardiac status. Thrombolysis with streptokinase may be needed in those with active coronary artery thrombosis. Serum Lipid Profile (SLIP) should be followed up in view of future coronary ischemia. Ophthalmology evaluation should be done in view of uveitis.

Fig. No. 24 (Plate 6)

CHAPTER 6

IMMUNITY AND ALLERGY

SECTION 6.4

AN 11-YEAR-OLD GIRL WITH SKIN RASH AND MUSCLE WEAKNESS

A 11-year-old girl presented with fever of 4 weeks duration, skin rash, abdominal pain and difficulty to walk and climb steps.

On examination: Febrile, rash + palpable purpura and bluish discolouration of nail beds, Induration, calcification and tenderness of muscles and periorbital facial oedema and malar flush +, erythema (violaceous) of eye lids +, hyper and hypopigmented skin lesions on the knee and elbow +, Proximal muscles weakness and inability to raise head in supine position and weakness of flexors of neck +, Gower's sign positive. Hb 9 g/dl, TC 14500, P 72, L 20, E 8, ESR 95, CPK 800 U/L, ANA + ve, RA –ve, EMG Neuropathic and Myopathic pattern.

DIAGNOSIS AND DISCUSSION

Dermatomyositis

Differential Diagnosis: SLE, polymyositis, myopathy, muscular dystrophy, GBS.

Dermatomyositis is a multi system autoimmune disorder in which lymphnokines destroy muscles. Muscles weakness and skin changes are pathognomonic. Violecious erythema of eyelids called 'heliotrope hue of eyelids', 'Grotton's papules' over knuckles, knee and ankle, vasculitis of nail beds and induration and calcification of muscles occur. Respiratory and cardiac muscle involvement may become fatal. Skin biopsy is diagnostic. Treatment includes corticosteroids. Methotrexate, cyclosporine and azathioprine alone or in combinations also may be tried.

Other Vasculitis Syndromes

1. **Small arteries:** Henoch-Schönlein purpura (HSP)/anaphylactoid purpura- palpable purpura especially in lower extremities in the absence of thrombocytopenia, arthritis, abdominal pain, nephritis, GI bleed (may be post streptococcal—ASO +ve).

2. **Medium arteries:** Polyarteritis nodosa (PAN)—palpable purpura, hypertension, mono neuritis multiplex, GI bleed, stroke, myocardial infarction.

3. **Large arteries:** Takayasu's/Pulseless Disease—absent upper limb pulsation and high BP in lower limb (reverse coarctation), renal, visual and joint involvement.

4. **Scleroderma:** Focal (Morphea), Linear/Systemic Sclerosis—hard skin with hide binding to deeper structure, hyperpigmentation/vitiligo, joint contractures.

Scleroedema Adultoum of Buschke is usually post streptococcal with inability to pinch the skin. **Sclerema** occurs in sick newborns and infants with advanced sepsis, where the skin becomes tight and non pinchable.

5. **Mixed connective tissue disease (MCTD):** This is an overlap syndrome with multi system involvement and positive anti RNP antibody. Anti DsDNA is pathognomonic of SLE, but may occur in MCTD and autoimmune hepatitis.

A BOY WITH VESICULOBULLOUS LESIONS

A 3-year-old boy with history of fever and medications from local hospital presented with vesiculobullous lesions of skin.

On examination: Target lesion +, mucus membrane of eye, mouth and urethra involved.

DIAGNOSIS AND DISCUSSION

Stevens-Johnson Syndrome (SJS)
Differential Diagnosis:

1. Erythema multiforme (EM)
2. Toxic epidermal necrolysis (TEN)
3. Staphylococcal scalded skin syndrome (SSSS)
4. Epidermolysis bullosa (EB)
5. Acrodermatitis enteropathica—usually no mucosal involvement, diarrhea+

(Refer Table 6.4).

SJS involves skin and at least 2 mucus membrane and may lead to corneal or oesophageal stricture. It is secondary to some antigens, usually drug or microbes. Cleavage is subepidermal with dermal infiltrations. 'Kobner phenomenon' leading to new lesions along the line of trauma +.

'Cutaneous pathergy' is sterile pustules developing after 24-48 hours at needle prick site seen in 'Bechet syndrome'.

'Erythema multiforme' involves skin and mucus membrane due to antigens like drug, toxin, virus or mycoplasma. Mucus membrane lesions are less severe and localized than SJS. Target lesions with dusky centre, pale, inner ring and red outer ring are seen in EM and SJS. Blister cleavage is intra epidermal and hence no scarring will occur.

TEN leads to skin tenderness and charred lesions, absent target lesions and full thickness epidermal necrosis. Blister cleavage is subepidermal with absent/minimal dermal inflammation. 'Nikolski sign' leading to denudation of skin from red areas on gentle pressure is noted. Mucosal involvement is less severe. Loss of nail and hair may occur. It is due to hypersensitivity to basal cells.

SSSS due to exfoliative toxin of staphylococci (exfoliatin of phase II), start around areas of staphylococcal colonisation sites like neck, axilla/groin or periorifical areas with tenderness and erythema. As cleavage is intra epidermal in stratum corneum, it is non scarring.

Epidermolysis Bullosa (EB) is a genetic disease. Usually congenital or may appear later .

1. **EB simplex:** Autosomal dominant, involves palms and soles, no scarring.
2. **Junctional EB:** AR, lethal with scarring
3. **Recessive Dystrophic EB:** AR, 'mitten scarring' of hand and feet, Squamous cell carcinoma may occur later.
4. **Dominant Dystrophic EB:** AD, hyperkeratotic lesions, prone for Ca. Skin.

Fixed Drug eruptions are localized lesions occurring at particular sites repeatedly during repeated usage of drugs. The usual drugs are sulpha, amoxicillin, pheno, carbamazepine, phenytoin, butazones, allopurinol etc.

Treatment includes supportive care, saline irrigation, antibiotics and antihistamines. Stoppage of the offending drug is mandatory. Care of the eye, mouth, genitalia etc. is also important. Corticosteroids may be used in non-responding or life threatening cases.

The Naranjo Adverse Drug Reaction probability scale is given in Table 6.5. The different allergic reactions are depicted in Table 6.6.

Table 6.1: Congenital immunodeficiency states

I. Primary B cell Deficiency
1. Selective IgA deficiency—Surface Tract infections like Respiratory, GIT
2. X-linked Agammaglobulinemia (XLA)/Bruton's disease
3. Heavy and Light chain immunoglobulin deletion
4. Combined variable immunodeficiency (CVID)
5. IgG subclass deficiencies
6. X-linked lymphoproliferative syndrome/Duncan disease (XLP)—EB Virus related.

II. Primary T cell Deficiency
1. Di George syndrome
2. CD_8 lymphocytopenia
3. T cell activation defects

III. Combined B and T cell Deficiency
1. Severe combined immunodeficiency (SCID)
2. Combined variable immunodeficiency (CVID)
3. Nezelof syndrome—combined immunodeficiency
4. Cartilage hair hypoplasia–short limbed dwarfism
5. Wiskott Aldrich syndrome (WAS) X linked recessive
6. Omenn syndrome–Autosomal recessive with exfoliative erythroderma and hypereosinophilia
7. Hyper IGE syndrome/Job Syndrome
8. Ataxia telangiectasia (AT)
9. Adenosine deaminase deficiency (ADA)
10. Defective expression of Major Histocompatibility (MCH) Antigen
11. Purine nucleoside phosphorylase deficiency.

IV. Complement Disorders—Urticaria

V. Phagocytic Disorders
1. Congenital neutropenia and cyclical neutropenia
2. Chronic granulomatous disease (CGD)
3. Neutrophil function defects: Pelger Huet, Alder Reily, May Hegglin etc.

Table 6.2: Criteria to diagnose SLE (4 or more)

1. Malar rash
2. Discoid rash
3. Photosensitive rash
4. Oral ulcer
5. Arthritis
6. Serositis
7. Nephritis
8. Neuropsychiatric disease–Seizure/Personality changes
9. Hematological—Pancytopenia, Hemolysis
10. Immunologic: Positive LE cell, Anti DsDNA and Anti Sm antibodies, False +ve VDRL due to APLA antibodies
11. Positive ANA in the absence of drug induced lupus.

Table 6.3: Diagnostic criteria of KD

1. Fever> 5 days

2. Any 4 out of the following 5 features:

   a. B/L non purulent conjunctivitis

   b. Mucosal changes like fissured lips, strawberry tongue, redness of pharynx

   c. Peripheral oedema

   d. Erythema, rash and later desquamation beginning perlingually in 2nd/3rd week

   e. Cervical lymphadenopathy—usually unilateral

3. Illness not explained by another known disease.

Table 6.4: Differential diagnosis of vesiculobullous lesions *

I. **Infections:**
   1. Viral: Varicella–'dew drop' vesicles more on trunk, Variola (Small Pox), Zoster occurring along dermatomes, Herpes Simplex – Type I Lips and II genitals, Coxsakie A16- Hand, foot, mouth, Molluscum (pox virus), ORF–fingers of sheep and goat rearers, Rickettsial
   2. Bacterial: Streptococcal, Staphylococcal–SSSS, bullous impetigo.

II. **Classification according to line of cleavage**
   A. Intraepidermal
      1. Epidermolysis Bullosa simplex–immunofluorescence
      2. Incontinentia Pigmenti–smear for eosinophils
      3. Insect bite reactions (IBR)
      4. Scabies—Scraping for Sarcoptes scabeii
      5. Viral——Herpes—multinucleated giant cells in **Tzanck smear**
   B. Subepidermal
      1. Bullous pemphigoid—immunofluorescence
      2. Dermatitis Herpetiformis—grouped vesicles (wheat induced)–immunofluorescence
      3. Chronic Bullous Dermatitis of Childhood–IgA mediated, may last for 2-4 years—linear vesicles
      4. Junctional Epidermolysis Bullosa–immunofluorescence
      5. Dystrophic EB—Dominant and Recessive—immunofluorescence
      6. Erythema multiforme
      7. TEN—frozen section biopsy
   C. Subcorneal—Transient Neonatal pustular melanosis
   D. Suprabasal—Pemphigus Vulgaris – painful oral and skin lesions–acanthocytes in Tzanck smear. Nikolski sign +, antigen involved is Desmoglein III, biopsy will show intra epidermal acanthocytes. Transfer of antibodies to fetus may lead to transient neonatal pemphigus vulgaris
   E. Granular layer—Bullous impetigo—Gram stain +ve, pemphigus foliaceous

* Vesicles are fluid filled collections <0.05 cm and bullae are >0.05 cm.

CHAPTER 6

IMMUNITY AND ALLERGY

Table 6.5: Naranjo Adverse Drug Reaction (ADR) Probability Scale

Clinicians often seek to determine whether an adverse event observed during the course of patient care is likely to be as a result of an adverse reaction to a drug. Although it is usually difficult to ascribe "cause and effect" definitely, careful analysis may help to elucidate the nature of possible adverse drug reactions. One approach that is recognized internationally is the use of the **Naranjo** ADR **Probability Scale**. The use of the **scale** involves answering a series of questions about the adverse event, and then calculating a final score that provides some indication of the overall **probability** that the adverse event represents an adverse reaction to a drug.

1. Are there previous conclusive reports on this reaction?
   Yes (+1) No (0) Don't know (0)
2. **Did the adverse event appear after the suspected drug was administered?**
   Yes (+2) No (-1) Don't know (0)
3. Did the adverse reaction improve when the drug was discontinued, or a specific antagonist was administered?
   Yes (+1) No (0) Don't know (0)
4. Did the adverse reaction reappear when the drug was readministered?
   Yes (+2) No (-1) Don't know (0)
5. **Are there alternative causes (other than the drug) that could on their own have caused the reaction?**
   Yes (-1) No (+2) Don't know (0)
6. Did the reaction reappear when a placebo was given?
   Yes (-1) No (+1) Don't know (0)
7. Was the drug detected in the blood (or other fluids) in concentrations known to be toxic?
   Yes (+1) No (0) Don't know (0)
8. Was the reaction more severe when the dose increased, or less severe when dose was decreased?
   Yes (+1) No (0) Don't know (0)
9. Did the patient have a similar reaction to the same or similar drug in any previous exposure?
   Yes (+1) No (0) Don't know (0)
10. **Was the adverse event confirmed by any objective evidence?**
    Yes (+1) No (0) Don't know (0)
    The final score allows some basis for an objective assessment of the likelihood that an ADR may have occurred:
    > 9 = highly probable
    > 5 - 8 = probable
    > 1 - 4 = possible
    = 0 = doubtful

Table 6.6: Types of allergic reactions

1. Type I: Anaphylaxis IgE Mediated—Penicillin anaphylaxis. Early 10-30 mts. Late 4-8 hours.
2. Type II: Cytotoxic e.g. drug induced hemolysis.
3. Type III: Arthus/Immune complex disease e.g. PSAGN.
4. Type IV: Cell mediated delayed hypersensitivity e.g. Mantoux positivity/Graft versus Host reaction.
   (Type V: Due to stimulating antibodies mediated disease—Long acting thyroid stimulator (LATS) antibody e.g. thyrotoxicosis—Types V & VI are no longer in use.
   Type VI: Lymphoid K Cell dependent antibody (LDA) mediated cytotoxicity e.g. Myasthenia gravis.)

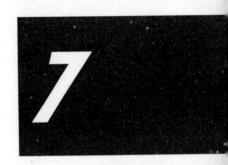

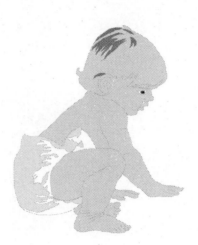

Gastrointestinal System

7

Gastrointestinal System

SECTION 7.1
A CHILD WITH RECURRENT ORAL ULCERS

A 10-year-old child with history of recurrent oral ulcers was admitted.

On examination: Fetor oris +, erythema and ulceration of gingiva and mouth +, greyish pseudomembrane + on the gums, cervical adenitis +.

DIAGNOSIS AND DISCUSSION

Herpetic Gingivo Stomatitis (HGS)

Differential Diagnosis: Aphthous ulcer/Aphthous stomatitis (AS), chemical burns, Vincent's Infection or Vincent's angina, A/c Necrotising ulcerative gingivitis (ANUG) due to anaerobes/spirochetes, Herpangina—Coxsackie A, Hand Foot Mouth Disease (HFMD) etc.

HGS is multiple ulcers and affects gingival and oral mucosa. ANUG is localized to gingiva. AS occur singly or in crops, secondary to stress, micronutrient deficiency, malabsorption or physiological conditions like menstruation. HFMD is vesicles in hand, foot, mouth, genitalia and buttocks due to coxsackie A 16 infection.

Treatment includes oral hygiene, hydrogen peroxide rinse, topical xylocaine, metronidazole, tetracycline pastes or powder. Micronutrients, antibiotics and metronidazole given orally and reassurance will work in most cases. Oral acyclovir may be given in severe cases of HGS for 7-14 days.

In Bechet syndrome, there is recurrent oral/genital and eye inflammation and ulcers. Arthritis, colitis and vasculitis may occur. 'Cutaneous pathergy' is sterile pustule noticed 24-48 hours at needle prick site in this condition.

In SLE, there will be oral ulcers and multisystem involvement. In SLE ulcers are painless, but in aphthous, these are very painful. Pemphigus may start as oral ulcers. HGS is a primary infection by herpes simplex virus. Oral ulcers may occur in inflammatory bowel disease also. Vincent's angina is another name for ANUG and is also called 'trench mouth'. It is a periodontal disease. Herpangina leads to posterior oropharyngeal vesicles/ulcers 1-15 in No. with high fever unlike herpetic gingivostomatitis with anterior lesions.

SECTION 7.2

AN INFANT WITH CONGENITAL ANOMALIES INVOLVING FACE

A 10-month-old baby brought with multiple congenital anomalies involving the face. Baby was born to non consanguineous parents.

On examination: Maxillary and mandibular hypoplasia, micrognathia, macrostomia, preauricular tags and pits on left side of cheek +, B/L microtia, scoliosis, B/L epibular dermoid + CHD-PDA, high arched palate + No cleft lip/palate and CHD-PDA.

DIAGNOSIS AND DISCUSSION

Goldenhar syndrome/Facio oculo auriculo vertebral dysplasia

The child has all features of the syndrome with facial, ocular, auricular, vertebral and cardiac defects.

Differential Diagnosis: Pierre Robin sequence—with micrognathia, glossoptosis, pseudomacro glossia, high arched/cleft palate. The facial features improve by six years of age. Nursing in prone position and temporary suturing of tongue to lower lip are beneficial.

Treacher Collins/Franceschetti Syndrome/ Mandibulo facial dysostosis—The features are antimongloid slant, coloboma of lower eye lids, deformed pinna, retrognathia (receding chin), macrostomia, hair growth towards cheek, facial cleft or fistula, high arched palate, deafness and facial malocclusion. CHD may occur. Inheritance is AD with variable expression. This is a first arch syndrome.

Brachial Arch Syndromes

Out of the embryonic 6 branchial arches, 1st and 2nd are prominent in humans. First arch includes maxillary and mandibular prominences that fuse in the midline. The 2nd is hyoid arch that also fuses in midline.

First Arch syndromes involve cleft lip, palate, sinus/fistula/cyst in the face, ear anomalies and deafness due to malformation of incus and malleolus. CHD may be associated. Cysts may be present at birth or may appear after birth. Examples are Treacher Collins, Goldenhar etc.

Second Arch syndromes lead to branchial fistula/sinus/cyst over the sternomastoid. Cyst may appear after birth. Cartilagineous remnants also may be seen. Vertebral anomalies are common in second arch syndromes. Sometimes 1st and 2nd arch syndromes may appear together.

Cleft palate may be posterior or may be submucus. So it is important to palpate the palate in suspected cases. Undiagnosed ones lead to feeding difficulty, vomiting, regurgitation, aspiration and failure to thrive.

Feeding plates called 'obturators' may be used to occlude the defect during feeding. The usage of this should be trained soon after birth. This will prevent feeding difficulty and regurgitation. The same can be procured from the dental specialists.

'Rule of 10' is useful to plan cleft lip and palate surgery (Table 7.1).

A YOUNG INFANT WITH FAILURE TO THRIVE, REGURGITATION AND VOMITING

SECTION 7.3

A two-month-old male baby with failure to thrive was brought with regurgitation and non-bilous vomiting. It started in newborn period. Baby was vomiting forcefully in the horizontal position itself before attempting burping. Birth weight 3 kg, present weight 2.4 kg.

DIAGNOSIS AND DISCUSSION

Gastro Esophageal Reflux Disease (GERD)/ Chalasia Cardia

This history is suggestive of gastro esophageal reflux disease (GERD). Non bilious vomiting in the horizontal position occurs in GERD. In reflux esophagitis, hemorrhage may also occur. It may also lead to aspiration pneumonia, apnoea and wheeze. In **Sandiffer syndrome**, there is associated intermittent stiff posturing of the neck or arching back during reflux. GER may occur occasionally in any baby, but GERD is pathological, recurrent and affects growth or causes respiratory symptoms.

Differential Diagnosis:

1. **Overfeeding**/lack of burping. In this condition, vomiting is usually in the upright position. This is called 'regurgitation'.

2. In **Achalasia cardia**, due to aganglionic gastro esophageal sphincter. There is esophageal dilatation and air fluid levels in upright X-ray chest.

3. In **congenital hypertrophic pyloric stenosis** (CHPS), it is more in first born male and may be familial. There will be projectile vomiting, dehydration and hypochloremic metabolic alkalosis. Tumor like mass in epigastrium and visible peristalsis may appear during feeding and resolve after vomiting.

4. **Congenital hernias**—Hiatus hernia may be a sliding hernia or para oesophageal hernia of the stomach into the thorax. Congenital diaphragmatic hernia (CDH) is usually on the left side through the foramen of Bochdalek. It is a pseudohernia as it is not covered with peritoneum. It usually presents in newborn period with shifted or dextropositioned heart, scaphoid abdomen and RDS due to hypoplastic and collapsed lung. CDH may also be intermittent leading to late diagnosis in some cases.

5. **Eosinophilic esophagitis** is another DD. It may be familial and leads to trachealisation of the esophagus, difficult swallowing, food impaction and erosions.

6. **Pyloric or duodenal atresia** proximal to Ampulla of Vater, antral webs and gastric duplications are other conditions that present with non-bilous vomiting.

Bilious Vomiting

Pseudo intestinal obstruction may occur due to congenital neuropathy or myopathy. It may run in families. It presents with failure to thrive and bilious vomiting without any anatomical obstruction. Biopsy is diagnostic.

Bilious vomiting occurs in Duodenal atresia (Double bubble appearance in newborn X-ray), Intestinal atresia (multiple fluid levels), Malrotation gut and intestinal obstruction. Hematochezia indicates bowel infarction.

Barium swallow and Barium Meal, PH studies, Radionuclide scans and cine oesophagogram are warranted in a baby with recurrent vomiting or regurgitation. Milk scan is a useful investigation.

Treatment includes positioning of the baby in left lateral/semi prone position, while resting, feeding in upright position, burping and thickened feeds prepared from milk and cereal flour. Prokinetic agents like cisapride (0.2 mg/kg/dose Q 6 H), metaclopramide (0.15 ml/kg/dose Q 6

H), antacids, proton pump inhibitors like omeprazole and H_2 receptors blockers are beneficial. Cisapride is useful, but is not safe due to associated cardiac events and deaths. The dose of omeprazole is 1-3 mg/kg/day Q 12 H before meals.

Oral bronchodilators are better avoided in GERD. Wheeze secondary to GERD will respond to the above drugs than bronchodilator. GERD usually resolves with age, but may be resistant in some neuro cases and Down syndrome. In such cases, **Nissen fundoplication** is indicated.

In achalasia, calcium channel blockers like nifedipine, balloon dilatation etc. may be tried. **Heller's operation** is done in Achalasia cardia, where mucosa is not cut, but the sphincter muscle alone is divided. **Ramstedt's operation** is done in CHPS. Endoscopic balloon dilatation also may be tried.

SECTION 7.4 A TODDLER WITH CHRONIC CONSTIPATION

A 3-year-old boy was brought with chronic constipation and progressive abdominal distension.

Growth and development normal, P/R examination revealed empty rectum with explosive passage of motion. There was a history of delayed passage of meconium. Occasionally, there were also blood streaking of stools.

DIAGNOSIS AND DISCUSSION

Congenital Aganglionic Megacolon/Hirschsprung's Disease

Differential Diagnosis:

1. *Acquired Megacolon/Habitual constipation:* It is due to lack of toilet training and painful passage of hard stools leading to voluntary holding. There may be associated fecal soiling (Encopresis) and P/R reveals loaded rectum as against empty rectum in congenital megacolon.
2. *Hypothyroidism:* There will be associated developmental retardation, puffy/coarse facies, increased sleepiness etc.
3. Anal stenosis/Ectopic anus also may present with constipation.
4. Anorectal malformation (ARM) should be considered in a newborn baby with delayed passage of meconium.
5. Anal fissure is a painful condition with bleeding P/R. There may be voluntary holding of motion due to pain. Polyposis of the intestine/colon/rectum present with painless bleeding.

ARM present with delayed passage of meconium more than 24 hours of birth and there may be associated fistula leading to passage of meconium through urethra or vagina. Inverted X-ray (Invertogram) taken in 'King Solomon's position' after 12 hours of delivery, ensuring time for passage of gas upto rectum, is helpful in the diagnosis. Gas shadow above the pubo coccygeal line denotes a 'high anomaly'. This line is above levator ani. Obstruction below this line denotes 'low anomaly'. Perineal anoplasty is done in low ARM and colostomy followed by abdominal pull through operation after 3-4 months is done in high ARM.

In Hirschsprung's disease, barium enema should be done. Funnel shaped dilated proximal segment may be seen in long segment diseases. The defect may be short segment/ultra short segment in some cases. Colostomy is followed by Duhamel operation or ileo anal anastomosis.

Habitual constipation is generally managed by proper toilet training and laxatives to make the act of defecation painless. High fibre diet and avoiding constipating agents like biscuit, banana, apple etc. are often beneficial. Conditioning the baby to go to the toilet is a rewarding exercise.

SECTION 7.5 A BABY WITH ACUTE ABDOMEN

A 5-month-old baby who was initiated on complementary feeds 2 days back was rushed to the casualty with excessive episodic crying, bilious vomiting, constipation followed by passage of blood and mucus.

Abdomen examination showed upper abdominal distension with a soft mass and an empty right iliac fossa.

DIAGNOSIS AND DISCUSSION

Intussusception

The history and C/F are typical of intussusception following weaning. It may also occur following diarrheal disease, Adeno virus infections, vasculitis, lymphoma/leukemia and abdominal surgery. There is telescoping of a loop of intestine into the colon. The ileo colic and ileo–ileo-colic are the common types. If not reduced without much delay, gangrene or auto amputation may occur.

'Red current jelly' is passage of fresh blood mixed with mucus. Right iliac fossa will be empty and sausage shaped mass may be palpable in right upper abdomen or epigastrium. USS will show 'doughnut or target appearance' in transverse cuts. Barium meal will show 'coil spring appearance'. Surgery is warranted only if hydrostatic saline or pneumatic pressure reduction fails. Saline reduction is undertaken under USS guidance. Recurrence may occur following saline reduction.

Differential Diagnosis: Acute Invasive Diarrhea/Dysentery.

In dysentery, there may be mild fever, increased frequency of stools, loose consistency mixed with blood and mucus. The child may have tenesmus and not colicky pain. Bilious vomiting and rapidly deteriorating course are unlikely in dysentery.

SECTION 7.6

A SCHOOL GIRL WITH RECURRENT ABDOMINAL PAIN (RAP)

A 10-year-old girl was brought with history of periumbilical RAP. She used to have it usually in the morning. It is less during week ends. Growth and development were normal. Bowel and bladder habits normal.

On examination: Abdomen soft, no organomegaly, no area of tenderness/palpable mass.

DIAGNOSIS AND DISCUSSION

Functional RAP/Psychosomatic Illness

Periumbilical without focal lesion/tenderness and improvement during week ends suggest Functional RAP. It is usually diagnosed >2 years of age.

Differential Diagnosis: Dyspepsia, gastric/duodenal ulcer, H pylori infection, Milk/food intolerance, psychosomatic illness, school phobia, physical/sexual abuse. Genitourinary infection, helminthiasis especially hook worm infection are the other conditions.

Abdominal migraine and abdominal epilepsy also come in the DD. **Abdominal epilepsy** manifests with cyclical vomiting, butterfly sensation in the abdomen with or without loss of consciousness (LOC)/motor activity. Family history of epilepsy may be obtained in some cases. Neuro cutaneous markers also should be looked for.

Inborn errors of metabolism like urea cycle disorders, Reye like encephalophrosis also come in the DD of cyclical vomiting.

'Apley's law' states that pain away from the umbilicus is usually organic. USS Abdomen may show cystitis, hydronephrosis, cholelithiasis, urolithiasis etc. when pain is away from the umbilicus.

Urine, blood, X-ray abdomen—erect, USS, psychological evaluation, neurological evaluation and H pylori IgG estimation are helpful. These investigations will help to exclude organic causes and thereby confirm functional RAP. Functional RAP is thought to be due to overperception of abdominal movements. H. pylori IgG is more useful than IgM as it is a chronic illness.

Deworming, antacids, counselling etc. are usually beneficial in the management of RAP. Mid cycle ovulation pain/cyclical calendar wise menstrual pain should also be considered in older girls. Mefenamic acid is effective in these conditions. It may also control excessive bleeding.

H. pylori infection is a common cause of dyspepsia, ulcer and RAP in children. These cases were previously thought to be psychosomatic. Triple therapy is beneficial in those who are H. pylori IgG +ve (Table 7.2).

CHAPTER 7

GASTROINTESTINAL SYSTEM

SECTION 7.7

A 7-YEAR-OLD CHILD WITH ACUTE ABDOMINAL PAIN (AAP)

A 7-year-old child was rushed to casualty with acute abdominal pain. The child was febrile and had vomited twice. She was pointing to umbilicus as the area with pain. She could not stand erect.

On examination: Febrile, tachypneic, tachycardia + tenderness Rt Iliac fossa +, Urine Alb Trace, Puscell 5-10/HPF.

DIAGNOSIS AND DISCUSSION

Acute Appendicitis

The triad of symptoms, fever, pain and vomiting and Mc Burney's point tenderness are diagnostic of A/c Appendicitis. Children may have difficulty in walking and standing erect. Appendix may be in ectopic sites with variable present action.

Differential Diagnosis: UTI—Frequency of micturition, dysuria and PC > 30/HPF and fever with chills and rigor are characteristic.

Peritonitis is associated with generalized tenderness and distension. In primary peritonitis, loose stools may be seen. It is more common in girls and those with nephrotic syndrome.

In **renal colic**, pain radiates to groin and in **gall stones/cholecystitis**, pain radiates to right shoulder. In **pancreatitis**, pain radiates to the back. **Basal pneumonia and pleurisy** also may present as AAP.

Meckel's diverticulitis may present similar to acute appendicitis, but with pain and tenderness in left iliac fossa. Ulceration and bleeding may occur from Meckel's during therapy with aspirin/NSAIDs and steroids due to presence of gastric mucosa. It is a remnant of Vitelline duct, which connects yolk sac to gut. It regresses by 7th week of gestation. It may persist in 2% of population, more common in boys, as a projection, 2 inch long (3-6 cm), 20 inches (50 cm), away from the ileo ceacal valve.

Approach to Acute Abdominal Pain

In Acute abdomen, the cause may be in the groin, abdomen, chest or CNS (Fig. 7.1). This can be represented as follows:

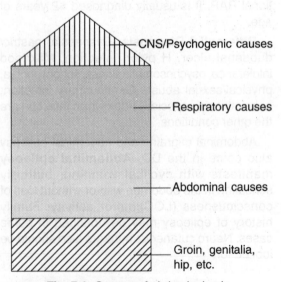

CNS/Psychogenic causes

Respiratory causes

Abdominal causes

Groin, genitalia, hip, etc.

Fig. 7.1: Causes of abdominal pain

SECTION 7.8

A 6-MONTH-OLD BABY WITH PERSISTENT DIARRHEA

A 6-month-old baby was admitted with persistent diarrhea. He had an episode of acute watery diarrhea 3 weeks back, which became persistent. It started following a travel to a far away sacred place for rice giving ceremony. Diarrhea was more during day time when feeds were given.

On examination: Some dehydration +, Development normal, grade I PEM. Systemic examination within normal limits. Perianal excoriation +.

DIAGNOSIS AND DISCUSSION

Persistent Diarrhea most probably osmotic diarrhea—Lactose intolerance with some dehydration and grade I PEM

Acute diarrhea usually stops in 4–5 days. It is the time taken for renewal of intestinal mucosa. **'Intermediate Diarrhea'** is the term used for diarrhea lasting for 7-14 days. **'Persistent Diarrhea'** is more than 14 days and usually is of infectious etiology.

'Chronic diarrhea' is the term reserved for recurrent or prolonged diarrhea which may be usually of non infectious etiology.

'Acute Invasive Diarrhea or (AID)' is due to dysentery with blood in stool. Chronic Invasive Diarrhoea is associated with amebiasis, whip worm colitis, cryptosporidium infection, immuno-deficiency, intestinal TB etc.

Watery diarrhea is divided in to Osmotic and Secretory. Osmotic is due to increased osmotic-ally active particles in the gut and is usually related to food intake and will stop during fasting trial. It is due to rotavirus infection or lactose intolerance. Secretory is due to toxins like cholera, enterotoxigenic E Coli (ETEC) or uncontrolled proliferation of immature crypt cells, that are secretory. Secretory is not related to food intake and may be there during sleep/fasting trial also. Osmotic diarrhea responds to dietary modification and anti secretory agents like rececadotril are beneficial in secretory diarrhea. Secretory diarrhea may crop upon osmotic diarrhea.

Watery Diarrhea

Osmotic: Acute: Rotavirus and Persistent: Lactose intolerance.

Secretory: Acute: Cholera/ETEC and Persistent: Crypt cell hyperplasia.

'Intestinal hurry' and rapid transit may lead to detection of sugar >1% in motion in infants with acute diarrhea. But classical symptoms of persistent diarrhea, sugar >1% and perianal excoriation due to acidic stool and pH < 6.5 on two different occasions will confirm lactose intolerances. Perianal excoriation without lactose intolerance may occur in acrodematitis entero-pathica.

Approach to persistent diarrhea is given in Figure 7.2. Dietary modification and various diets and commercial preparations are given in Tables 7.3 and 7.4.

CHAPTER 7

GASTROINTESTINAL SYSTEM

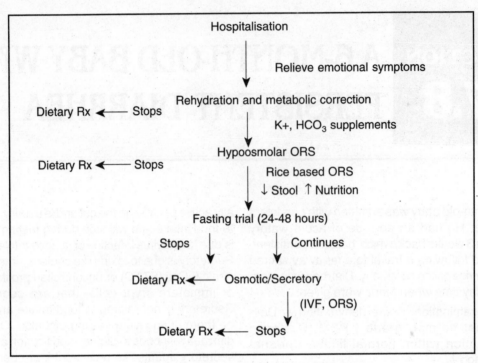

Fig. 7.2: Approach to persistent diarrhea

SECTION 7.9

A CHILD WITH CHRONIC DIARRHEA AND MAL-ABSORPTION

A 2-year-old child was brought with history of chronic diarrhea since infancy, first noticed during weaning phase. Motion was foul smelling with an oil slick in the toilet. Nausea and vomiting +. Child used to eat eagerly, but had Grade IV PEM and II degree stunting. Growth retardation +, Loose skin folds in axilla, groin, thigh, buttocks, chest and cheeks. No edema, clubbing +, pallor +, stool ova, Amoeba, parasites negative. Fat globules >8/LPF in smear after mixing with water and staining with Sudan Red. Sweat chloride test was ordered.

DIAGNOSIS AND DISCUSSION

Cystic Fibrosis (CF), Gluten Enteropathy/Celiac sprue

Chronic diarrhea with malnutrition and steatorrhea is suggestive of fat malabsorption. Fat globules >8/Low powder field seen towards the edge of the slide suggests fat malabsorption. This test can even replace 24 or 72 hours total fat estimation, which is very cumbersome. In mild steatorrhea, stool may appear normal. Passage of muscle fibres on taking meat or chicken, suggest protein malabsorption, called **creatorrhea**.

1. **Cystic fibrosis:** Increased sweat chloride >60 mEq/L indicates severe CF. 40-60 is noted in mild disease. CF is an autosomal recessive condition and the CF mutant gene is a common 'mutant gene' seen in many communities like the Caucasians and hence may occur even in offsprings born to non consanguinous parents.

CF is characterized by chronic lung disease like bronchiectasis and pancreatic insufficiency. Insulin dependent DM may also occur later on. Mutation in CF transmembrane regulator protein (CFTR) is the abnormality. Pseudomonas infection is very common in this condition. Stool pancreatic elastase 1 level <100 mg/g indicates severe deficiency. Immunoreactive trypsinogen which is initially high is used for newborn screening. This level will decrease by 5 years of age. Hydration, free access to salt, mucolytic and antibiotic therapy are indicated. Medium chain triglycerides (MCT) oils like coconut oil and cotton seed oil that are absorbed straight into the portal vein bypassing the chylomicron formation and lymphatics are useful. Micronutrient supplements are also beneficial. In pancreatic enzyme replacement therapy (PERT), the dose of Lipase is adjusted to 10,000 IU/kg/day or 1500 IU/kg/dose/meal. Pancreatin/Creon is given mixed with small quantity of food or drink before feeding. Mickeys gastrostomy, that can be inserted laparoscopically, will ensure continued feeding usually in the night and normal activity during day time. This is a blessing to those with severe cases. Parenteral nutrition is needed in severe cases to promote optimum growth. Celiac disease complicating CF has been described in some children.

2. **Celiac disease:** It is a small bowel disease due to gluten hypersensitivity, usually starting during weaning phase, when items like wheat,

rye, barley and oats are introduced. Certain amino acid sequences, called 'motifs' present in the gliadin fraction of gluten, cause the hypersensitivity. Genetic predisposition and environmental factors are responsible for the disease. There is villous atrophy leading to malabsorption, crypt hyperplasia leading to secretory diarrhea, reduced cholecystokinin and secretin levels that are secreted by the intestine and pancreatic insufficiency. Clubbing and rectal prolapse may occur. Serum Ig A—endomysial antibody is diagnostic, but Antigliadin antibodies are not reliable. Gluten free diet and oral prednisolone are beneficial. Bowel lymphoma may occur in this condition. Gluten containing items are wheat, rye, barley and oats.

3. **Tropical sprue:** It is a small bowel disease seen in tropical countries, probably due to bacterial overgrowth. It presents like celiac sprue, but may respond to B_{12} and folic acid supplements and Tetracycline or Sulpha drugs for 3-4 weeks.

4. **Blind loop syndrome** is due to partial intestinal obstruction and bacterial overgrowth. Bacteria deconjugate bile salts and cause steatorrhea.

5. **Short bowel syndrome** occurs when 50% of absorptive surface is surgically removed due to atresia, volvulus or worm mass obstruction. 15 cm of bowel with ileocecal valve or more than 20 cm bowel without valve may lead to subsequent adaptation and decrease in diarrhea in about 2 years time. Many cases may need TPN for survival. Upper GI malabsorption is diagnosed by D Xylose test and lower GI malabsorption by B_{12} malabsorption (Schillig test). Hydrogen breath test will be positive in carbohydrate malabsorption. B_{12} stores at birth may be sufficient for a decade in most cases. Once a month B_{12} injections are beneficial to prevent overt deficiency.

7. **Other malabsorptions:** In abetalipoproteinemia, Wolman disease and intestinal lymphangiectasia, steatorrhea can occur.

Oxaluria and oxalate stones may occur in chronic steatorrhea. In malabsorption states, twice the requirements of water soluble vitamins and 5 times of requirements of fat soluble vitamin may be needed. Aqueous forms of Vitamin A 10,000-15,000 IU/day, Vitamin E 50-400 IU/day, Vitamin D-5000-8000 IU/kg/day, Vitamin K 1 mg/year of age (upto 10 mg) every 2-4 weeks are needed in addition to water soluble vitamins. Cryptosporidium is the usual pathogen associated with HIV/AIDS.

In conditions like antibiotic associated diarrhea/persistent diarrhea with alteration in intestinal microflora, **probiotics** (lactobacilli/sachromyces) and synbiotics that contain both pro and prebiotics (lactobacilli + inulin/oligofructo saccharides) are useful. In secretory diarrhea, anti secretory agents like rececadotril are useful.

Protracted diarrhea syndrome of infancy (PDSI) is an intractable type of persistent diarrhea with high mortality in spite of TPN/PPN.

Other Chronic Diarrheas (Table 7.5)

Congenital microvillus atrophy is an autosomal recessive condition with profuse diarrhea. It may respond to octreotide infusion.

In **primary lactose intolerance**, milk is not tolerated including breast milk.

In **enterokinase deficiency,** pancreatic trypsinogens are not activated leading to creatorrhea.

Whip worm colitis and eosinophilic enteropathy: In these conditions, bloody diarrhea may occur. In **giardiasis,** malabsorption may occur. **Intestinal TB, amebiasis and cryptosporidium infection** may result in chronic diarrhea.

Acrodematitis entropathica, congenital or acquired immunodeficiency states, carcinoid syndrome and neuro-endocrine tumors and congenital chloride/sodium transport defects also come in the DD.

Irritable bowel syndrome (IBS) and inflammatory bowel disease (IBD): These are not uncommon in children. **Ulcerative colitis** present with colitis and crampy abdominal pain and extraintestinal signs like hepatitis, spondylitis. Anti neutrophil cytoplasmic antibodies (ANCA) may be positive. 'Lead pipe' colon in Barium enema is diagnostic. Terminal ileum may show 'back wash ileitis' and dilatations. Treatment of ulcerative colitis includes sulfasalazine 50 mg/kg/day Q 12 H or prednisolone/azathioprine. Folic acid should be supplemented with sulfasalazine. There is increased risk of colon cancers in this condition.

Crohn's Disease or Regional Enteritis is characterized by, 'skip lesions', involving different parts of the GIT from mouth to anus. Transmural involvement is seen in Crohn's disease as against transmucosal lesion in ulcerative colitis. Extra intestinal symptoms are aphthous ulcer, arthritis, clubbing, episcleritis and renal/gall stones. Skip area, strictures and linear ulcers leading to 'cobblestone appearance' are seen in barium studies. Treatment is similar to ulcerative colitis. Monthly B_{12} injections are also needed.

Whip worm colitis is treated with oral albendazole or mebendozole retention enema. 6 tablets in 100 ml saline may be given as a single dose or 2 tabs/day for 3 days.

In **pseudomembranous colitis**, there is anaerobic infection by Clostridium difficile leading to severe diarrhea. Antibiotic therapy may lead to overgrowth of anaerobes resulting in this condition. It may also be a nosocomial infection. Hemorrhagic colitis, toxic megacolon, bowel perforation and septicemia may occur in this condition. Oral vancomycin is effective. Metro-nidazole 20-40 mg/kg/24 hours divided q 6-8 hours PO is another treatment option. Probiotics like saccharomyces boularidii 250 mg bd for 1-2 weeks is also effective.

Irritable bowel syndrome is recurrent urge to pass motion due to stress, anxiety etc. Bowel binding agents like loperamide may be beneficial.

Commercial preparations for enteral nutrition are given in Table 7.4.

CHAPTER 7

GASTROINTESTINAL SYSTEM

A BOY WITH RECURRENT MILD JAUNDICE

A 10-year-old child was brought with history of mild intermittent jaundice. This became evident during intercurrent infections. No constitutional symptoms.

On examination: Growth and development normal. No organomegaly. Blood Exam: Hb 11 g/dl, no evidence of hemolysis, blood counts normal, LFT: S. Br. 7 mg/dl, Direct 0.2 mg/dl, Liver enzymes SGOT/SGPT 33/32, S. Alkaline Phosphatase 550 IU/L, S. Protein, S. Alb normal. Prothrombin Time normal, Viral Markers Negative, Thyroid Function Test Normal.

DIAGNOSIS AND DISCUSSION

Gilbert's Disease

This is a case of mild recurrent unconjugated hyperbilirubinemia. It is a benign disorder due to mutation of transferase gene. Mild jaundice without hemolysis, becoming overt during infections or stress is diagnostic.

In the immediate newborn period, **breast milk jaundice** comes in the DD. The various causes of jaundice in the newborn are discussed in Table 7.6 (Also refer Table 4.5).

Indirect hyperbilirubinemias that manifest in newborn period are:

1. **Crigler-Najjar syndrome**

   Type II is an Autosomal Dominant condition with variable expressions. It is less severe than type I and is due to deficiency of hepatic glucuronyl transferase enzyme. In type I, there is severe deficiency manifesting in newborn period with chance for kernicterus. In type I, bile bilirubin is less than 10 mg/dl compared to normal bile bilirubin - 50-100 mg/dl, seen in type II. Type II may respond to phenobarbitone 5 mg/kg/day.

2. **Lucey Driscoll syndrome** is yet another condition with unconjugated hyperbilirubinemia. It may be severe, but is transient in the newborn period due to placental transfer of glucuronyl transferase inhibiting substance, called ortho-aminophenol. It may need exchange transfusion to prevent kernicterus in severe cases.

SECTION 7.11

A CHILD WITH CONJUGATED HYPERBILIRUBINEMIA

A 3-year-old child born to 3rd degree consaguineous parents presented with prolonged deep jaundice, itching and xanthomas. He had pale stools. Birth weight was normal.

On examination: Grade II malnutrition and 2nd degree stunting present. Liver palpable 3 cm. His S bilirubin was 12 mg/dl, Direct 5 mg/dl, Liver enzymes normal, Viral markers negative. Prothrombin time normal, thyroid function normal.

DIAGNOSIS AND DISCUSSION

Dubin Johnson syndrome

It is a case of direct hyperbilirubinemia with cholestasis as evident by Direct bilirubin > 20% of the total. Normal liver enzymes rule out obstructive phase of hepatitis. Liver biopsy is diagnostic and shows black pigment and there is associated defect in porphyrin metabolism and abnormal gall bladder roentgenography.

DD include the following (Table 7.6):

1. **Rotor syndrome:** There is no black pigment in the liver and gall bladder roentgenography is normal.

2. **Intrauterine infection (TORCH)**–Manifest in newborn.

3. **Neonatal hepatitis**–Manifest in newborn period. Liver enzymes will be abnormal.

4. **Extrahepatic biliary atresia** is also unlikely, as it manifests in newborn period and progress to early biliary cirrhosis and death unless operated before 2-3 months of age. The surgery includes **Kasai procedure** (porto-duodenal enterostomy).

Those with persistent cholestasis may benefit with high dose vitamins especially fat soluble vitamins. Anti histaminics may be given for extreme pruritus with caution. Cholestyramine is useful to bind bile acids in severely symptomatic patients.

SECTION 7.12 — A CHILD WITH ACUTE HEPATIC FAILURE

An 8-year-old child was admitted with jaundice and melena of 5 days duration. She had fever, nausea and lethargy. She had hepatitis B vaccination in childhood. There was history of a few cases of jaundice in the locality.

On examination: Growth and development normal, Icterus+, liver+2 cm below right costal margin, spleen palpable 2.5 cm, No ascites, sensorium—confused and drowsy, increased sleepiness+, DTR Brisk, Plantar B/L upgoing, asterixis (flapping tremor) +, fetor hepaticus +, S.Bilirubin 18 mg/dl, Direct 2 mg/dl, SGOT 1995 and SGPT 2004, S.AP 600 IU, Prothrombin time 50 seconds, control 13 seconds, HBsAg negative.

DIAGNOSIS AND DISCUSSION

Viral hepatitis A or E with Hepatic Encephalopathy – Stage III

A and E Hepatitis are the enteral route viral hepatitis, that manifest with constitutional symptoms and occur as small outbreaks. C, B and D Hepatitis are usually acquired through parenteral route and have an insidious onset without constitutional symptoms. Bleeding manifestation occurs due to prolonged prothrombine time (PT). In acute viral hepatitis, palpable liver is a good sign. Splenomegaly may occur in 20% cases. Acute yellow atrophy leading to shrinkage of liver may result in acute decompensation and may result in a fatal outcome. S.Br >17.5 mg/dl (300 micromol/L) and PT > 50 seconds are usually bad prognostic factors. Fetor hepaticus is due to mercaptens.

Vaccination can protect against HAV, HBV and HDV. D is usually a coinfection with B. The complications are hypoglycemia, electrolyte imbalance and acid base imbalance. The staging of encephalopathy is given in Table 7.7.

Treatment includes (1) supportive care, (2) hepatic drip, (3) fresh frozen plasma, (4) injection Vitamin K (Natural Kenadion is preferred to synthetic Menadion) 1 mg/year of age upto 10 mg/dose for 3 days, (5) bowel sterilization with ampicillin, (6) Ryles tube aspiration, and (7) bowel wash. The use of Neomycin is discouraged due to nephrotoxicity. Broad spectrum systemic antibiotic also may be beneficial in case of associated septicemia.

Lactulose 1 ml/kg/day or more to produce osmotic diarrhea is beneficial. It is an unabsorbed disaccharide (Beta galactoside fructose), that will reduce ammonia production, ammonia absorption and cause osmotic diarrhea. Oral lactilol (Beta galactoside sorbitol) in a dose of 30-40 g/day is better tolerated than lactulose.

In patients with cirrhosis, eradication of H Pylori should be undertaken as it generates ammonia in stomach via urease enzyme. Magnesium sulphate or lactulose enema is useful to clear bowels.

Flumazenil is imidazo benzodiazepine, that acts as benzodiazepine antagonist, via binding to the receptors. It is given in a dose of 0.01 mg/kg/day upto 2 mg as slow IV infusion.

Lamivudine 3 - 8 mg/kg/day is beneficial in HBV. It may be given till liver enzymes become normal and/or HBsAg becomes negative. Interferon is useful in HCV.

Avoidance of hepatotoxic drugs and restriction of protein by mouth are mandatory. Mannitol and flumazenil are beneficial in reducing cerebral edema and controlling seizures. Diazepam may displace bilirubin from binding sites and hence not preferred. Phenobarbitone may increase drowsiness but is useful. Phenytoin is hepatotoxic.

Glucagon 0.03 mg/kg/day upto 1 mg/day 3 days may help to tackle hypoglycemia and to promote liver regeneration. L ornithine - L aspartate (Hepamerz) 5-10 mg 2-3 times/day orally, will help to convert ammonia to urea and glutamate. Sodium benzoate 10 g/day may react with glycine to form hippuric acid and prove beneficial in hyperammonemia. IV Branched chain amino acids (proteinsteril Hepa/astymin Hepa) may also be helpful. Silimarin is useful in toxic hepatitis. Sorbilin and urso deoxy cholic acid (UDCA) are useful in increasing bile flow. UDCA is also useful in acalculous cholecystitiis due to cholesterol stones. When renal failure is associated with hepatic failure, it is called hepato renal syndrome.

Pathogenesis of HE

In hepatic encephalopathy, there will be abnormal shunting of toxic metabolites into the brain without hepatic detoxification. This is called 'porto-systemic shunting'. In cirrhosis, there may also be internal shunt, through large natural collaterals/portal – hepatic vein anastomosis around the nodules. Ammonia plays the key role in patho-genesis of HE. It combines with alpha glutarate to form glutamic acid, thus removing an important link in Kreb's citric acid cycle, which is vital for brain metabolism. Ammonia is also toxic to brain cell membrane and depresses cerebral blood flow and glucose metabolism. Aromatic amino acids may cross the blood brain barrier (BBB) and result in formation of false neurotransmitters (NT). False neurotransmitters like octopamine, produced by colonic bacteria may replace normal NTs like dopamine and nor adrenaline and add to the pathogenesis of HE. GABA is the inhibitory NT, that is also produced by enteric bacteria and there will be upregulation of GABA receptors in the brain. Benzodiazepine like endogenous substances may activate GABA system leading to aggravation. GABA Benzodiazepine complex plays an important role in HE. Other factors are hypokalemia, alkalosis, hypoxia and hypocapnea, due to stimulation of respiratory centre and reduced cerebral blood flow.

The factors that precipitate HE are GI bleed, infections, spontaneous bacterial peritonitis, vomiting, diarrhea, electrolyte imbalance, diuretics, hepatotoxic drugs, constipation, proteins by mouth and surgical procedures.

The composition of hepatic drip is as follows:

Item	Quantity
10% Glucose	400 ml
N Saline	100 ml
15% KCl	5 ml
10% Ca Gluconate	5 ml
Multi Vitamin Infusion (MVI)	2 ml

SECTION 7.13 A CHILD WITH PROLONGED LIVER DISEASE

An 8-year-old child was admitted with prolonged jaundice of 1 year duration. History of occasional melena +, history of joint swelling +.

On examination: Grade 2 PEM, 2° stunting and hepatosplenomegaly +, pallor + HBs Ag negative, Hb 9 g/dl. No evidence of haemolysis. S.Br. 7 mg/dl, SGOT/SGPT 605/700, SAP 600 IU/L, PT-20 seconds, control 13 seconds, S. Protein 6 mg, S. Alb. 3.5 g/dl.

DIAGNOSIS AND DISCUSSION

Chronic Active Hepatitis/Chronic Liver Disease (CLD)

Differential Diagnosis: Cirrhosis, Wilson disease:

Cirrhosis is unlikely as albumin globulin ratio is normal. Albumin globulin ratio will be reversed in cirrhosis due to markedly reduced albumin production. Jaundice and or elevated liver enzymes lasting for more than 6 months indicates chronic hepatitis. Based on histology, it will be divided into chronic persistent hepatitis (CPH) and chronic active hepatitis (CAH). In CPH, the inflammation is limited to portal triad and architecture is maintained, but in CAH, the inflammation is extensive and architecture is distorted and it will usually progress to cirrhosis.

Liver biopsy should be done after correcting prothrombin time. It can be achieved by giving Vit. K and FFP. Single donor plasma (SDP) is a colloid and it helps in volume expansion and in supplying albumin, whereas fresh frozen plasma (FFP) will provide coagulation factors and is useful in liver diseases, DIC, hemophilia etc. Abdominal girth and vital signs should be observed after biopsy to look for intra abdominal bleeding. Liver biopsy should be done only through the intercostal space. Subcostal procedure may lead to intractable biliary peritonitis.

Chronic persistent hepatitis is usually seen in HBV and HCV. Lamivudine in a dose of 2-4 mg/kg/day and Interferon alpha in HCV may be beneficial. CAH may be post hepatitic or due to auto immune/unknown reasons. Post hepatic/post necrotic lead to micronodular cirrhosis. Lupoid/Auto immune hepatitis (AIH) shows positive Antinuclear (ANA), Anti Liver Kidney Microsomal antibodies and anti smooth muscle antibodies (ASmA). Anti DsDNA antibody may be rarely positive in AIH.

Extrahepatic manifestations of CAH include rash, arthritis, arthralgia, Coomb's positive hemolytic anemia etc. It may be direct Coomb's positive or indirect Coomb's positive hemolytic anemia. When antibodies are coated on RBCs, the test becomes direct positive and when it is freely circulating, it will be indirect Coomb's positive anemia.

In **Wilson's disease,** KF (Kayser Fleicher) ring will be positive in the Descemet's membrane of the eye. It may be visible with naked eyes or slit lamp. In this disease, copper excretion will be increased. It may be better tested after giving penicillamine challenge, that will increase excretion. Serum ceruloplasmin will be low. This disease was called 'unlucky disease' as the defect was located on chromosome 13. It is hereditary hypercuprosis. In the young child, it presents with chronic liver disease, but in young adults, more neuropsychiatric manifestations will be seen. Zinc sulphate may be given to reduce copper absorption and copper chelation can be achieved by giving penicillamine. Vitamin B_6 should be given along with penicillamine. Zinc is also beneficial in all cases of cirrhosis due to zincuria and deficiency of zinc dependent enzymes.

Alcoholic cirrhosis is characterized by SGOT/SGPT ratio > 2, unlike other liver conditions. This is due to inability to synthesize SGPT, subsequent to enzyme blockade in alcoholic cirrhosis.

CAH usually progress to cirrhosis. In cirrhosis, histology is typical and there will be reversal of albumin globulin ratio. In cirrhosis, treatment is only symptomatic. The treatment of CAH include steroids or azathioprine to keep the SGPT (ALT) enzyme value <100 (double the normal). Silymarin is an antiprostaglandin drug given in a dose of 10-20 mg/kg/day in 2-3 divided doses.

The different causes of CLD are given in Table 7.8.

SECTION 7.14 A CHILD WITH MASSIVE HEMATEMESIS

A 10-year-old child was admitted with repeated bouts of massive hematemesis. No history of liver disease in the past.

On examination: No hepatosplenomegaly, growth and development normal, no icterus.

DIAGNOSIS AND DISCUSSION

Extrahepatic Portal Hypertension with Esophageal Varices

Differential Diagnosis: Congenital portal fibrosis, erosive gastritis/peptic ulcer.

Intrahepatic PH is more common than EHPH and is due to cirrhosis liver or hepatic fibrosis. Extrahepatic is due to portal vein obstruction following umbilical procedures, sepsis or thrombosis. Post hepatic PH is seen in Veno occlusive disease and Budd Chiari syndrome

Extrahepatic PH and portal vein thrombosis may also occur in hypercoagulable states like protein C or S deficiency. Normal portal pressure is 7 mm/Hg and size is < 10 mm. 10-12 mm is mild and >20 is severe PH. Esophageal varices

bleed spontaneously or with NSAIDs intake. Spleen which is enlarged may shrink after massive bleed. This is called **'Howard Smith sign'**, but spleen will reappear later.

LFT is usually normal in extrahepatic PH. USS Abdomen, Doppler and endoscopy are diagnostic of PH and varices. Endoscopy may be combined with sclerosant therapy. Red spots noted on endoscopy predicts future bleeds. Crystalloids, blood, FFP, Vitamin K are helpful to control bleed.

Vasopressin and octreotide are also beneficial. Octreotide is a vasopressin analogue, that is given in a dose of 25 mcg bolus, followed by same dose hourly till bleeding stops. Propranolol is beneficial to reduce splanchnic blood flow. Surgical Porto-Caval/Spleno-Renal shunts are needed in some cases. Cold saline stomach wash and H_2 receptor blockers are useful in acute cases.

Hepatic encephalopathy is rare in extrahepatic PH, but sometimes it may occur in spite of normal LFT, due to porto systemic shunting of ammonia and other toxic products.

SECTION 7.15

A GIRL WITH ABDOMINAL PAIN AND LOOSE STOOLS

A 11-year-old girl was admitted with fever abdominal pain and diarrhea. On examination: Sick and toxic, with diffuse abdominal tenderness and decreased bowel sounds. Mc Burney's area tenderness not elicited. Mild ascites +.

DIAGNOSIS AND DISCUSSION

Primary Peritonitis: PP

Differential Diagnosis: Acute diarrheal disease.

PP is more common in girls after 6 years of age. X-ray abdomen will show "shaggy fat line" with dilated bowel loops and bowel edema. Ascitic tap will show exudate with increased pus cells. Treatment includes supportive care and penicillin/ Cefotaxime for gram positive organisms like pneumococci, an aminoglycoside to cover gram negative organisms and metronidazole to cover anaerobes. For anerobic infections, above the diaphragm, CP and below the diaphragm, Metronidazole is preferred. It is most common in those with nephrotic syndrome and asplenia. Secondary peritonitis is seen in bowel perforation, appendicitis etc. Surgical drainage may be needed in some cases.

Serum to Ascitic Albumin Gradient (SAAG) is useful to differentiate between certain conditions of ascites. It is not useful to differentiate between exudates and transudate. Serum Albumin–Ascitic Albumin > 1.1 is seen in portal hypertension. It is <1.1 in other conditions like inflammatory exudates (Table 7.9), i.e., low gradient/Ascites.

Ascitic fluid amylase is high in pancreatic ascites and adenosine deaminase is high in TB and lymphoma with high lymphocyte count. Cholesterol > 50 mg/dl in malignancy, fibronectin > 75 in malignancy, bilirubin > 6 mg/dl in upper gut/biliary perforation are other useful clues for diagnosis. Cytology is important in malignancy and differential cell count in bacterial infections along with gram stain and culture are also useful.

Table 7.1: Rule of 10 in cleft lip and palate surgery

- **Rule of 10 for cleft lip**
- 10 weeks of age, around 10 pound weight and 10 g Hb
- **Rule of 10 for cleft palate**
- 10 months of age, around 10 kg weight and 10 g Hb
- Screen for CHD, other malformations and chromosomal anomalies before surgery.

Table 7.3: Dietary modification in persistent osmotic diarrhea

Level I/Diet A–Low Milk Diet

Milk 50 ml/kg/day as Curd, Rice/Sooji gruel with milk

Level II/Diet B—Milk free diet—Lactose free–Cereal pulse gruel without milk

Level III/Diet C Lactose, Sucorse and Starch free diet—Soyabased/Chicken based diet/Elemental diet

Zn SO_4 20 mg/day x 2 weeks (< 1 year —10 mg/day)

Vita A concentrate—1-2 lakh/dose

Convalescence—Give one extra meal/day 2-4 weeks

Amylase Rich Food (ARF)—germinated grains, sun dried and powdered.

Table 7.2: Treatment of H pylori infection (triple therapy)

Acid suppression	Antibiotic 1	Antibiotic 2	Duration	Remarks
Omeprazole	Clarithromycin	Metronidazole	7 days	>90% cure
Omeprazole	Clarithromycin	Amoxycillin	10 days	In metronidazole resistance
Lansoprazole	Clarithromycin	Amoxycillin	7 days	First line
Lansoprazole	Amoxycillin	Metronidazole	7 days	Second line

Table 7.4: Various diets in diarrhea

1. Diet A/	Low milk diet (50 mL/kg/day)
Level I diet	Curd, rice/sooji gruel with milk
2. Diet B/	Milk-free diet—cereal—pulse mix/gruel, amylase
Level II diet	rich food
3. Diet C/	Lactose-Sucrose/starch-free diet
Level III diet	Soya based, chicken based, egg

A. Low lactose diet (level I) cereal-based diet with little milk

Ingredients	Amount	Kcal	Prot (g)
Milk	75 mL	52	2.6
Rice	10 g	34	0.8
Sugar	2.5 g	10	—
Water q.s.	100 mL	—	—
Total	100 mL	96	3.4

- Liquid consistency 1 kcal/mL, volume 100 mL; lactose 3.4 g.
- Suji, or broken wheat (dalia), jaggery and green leafy vegetable can also be added.
- Calorie density of the feed can be increased by adding more sugar (but more than 6% may cause osmotic diarrhea) and oil (upto 3% is well accepted by children).

B. Lactose free diet (level 2) Milk-free cereal-based diet

Ingredient	Amount	Kcal	Prot (g)
Rice	15 g	48	1.2
Cooked moong dal	5.0 g	17	1.1
Sugar	2.5 g	10	—
Coconut oil	2.5 g	22	—
Water q.s.	100 mL	—	—
Total	100 mL	97	2.3

C. Lactose and sucrose free diet (level 3) Chicken glucose puree (For infants and children with severe persistent diarrhea and malabsorption of disaccharides)

Ingredients	Amount	Kcal	Prot (g)
Chicken	150 g	165	39
Glucose	100 g	400	—
Coconut oil	50 g	440	—
15% KCl	10 mL	—	—
7.5% NaCHO$_3$	20 mL	—	—
Water upto	1000 mL	1005	39

The quantity of chicken can be increased according to the protein requirement of the child.

Contd.

CHAPTER 7

GASTROINTESTINAL SYSTEM

Contd.

D. Commercial formula (lactose free)

Proprietary name (manufacturer)	Composition per 100 g powder (fortified with vitamins and minerals)				
	Protein (g%)	Carbohydrate(g%)	Fat (g%)	Cal(Kcal)	Remarks
Isomil*	Soya protein 14	52	28	517	Lactose free Sucrose (40%)
Soyal	Soya solid 18.0	Sucrose 5.0	Vegetable oil 18.0	466	Lactose free
Prosoyal (FDC Ltd)	Soya protein isolate	Maltodextrin 15.6	Vegetable oil 24.0	506	Lactose free Sucrose free
Zerolac (Raptakos Bret)	Soya protein isolate 15.0	Maltodextrin 58.0	Vegetable oil 20.0	472	Lactose free Sucrose free
Nusobee-18 (Wockhardt)	Soya + Casein 18.0	Maltodextrin + Sucrose 56.9	Vegetable 20.0	480	Lactose free
Nusobee (Wockhardt)	Soyaprotein 15.6	Maltodextrin 50.0	Vegetable oil 20.0	412	Lactose free Sucrose free
Simyl MCT** (FDC Ltd)	Casein 14.0	Maltodextrin 61.4	Vegetable oil 18.0	412	Lactose free Sucrose free
Pregestimil*** (Mead Johnson)	Hydrolysed casein 19.0	Tapioca starch 90.0	Corn oil 27.4	453	Lactose free Sucrose free

* With methionine, safflower oil 42%, coconut oil 30%, and soy oil 28%.

** With medium chain triglyceride, carnitine, taurine.

*** With tyrosine, tryptophan, lecithin and medium chain triglyceride.

Table 7.5: Causes of chronic diarrhea	
Osmotic	
1. Maldigestion	PEM, pancreatic insufficiency, cystic fibrosis, intestinal enzyme deficiencies, cholestatic syndromes, short bowel syndrome, bacterial overgrowth
2. Disaccharidase deficiency	Congenital or acquired lactose/sucrose maltase/isomaltose deficiency
3. Other malabsorptions	Glucose-galactose malabsorption
4. Ongoing infections	Bacterial, viral, parasitic, opportunistic, HIV/AIDS, immunodeficiency
5. Inflammatory conditions	Celiac sprue, tropical sprue, cow milk protein intolerance (CMPI), soya protein intolerance (SPI), Eosinophilic gastroenteropathy. Auto immune enteropathy, ulcerative colitis, Crohn disease
6. Motility disorders	Toddlers diarrhea, irritable bowel syndrome
7. Lymphatic stasis/obstruction	Intestinal lymphangiectasia, Wolman disease
8. Neuro endocrine conditions	Hyperthyroidism, Carcinoid syndrome, Vasoactive intestinal peptide (VIP) mediated diarrhea
9. Drug induced	Antibiotics, laxatives, cytotoxic drugs
10. Mulifactorial	PEM
Secretory	
1. Congenital transport defects	Congenital chloride/sodium diarrhea bile acid malabsorption
2. Villous atrophy and crypt hyperplasia	Congenital microvillous atrophy
3. Ongoing infection	HIV/AIDS, immunodeficiency
4. Neural crest tumors	

Table 7.6: Causes of jaundice in the newborn		
Within 24 hrs	*24-72 hrs*	*After 72 hrs*
Rh, ABO, minor group Incompatibilities	Physiological jaundice	Septicemia
Intrauterine infections STORCH	EONS (early onset neonatal sepsis)	IU Infections LONS (late onset neonatal sepsis)
Hemolytic anemias	Prematurity	Extra hepatic biliary atresia/
Red cell membrane/ enzyme defects		Neonatal hepatitis
Crigler-Najjar syndrome	Hypothyroidism	Breast milk jaundice
Lucey Driscoll syndrome	Cephal hematoma/cerebral bleeding	Hypothyroidism
Maternal drugs Vit K, sulpha, aspirin	Birth asphyxia, acidosis, hypothermia, hypoglycemia	Intestinal obstruction, pyloric stenosis
Homozygous alpha thalassemia	Polycythemia, high altitude	Metabolic disorders

Table 7.7. Clinical staging of hepatic encephalopathy

Grade	Features
I	Lethargy with intermittent euphoria, alteration in sleep pattern, apraxia, EEG - Normal
II	Drowsy, agitated, disoriented, fetor hepaticus, asterixis, incontinence, EEG-Slowing with theta waves
III	Stupor, confusion, delirium, asterixis, hyperreflexia, extensor plantar, EEG abnormal with triphasic waves
IV	Coma, areflexia, flaccidity, no asterixis, EEG slowing/delta waves or electrical silence
IV A	Response to painful stimulus +
IV B	No response to painful stimulus

Table 7.8: Causes of chronic persistent/chronic active hepatitis

1. Ongoing infections	–	Hepatitis B,C,D
2. Auto immune hepatitis (AIH)/ lupoid hepatitis	–	SLE, Anti Liver KidneyMicrosomal antibodies (LKM) and anti smooth muscle (Anti Actin) and Anti nuclear antibodies (ANA) +ve
3. Drug Toxin induced hepatitis	–	INH, Methyldopa, sulpha, Nitrofurantoin, Alcohol
4. Metabolic	–	Wilson's, Anti Apha I antitrypsin deficiency, tyrosinemia, cystic fibrosis, glycogen storage disease type IV, Niemann Pick type II etc.
5. Crytogenic	–	Non infective, non-alcoholic

Table 7.9: Classification of ascites based on SAAG

High gradient ascites (>1.1 g/dl)	Low gradient ascites (< 1.1 g/dl)
Portal vein thrombosis	TB ascites
Cirrhosis	Nephrotic syndrome
Hepatic failure	Pancreatic ascites
Budd-Chiari	Chylous ascites
Veno occlusive disease	Biliary ascites
Cardiac ascites Liver metastasis	Collagen vascular disease with serositis Peritoneal metastasis
Mixed ascites-portal	Bowel obstruction/infarction
Hypertension + other causes like Cirrhosis + TB peritonitis	Post operative lymphatic leak

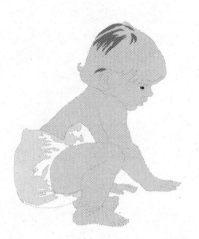

8

Respiratory System

SECTION 8.1

A CHILD WITH FEVER AND DROOLING

A 2-year-old child presented with fever, throat pain, inability to feed and drooling of saliva of 2 days duration.

On examination: Febrile, irritable, hyperextension of head +, pooling of secretion +, no palatal palsy, bulge in the posterior pharyngeal wall+, growth and development normal.

Hb 10 g/dl, TC- 13,000/cumm, P 76%, L 23%, E 1%, ESR 78 mm/1st hour.

DIAGNOSIS AND DISCUSSION

Retropharyngeal Abscess

The C/F and bulge in the posterior pharyngeal wall suggest the diagnosis. Lateral X-ray neck will show a soft tissue shadow. The space between vertebra and the tracheal shadow will appear wide, i.e., more than the width of one vertebral body. Antibiotics for Streptcoccal and staphyloccal cover namely Ampicillin/Cefotaxim and Cloxacillin and anti-inflammatory drugs like serratio peptidase should be started. Incision and drainage should be done whenever indicated in consultation with Ped. Surgeon/ENT Surgeon. The differential diagnosis are:

1. **Quinsy/Peritonsillar abscess:** The abscess is around the tonsil and not on the posterior pharyngeal wall. It often will need surgical drainage with or without tonsillectomy.

2. **Ludwig's angina:** It is a cellulitis of the submandibular or submental area unrelated to lymphadenopathy.

3. **Tonsillitis/Pharyngitis:** It may be viral or bacterial. Viral involvement produces exudates in follicles with or without lymphadenopathy and there may be associated rhinitis and conjunctivitis. Bacterial especially streptococcal will have high fever, exudates in tonsil and tender lymphadenopathy.

4. **Diphtheria:** Large lymphadenopathy called 'bull's neck' and greyish white pseudo membrane which bleeds on removal are characteristic. Conjunctival, pharyngeal and laryngeal involvement can occur. Toxic neuritis and myocarditis occurs during the course. **Local pharyngeal or palatal** paralysis occurs early in the course followed by **focal ocular paralysis. Generalized and symme-tric Post diphtheritic paralysis (PDP)** occurs later after a latent period of 2 weeks. Myocar-ditis occurs in the 2nd week (Refer Section 5.4).

5. **A/C Epiglottitis:** High fever, air hunger, drooling, dysphagia and shock may be noted in this condition. The child prefers to sit up leaning forward. It may be a fatal condition. Lateral neck X-ray may show inf lamed epiglottis as 'thumb's up' sign. Direct laryngoscopy will confirm the diagnosis. Intubation/tracheostomy may be life saving. Antibiotics to cover H. Influenza B (Ampicillin/ Cefotaxim) and steroids are indicated along with supportive care.

CHAPTER 8

RESPIRATORY SYSTEM

Indications for adeno-tonsillectomy are recurrent tonsillitis and pharyngitis presenting as recurrent fever and missing of school, chronic mouth breathing, respiratory obstruction with adenoid facies/nasal twang of voice, snoring, repeated otitis media and deafness. Tonsils tend to be large in children upto puberty age due to rapid lymphoid growth phase. Regression occurs in later age. Large tonsils meeting in the midline are called 'Kissing tonsils'.

8.1 DROOLING

SECTION 8.2 AN INFANT WITH STRIDOR

A 2-month-old baby was brought with failure to thrive, tachypnea and noisy breathing of one month duration. The symptoms used to get aggravated during nasal block, URI and cough. BW was 2.6 kg.

On examination: Growth below 3rd centile, social smile +, RR-58/mt, HR- 108/mt, Suprasternal and subcostal retractions + No cardiomegaly, Basal ejection systolic murmur with widely split second sound in pulmonary area, liver and spleen palpable, liver span 5 cm.

DIAGNOSIS AND DISCUSSION

Congenital laryngeal stridor (CLS) due to laryngo-tracheomalacia, FTT with severe malnutrition and CHD–ASD with no evidence of congestive cardiac failure.

Palpable liver and spleen are the pushed down organs. The stridor is due to congenital flabbiness or dilatation of larynx and trachea leading to collapse of the airways. This manifests within the first 2 weeks to 2 months of life and persists for 1-2 years. So, improvement will be noted with age. Apart from the stridor, baby will be comfortable, feeding and sleeping well. Chest deformity may also occur. The babies may be more comfortable in the prone/lateral position. Associated conditions are FTT and CHD, usually ASD. Treatment includes reassurance and proper nutrition. Direct laryngoscopy may be done to rule out laryngeal webs/tumors, which will show a progressive course.

ASD should be looked for in babies who are more symptomatic or when X-ray/ECG is suggestive. In isolated CLS, child will be feeding well, sleeping well and thriving well in spite of the noisy breathing.

Laryngeal web, cleft/vascular anomalies or tumor: Aggravation of stridor or distress in certain positions of the neck and no improvement with increasing age occur in these conditions. This is unlike CLS, which improves with age.

SECTION 8.3   A CHILD WITH FEVER AND ACUTE STRIDOR

A 3-year-old boy, who was on treatment for fever and cough for 2 days, was rushed to the casualty in the night with acute stridor.

On examination: He was in distress, hypoxic, unable to drink and had tachycardia and tachypnea. Growth and development normal.

DIAGNOSIS AND DISCUSSION

A/C Laryngo-Tracheo Bronchitis (ALTB)/ Croup

A child having URI, developing stridor in the night is characteristic of ALTB. Viral infections or bacterial infections like H. influenza B (HIB) are responsible for croup. The treatment includes reassurance, antibiotics like ampicillin/cephalosporin to cover HIB, steroids and humidified oxygen. Sore throat and hoarseness of voice will occur in associated laryngitis. X-ray may show 'steeple' sign. This is due to the typical subglottic narrowing. IV fluids and humidified oxygen should be given in acute cases.

Differential Diagnosis includes malformations/tumors becoming symptomatic with infections, laryngeal edema due to food/drug allergy etc.

Other causes of stridor are recurrent spasmodic cough, psychogenic cough, allergic edema, epiglottitis and GERD (gastroesophageal reflux disease).

SECTION 8.4

A CHILD WITH HISTORY OF CHOKING AND EPISODIC COUGH

A 2½-year-old child was brought with episodic cough and mild fever of one week duration. He gave history of choking while taking peanuts 3 days back. Growth and development normal, R.R 42/mt, HR-120 /mt, Temp 101°F, CFT normal, air entry decreased in the Rt infrascapular area with resonant percussion note. No mediastinal shift. X-ray chest showed localized emphysema in Rt Lower Lobe.

DIAGNOSIS AND DISCUSSION

Foreign body aspiration leading to 'ball valve type' of obstructive emphysema—Rt lower lobe

Differential Diagnosis: Pneumothorax (Rt).

Right lower lobe bronchus is more commonly affected in foreign body aspiration due to its position. Foreign body aspiration can also occur into right middle lobe or left lower lobe. Non obstructive foreign bodies may remain silent for many days before becoming symptomatic. Only repeated questioning may yield the history of peanut ingestion or choking while eating in some cases. Elder sibling may give peanuts to younger sibling without the notice of the parents. Vegetable foreign bodies may swell up absorbing moisture and may get infected. Most of the foreign bodies are not radio opaque, but X-ray will show localized emphysema or atelectasis in case of complete obstruction.

Complete obstruction of a bronchus will lead to atelectasis or collapse and mild incomplete obstruction will act like a 'bypass valve' allowing air passage in both directions and case localized wheeze. Moderate obstruction will act like a 'ball valve' that allows air to enter during inspiration, but prevents escape of air during expiration leading to obstructive emphysema. Bronchoscopy and antibiotics are indicated. Steroids for a few days may be useful to reduce post procedure edema.

In pneumothorax, there will be reduced air entry and hyperresonant percussion note. Mediastinal shift to the opposite side will be seen in tension pneumothorax. X-ray will show air in the pleural cavity with no bronchovascular markings and mediastinal shift. Collapsed lung may also be seen towards the heart.

CHAPTER 8

RESPIRATORY SYSTEM

SECTION 8.5

A CHILD WITH UNRESOLVED CHEST INFECTION

A 4-year-old child was brought with history of unresolved pneumonia, treated in various hospitals. Previous X-rays showed opacity in the left hemithorax and present X-ray showed air fluid level in the left hemithorax.

On examination: Growth below 3rd centile, development normal, No clubbing, halitosis +, RR 42/mt, pulse 110/mt, temp 101°F, air entry decreased in left infrascapular area with impaired percussion note. No mediastinal shift, HIV-ELISA Negative, Mantoux test Negative, Blood counts Hb 9.5 g/dl, leukocytosis with neutrophilia, ESR 45 mm/1st hour.

DIAGNOSIS AND DISCUSSION: LUNG ABSCESS (LT)

Differential Diagnosis:

1. Pneumonia (Lt)
2. Empyema (Lt)
3. Sequestration lung left and severe malnutrition.
4. Acquired/Congenital immunodeficiency (Hypergammaglobulinemia is seen in Acquired and Hypogammaglobulinemia in Congenital).

Reduced air entry and impaired note suggests pneumonia. History of repeated admissions with pathology on the same side favour the possibility of sequestration lung. Air fluid level in X-ray favours the diagnosis of lung abscess.

Extralobar sequestration is more common on the left side compared to intralobar type. It becomes symptomatic with infection. Sequestration is due to aberrant blood supply from the aorta. Systemic feeding artery demonstrated by contrast CT or aortography is diagnostic. **Intralobar sequestration may also occur with cystadenomatoid malformation.** Sequestration requires surgical resection after identifying the blood supply.

Treatment includes antibiotics and supportive care irrespective of the final diagnosis.

Mycoplasma pneumonia and pleuro pneumonia like organism (PPLO) infection usually occur in school going children > 4 years of age. The patient may be afebrile and cold agglutinin test positive in mycoplasma. It is also called 'walking pneumonia'. Treatment of choice is macrolides. Azithromycin can be given orally or IV.

Lung abscess is a chronic suppurative lung lesion with abscess formation in the infected lung. The duration is usually more than 1 month. Clubbing may be evident by 2-4 weeks. **Posterior segments of the upper lobe and superior segments of the lower lobe are the usual sites for lung abscess.** Staphylococcal infection produces multiple breaking down lesions and small abscess, emphysema and pneumatocele. **Klebsiella pneumonia involves right upper lobe leading to bulging horizontal fissure.** Anaerobic infections and immunodeficiency states may also be the cause for lung abscess. It may be associated with septic embolization from thrombophlebitis and bacterial endocarditis. There may be history of foul smelling sputum or blood stained sputum. X-ray chest Erect and Lateral views and CT chest will show air fluid level and will be diagnostic of lung abscess. Treatment includes appropriate antibiotics after culture and sensitivity for 4-6 weeks. Cefotaxime or ceftazidime and aminoglycoside plus penicillin and or metronidazole will cover gram positive, gram negative and anaerobic infections. For anaerobic cover, penicillin is preferred for infections above the diaphragm and metronidazole for infections below the diaphragm like peritonitis/retroperitoneal or liver abscess. In immunosuppressed children/those with cystic fibrosis, pseudomonas cover is imperative. Drugs as per culture and sensitivity of sputum should be started as soon as the results are available. Other drugs like chloramphenicol, clindamycin or vancomycin may be tried in non responders. Those who respond will become afebrile within one week time. Bronchoscopic aspiration of pus and culture may

also be done if the response is poor. Lobectomy is indicated in recurrent hemoptysis or broncho pleural fistula.

DD also includes Mass/space occupying lesions (SOL) of the chest. Heterogenous mass lesions and solid tumors of pleura, lung and mediastinum can be diagnosed by CT chest.

Lung malformations should be considered in persisting lung shadows. CT scan with contrast will be useful in the diagnosis. These include the following: **Congenital lobar emphysema (CLE)** presents with distress, reduced air entry and resonant percussion note. X-ray will show emphysema on one side, more common on left side with visible bronchovascular markings unlike in pneumothorax. Herniation of emphysematous lung may occur to the opposite side. **Lung cyst** is usually solitary cyst with no bronchovascular markings. **Congenital Cystadenomatoid malformation (CCAM)** may be microcystic (good prognosis), macrocystic or solid. **Pulmonary lymphangiectasia** is rare, but has poor outcome.

SECTION 8.6 A CHILD WITH CHRONIC LUNG INFECTION

A 10-year-old boy was admitted with cough, copious purulent foul smelling sputum and weight loss of 1 year duration and hemoptysis of 1 week duration. Cough gets aggravated during lying down.

On examination: Grade III PEM, 2nd degree stunting, clubbing +, RR 38 /mt, pulse 100/mt, coarse crepitations on the right infrascapular area, occasional rhonchi and creps on the left side.

DIAGNOSIS AND DISCUSSION

Bronchiectasis Rt Lower Lobe

Long duration, copious foul smelling sputum, hemoptysis, clubbing and coarse crepetations suggest the diagnosis of brochiectasis. **It is a chronic suppurative lung disease with inflammatory destruction and dilatation of bronchi. It occurs following unresolved pneumonia and bronchial obstruction secondary to lymphadenopathy, TB or foreign body. Reversible or pseudo bronchiectasis occur in pertussis. The usually sites are right middle lobe, lingular segments and basal segments of lower lobe. In TB, Rt middle lobe is more commonly affected compared to Rt lower lobe seen in foreign body aspiration. Cystic fibrosis affects all lobes.**

Clubbing indicates illness lasting for more than 1 year. X-ray chest will show streaky opacities called **'rail road tracks'** and crowding of ribs due to loss of lung volume. Bronchogram will show

'honey comb appearance'. CT scan is also useful in delineating the affected area. Bronchoscopy is diagnostic and can help to suck out secretions and granulomas and to take cultures/ specimen for HPE. It also may be curative.

Antibiotics like Cefotaxime and aminoglycoside with penicillin and or metronidazole are useful to cover gram positive, negative and anerobic infections. Duration is usually 2-3 weeks. Pseudomonas cover is essential in CF (cefta-zidime, amikacin or piperacillin). Chest physio is beneficial in getting rid of collections and to ensure chest expansion. Saline nebulizations may be done prior to chest physio to enhance efficacy. Bronchoalveolar lavage (BAL) can obtain specimen for culture and help for clearing secretions.

Lobectomy may be rarely needed in localized cases.

Differential Diagnosis:

1. **Cystic fibrosis (CF):** Sweat chloride > 40-60 mEq/L indicates mild disease and >60 indicates severe disease. Significant malabsorption and CF associated diabetes may also be noted along with chronic lung disease. In mild steatorrhea, stool may appear normal. Pseudomonas cover including ceftazidine and Amikacin are the antibiotics of choice. **CF transmembrane regulator (CFTR) protein is abnormal.** It is an autosomal recessive condition. It may be seen in non consanguinous couples due to fresh mutation or clustering

of this mutant gene in many families as seen among Caucasians. Pancreatic enzyme replacement will be helpful in malabsorption states.

2. **Alpha 1 Antitrypsin deficiency:** It is an autosomal recessive condition, characterized by chronic liver and lung disease. Cough, wheeze and emphysema are the usual manifestations. Environmental triggers like smoking will aggravate the condition. Danazole, a testosterone analog and recombinant Alpha 1 antitrypsin aerosoles are useful along with supportive care like antibiotics and bronchodilator.

3. **Immunodeficiency states, both congenital and acquired lead to chronic lung disease. Pulmonary hypertension and corpulmonale may occur in HIV AIDS.**

4. **Congenital bronchiectasis: Tracheobronchomegaly and cystadenomatoid malformation may lead to bronchiectasis.**

5. **Immotile cilia syndrome** may be the pathology in some cases. **In Kartagener syndrome,** there is chronic sinusitis and bronchiectases and situs inversus. Sterility may also occur. **In Young syndrome,** there is chronic sinusitis and bronchiectasis with azoospermia.

GOLD is the Global Initiative for Chronic Obstructive Lung Disease compared to GINA (Global Initiative for Asthma).

CHAPTER 8

RESPIRATORY SYSTEM

SECTION 8.7

A CHILD WITH ABSCESS SCALP AND CHEST INFECTION

A 10-month-old baby was admitted with high fever and tachypnea of 3 days duration. The baby had an abscess on the scalp, which was treated in local hospital with local antibiotics.

On examination: Growth and development normal, RR. 58/mt, HR 120/mt, Temp 103° F, indrawing of lower chest +, edema and fullness + on Rt side chest wall, percussion note—stony dull with decressed air entry Rt side, VF and VR decreased in the same area, trachea shifted to the left, apex beat in the 5th left intercostal space outside mild clavicular line. Blood counts—polymorphonuclear leukocytosis with ESR 85 mm/1st hour.

DIAGNOSIS AND DISCUSSION

Empyema Rt with Mediastinal Shift, Probably due to Staphylococcal Pneumonia

Abscess scalp prior to the respiratory problem is suggestive of staph. infection. High fever, toxic look, intercostal oedema, tenderness, fullness with shift of mediastinum to opposite side and stony dullness with reduced air entry, reduced VF and VR suggest empyema. Empyema dissecting through the chest wall is called 'empyema necessitans'.

In pleural effusion, the patient may not be looking toxic unlike in empyema. Intercostal wall edema, tenderness and fullness are also unlikely. Air above the level of pus indicates pyopneumo-thorax. Staph. infection causes breaking down abscess and pneumatocele which may rupture

into the pleura causing empyema/pyopenu-mothorax. **Syn-pneumonic effusion usually occurs with pneumococcal and H. Influenza B infections, straw coloured effusion occurs in TB, chylous and hemorrhagic effusions occur in malignancies/post operative cases.** Gram stain and culture of pleural fluid will help to differentiate the organism. It is important to differentiate between transudate, exudates and TB effusions (Table 8.1).

Treatment includes cloxacillin for 3-4 weeks with intercostal drainage usually through the 4th space. ICD tube should be kept in situ for 5-7 days and should be removed only after lung expansion. In case of thin pus or transudate, repeated taps may be done instead of ICD tube.

The complications are septicemia, broncho pleural fistula and lung abscess. In methicillin resistant Staph aureus (MRSA), Vancomycin is the drug of choice. In Vancomycin intermediate sensitive SA (VISA), teicoplanin can be given. In Glycopeptide intermediate sensitive SA (GISA), linezolid is indicated.

In **encysted effusions**, streptokinase or urokinase may be instilled into the pleural space before planning decortication. Treatment of encysted effusion is by instilling streptokinase in a dose of 2.5 lakh/day for 6 days (1 vial =15 lakh units). It is diluted with 30 ml N. saline and is instilled through ICD and the tube should be clamped for 4 hours. **Decortication** may be needed in non responding cases. USS Chest will be helpful to diagnose encysted collection due to the presence of loculations. CT Chest is useful in differentiating collections in pleura versus lung (pleural based collections). Video assisted thoracoscopy (VAT) is very useful in tackling resistant and encysted effusions.

In pneumothorax, ICD is done in the 2nd space anteriorly. ICD tube is usually kept in situ for 2-3 days. Small air leak leading to mild pneumothorax may resolve by itself. In refractory cases, pleural stripping may be needed.

Pneumothorax and subcutaneous emphysema can occur in post thoracotomy cases, asthma or staphylococcal infection with pneumatocele formation. Subcutaneous emphysema usually resolves by itself. The child should receive oxygen and needs close monitoring. In mediastinal air leak, air will be seen around the mediastinum and below the cardiac shadow.

CHAPTER 8

RESPIRATORY SYSTEM

SECTION 8.8 — A CHILD WITH CHRONIC WHEEZE

A 7-year-old boy was admitted with acute air hunger, neck swelling noticed 2 hours back and respiratory distress. He gave history of wheeze since childhood.

On examination: RR 50/mt, HR 120/mt. Pulsus paradoxus > 10 mm of Hg, crepitus + on chest wall and neck, dusky nails, strap muscles acting with flaring of ala nasi. Growth <3rd centile, barrel shaped chest +, pectus carinatum +, percussion note—tympanic on both sides, Air entry reduced bilaterally. Oxygen saturation 89% without oxygen, X-ray B/L streaky opacities, B/L air trapping, S/C emphysema +.

DIAGNOSIS AND DISCUSSION

A/C severe asthma with chronic emphysema and S/C emphysema

Differential Diagnosis: Pneumothorax.

Wheezing is a very common symptom in children. In the very young, it should be differentiated from **bronchiolitis,** which is usually a single episode due to Respiratory Syncytial Virus (RSV) infection, starting as URI and proceeding to wheeze and feeding difficulty. There will be other family members having URI and blood counts will show lymphocyte predominance. X-ray will show air trapping. In **bronchopneumonia with wheeze or wheeze associated LRI (WALRI)**, there will be fever, tachypnea, intercostal retractions, grunt, polymorphonuclear leukocytosis and consolidation on X-ray with no previous history of asthma.

In asthma, there will be history of previous episodes and reversibility with bronchodilators. In **atopic asthma**, there will be history of allergy/atopy, symmetric skin lesions, positive family history of atopy/asthma. In **non atopic type**, previous episodes may be the only clue. Another cause of wheezing is anatomical defects like GERD, tracheo-bronchomalacia etc.These are the so called **'anatomical wheezers'**.

Early onset wheeze (< 3 years)	Late onset wheeze (> 3 years)
Bronchiolitis	Atopic asthma
WALRI	Non atopic asthma
Anatomical wheezer	
Transient hyperreactive airway disease	
Atopic asthma	

Acute attack should be managed as per the algorithm (Fig. 8.1).

The inhalor devices are **metered dose inhaler (MDI)** with or without spacer and baby mask, **dry powder inhaler (DPI—rotahalor)** and **nebulizers. MDI without spacer and DPI are suitable for children above 6-8 years. Below 3 years, baby mask with spacer is used.**

Long-term management depends on categorization of asthma as per **GINA guidelines** (Table 8.2). During follow up, asthma is categorized as well controlled, poorly controlled and uncontrolled asthma. In exercise induced asthma, salmeterol (LABA) is given as MDI before exercise. Severity of an acute attack can be assessed by pulmonary score (Table 8.3).

In life threatening cases, there will be inability to speak, count/drink, pulses paradoxus > 15 mm of Hg, cyanosis, altered sensorium, respiratory muscle fatigue with abdominal paradox, pneumothorax and silent chest. Wheeze may become audible only after nebulization.

O2+ Nebulization

Salbutamol 0.03 ml/kg/dose diluted in 2-3 ml N saline with oxygen

Repeat 3 times at 20 minutes interval– observe for 1 hour

If better, may be discharged on Oral/inhaled salbutamol with or with out steroids x 3 days, Steroid given in persistent Asthma/history of life threatening episodes/ ICU admission

If not better, Admit→continuous salbutamol nebulization—0.1 ml/kg in 9 ml N. saline 1st Hr/triple nebulization (salbutamol + budesonide + Ipatropium bromide)+, **Antibiotics**

Others: Terbutaline 0.01ml/kg/SC or IV infusion 10 mcg/kg bolus followed by 1 mcg/kg/mt, IV Efcorlin 10 mg/kg followed by 5 mg/kg Q6H, Aminophylline 5 mg/kg bolous followed by I mg/kg/hr

Other options before ventilatory care: IV methyl prednisolone 2-3 mg/kg/ dose Q8H, IV 50% Mg sulphate 0.2 ml/kg in 30 ml N. saline

No improvement: Early Ventilatory care

Fig. 8.1: Algorithm for A/C asthma management

Dose of Salbutamol 0.15 mg/kg or 0.03 ml/kg (Infants—maximum 2.5 mg or 0.5 ml/dose and older children 5 mg or/ml/dose) (1 ml= 5 mg).

Budesonide 0. 25 mg/dose in young child and 0.5 mg/dose in older child (1 ml=0.25mg/0.5 mg).

Ipatropium 125-250 mcg/dose <1 year-125 mcg (1 ml=250 mcg).

Fig. Nos. 25-34 (Plates 6 to 8) for various chest and lung conditions and X-rays.

CHAPTER 8

RESPIRATORY SYSTEM

Table 8.1: Differences between transudate, exudate and TB effusion

Item	Tansudate	Exudates	TB
Macroscopy	Clear	Purulent	Straw colour
Protein	< 3 g/dl	> 3 g/dl	> 3 g/dl
Glucose	> 40 mg/dl	<40 mg/dl	<40 mg/dl
Pleural Fluid/ Serum LDH ratio	<0.6	>0.6	>0.6
Pleural Fluid PH	>7.2	<7.2	<7.2
Microscopy	No cells	Polymorphs predominant	Lymphocytes predominant
Microbes	NIL	Gram stain +ve	AFB +ve

Table 8.2: Global initiative for asthma (GINA) guidelines for categorization

Category	Day time symptoms	Night time symptoms	PEFR	Treatment
Step I Intermittent	<1 time/week	< 2 time/month	> 80%, <20% variability PEFR normal in between attacks	Oral/inhaled short acting beta agonist (SABA)-salbutamol during attack
Step II Mild persistent	>1 time/week < 1time/day	>2 time/month	>80% variability 20-30%	1. Steroid 400 mcg/day 2. Chromai 5-10 mg Q 6 H 3. Time release deriphylline (TRD) 10-15 mg/day 12 H
Step III Moderate persistent	Daily	>1 time/week	60-80 variability	1. 800 mcg/day Q 12 H or 2. 400 mcg mg/day Q 12 H+(LABA) salmeterol 3. TRD if poor compliance to inhalations
Step IV Severe persistent	Continuous with limited physical activity	Frequent	<60% variability >30%	Steroid & LABA + Add on drug TRD, oral steroid, montelkast

SABA—— Short acting beta agonist

TRD—— Time release deriphylline

LABA—— Long acting beta agonist

* **Exercise induced asthma–LABA before exercise**

Table 8.3: Pulmonary scoring for severity of asthma				
Score	Resp rate < 6 years	Resp rate > 6 years	Wheeze	Accessory muscles acting
0	< 30	< 20	None	No apparent activity
1	31-45	21-35	Terminal expiratory, audible with steth	Mild/ questionable
2	46-60	36-50	Entire expiratory, audible with steth	Apparent activity
3	>60	>50	Inspiratory and expiratory audible without steth	Maximum activity

Pulmonary Score: 0-3—Mild, 4-6—Moderate, >6—Severe.

CHAPTER 8

RESPIRATORY SYSTEM

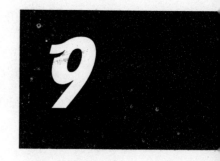

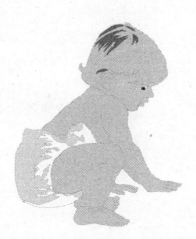

Cardiovascular System

9

A TWO-MONTH-OLD BABY WITH CCF

A two-month-old baby was admitted with cough and feeding difficulty of 2 weeks duration. History of excessive head sweat+, BW 2.6 kg.

On examination: Wt 3.2 kg, RR 56/mt, HR. 150/mt, CFT 2 seconds, pallor +, no edema. No cyanosis. All peripheral puses felt, subcostal retraction +, Resp system: bilateral creps and rhonchi +, Air entry equal. CVS: apex beat-4th Lt intercostal space outside mid clavicular line, forceful in nature, systolic thrill left sternal border with pansystolic murmur (Grade V/VI) best heard in the 3rd, 4th space close to sternum, same murmur heard in all areas with less intensity. Mid diastolic murmur + at the apex, P2 loud. Liver palpable 4 cm below costal margin, span 9 cm. Spleen palpable 2 cm. weight < 3rd centile, development: social smile +.

DIAGNOSIS AND DISCUSSION

Congenital Heart Disease left to right shunt, large ventricular septal defect with congestive heart failure and failure to thrive

Left to right shunts usually manifest around 6 weeks of age when pulmonary pressure reduce and lungs get flooded. The exceptions to the rule are premature/low birth weight (LBW) babies manifesting earlier due to more rapid fall of pulmonary pressure and those with complex heart disease, e.g., ostium primum ASD, VSD + PDA, VSD + AR etc.

In VSD, the murmur is usually best heard in 3rd and 4th space, but in supracristal (Subpulmo-nic) or subaortic VSD, the murmur may be best heard in 2nd and 3rd space. The most important sign of CHF in infants and children is tender hepatomegaly. Tenderness may not be elicited in those who are on decongestives or those with chronic CHF. Raised JVP is difficult to assess in young infants. Pedal edema may not be evident due to frequent change of posture, but paraspinal edema may be present. Orthopnea may be diagnosed if baby becomes more comfortable in the mother's shoulder in the upright posture.

In TOF like physiology, initially pulmonary stenosis is mild and left to right shunt is more and may be diagnosed initially as VSD only. Cyanosis may become evident only in the second half of infancy. Acquired pulmonary stenosis with VSD called **Gassul VSD**, also should be looked for during follow up. In pulmonary stenosis, P2 becomes soft or may be absent, with a single second sound (A2) in pulmonary area. In pulmonary hypertension, P_2 becomes loud and booming. The dullness in second space widens beyond 2 cm (Positive Ribbons sign) and Rt parasternal heave appears due to Rt ventricular hypertrophy. Subsequently reversal of shunt may occur leading to **Eisenmenger syndrome**. Supracristal VSD is between pulmonary valve and crista supraventricularis. Infracristal VSD is between papillary muscle of the conus and supraventricularis. **Supracristal VSD may be associated with aortic regurgitation and infracristal VSD may be associated with pulmonary stenosis/TOF. Muscular VSD is**

CHAPTER 9

CARDIOVASCULAR SYSTEM

usually multiple leading to 'swiss cheese septum' appearance. 'Malady-de-Roger' (Roger's Malady) is small asymptomatic VSD which produces a very loud murmur.

The left to right shunt depends on the size of the defect and degree of pulmonary resistance. When pulmonary to systemic flow is >2.5:1 there will be cardiomegaly, pulmonary hypertension and mitral diastolic flow murmur as in this case. Mid diastolic murmur indicate >2:1 shunt.

In ASD with left to right shunt, the flow murmur is heard in the tricupid area. When pulmonary to systemic flow is <1.75.1, cardiac size and pulmonary vasculature may be normal. When both pressure equities to 1:1 the shunt may be bidirectional leading to cyanosis. Small defects < 0.5 cm^2 is called **restrictive VSD** and large defects >1cm^2 are called **non-restrictive VSD.**

Small VSDs are asymptomatic with normal hemodynamic parameters, usually detected during routine medical check up. Moderate VSDs are symptomatic with increased respiratory infection and CHF in infancy, but responds to medical management. Large VSDs are refractory to treatment and cause failure to thrive. Head sweats are due to increased sympathetic drive due to stress and CHF.

X-rays may be normal in small VSD. In moderate VSD, there will be cardiomegaly, increased venous markings in the upper lobes initially followed by arterial markings in the lower lobes and pulmonary plethora and prominent pulmonary artery and left atrium. In Eisenmenger syndrome, pulmonary vasculature will show **'pruning'** beyond the medial one third of hemithorax and cardiomegaly will resolve. ECG may be normal in small VSD or it may show biventricular hypertrophy (BVH). In Eisenmenger, RVH may be marked. Katz Watchel's sign is noted in BVH showing tall R and deep S almost filling and spilling the ECG paper in mid chest leads (V2 and V3). ECHO and pulse Doppler ECHO will delineate shunt and ventricular function and hence invasive methods like catheterization are not usually needed for evaluation.

Natural History of VSD

30-50% of small defects close in 1-4 years due to growth of the septum and aneurysm formation. Infective endocarditis (IE) is rare below 2 years of age. Small VSDs may be left alone with IE prophylaxis or may be closed optionally. Closure will enable the child to be normal and fit for any physical or competitive test. As operative mortality is negligible, it is optional as per affordability. Device or patch closure may also be done. Those who are not operated should have yearly follow up to look for appearance of pulmonary hypertension or acquired pulmonary stenosis. Moderate defects are very symptomatic during infancy due to recurrent lung infection and CHF. But they respond to medical management and usually become asymptomatic after infancy due to reduction in the size of the defect and increasing pulmonary pressure. If the defects do not spontaneously close, or are not taken up for surgery, they should be systematically followed up to look for development of pulmonary hypertension and Eisenmenger syndrome. Many may be lost to follow up as they are not symptomatic, but to return later with inoperable stage. Large VSDs have refractory CHF and failure to thrive and may need early surgery. Primary single stage closure is now preferred to two-stage operation, namely pulmonary artery banding to reduce pulmonary flow followed by patch closure.

Differential Diagnosis:

Other CHDs

1. **Patent Ductus Arteriosus (PDA):** Murmur is continuous in 2nd space with high volume bounding pulse.

2. **Ostium primum ASD:** Ejection systolic murmur with wide fixed split of S2 in pulmonary area and associated mitral regurgitation evidenced by pansystolic murmur conducted to axilla.

3. **AV canal defect (AVCD) or Endocardial cushion defect (ECD):** There is atrial and ventricular septal defect and AV valvular regurgitation. AVCD is usually associated with Down syndrome. ECG will show extreme left axis deviation (LAD), BVH, tall P waves and RV conduction defects with rSR pattern in V1,V3R and V4R. Angiography will show **'goose neck'** deformity.

4. **Ostium Secundum ASD:** It is rarely symptomatic till adulthood. It produces ejection systolic murmur with wide fixed split of pulmonary second sound. Small ASD/PFO usually close by 3 months of age.

The baby needs prompt control of CCF (Table 9.1) and IE prophylaxis (Table 9.2). Dietary supplements should be advised. Breast milk is a low salt diet compared to formula feeds. Expressed breast milk (EBM), human milk fortifiers (HMF), oil supplements etc can be tried in very young babies. In refractory cases, correction of electrolyte imbalance like hypokalemia and ACE inhibitors are useful. Treatment of IE is given in Table 9.3.

CHD may be syndromic or non-syndromic. The various syndromes associated with CHD are given in Table 9.4.

SECTION 9.2

A CHILD WITH CONTINUOUS MURMUR AT THE BASE OF THE HEART

A 3-year-old child was seen in O.P.D. with history of exertional dyspnea and mild pedal edema.

On examination: Growth—Grade II PEM, 1° stunting, Development: normal, Pallor +, No cyanosis/clubbing, RR 40/mt, HR 120/mt, CFT 2 seconds, high volume collapsing pulse, all peripheral pulses felt bounding, Apex 5th left intercostal space in the mid clavicular line, heaving apex, continuous systolo—diastolic murmur below the clavicle conducted to the clavicle and left sternal border. Both heart sounds heard in all areas. Liver palpable 2.5 cm tender, span 11 cm. Spleen not palpable, pitting pedal edema +, JVP raised and visible, hepatojugular reflux +.

DIAGNOSIS AND DISCUSSION

Congenital heart disease, left to right shunt, patent ductus arteriosus (PDA), CHF, Grade II PEM, 1° stunting

PDA leads to left to right shunt. The aortic end is distal to origin of subclavian artery and pulmonary end at the bifurcation of pulmonary artery and up to 70% of the cardiac output may be shunted to the pulmonary artery. Mid diastolic flow murmur may be heard in the mitral area in large shunts. Small PDAs are asymptomatic, but large PDAs lead to growth retardation, LVH, mitral flow murmur, CHF, recurrent respiratory infection and infective endarteritis.

With increasing pulmonary hypertension, there may be reversal of shunt **(Eisenmenger comp-** lex) with **differential cyanosis** of lower limbs with sparing of face and the upper limps. The murmur may be systolic initially, later becoming **continuous cresento-decresento systolo-diastolic murmur. This is described as** *machinery murmur, rolling thunder, humming top or train in the tunnel murmur.* With development of pulmonary hypertension, when diastolic flow is negligible, the murmur may become systolic. High bounding pulse is due to aortic leak through the ductus.

Ductus arteriosus usually closes by 15 hours of delivery, but may remain open in preterm babies leading to CHF. Indomethacin given orally or IV 0.2 mg/kg/dose Q 12Hx 3 doses may help closure of PDA in symptomatic babies. Others may need device or surgical closure if symptomatic in the newborn period or later. Closure of PDA will promote growth in growth retarded children. Small defects are suitable for coil or device closure. Large defects need surgical ligation and division. It is a relatively easy operation as heart lung bypass is not needed.

In PDA, ECG may be normal or may show LVH/BVH. Echocardiogram will show dilated left atrium and LA to Aorta ratio is usually quantified to measure LA dilatation. Doppler will show systolic/continuous retrograde turbulent flow. Invasive cardiac catheterisation is rarely needed as Doppler study will give useful information.

PDA can occur in high altitude and may run in families. Ductus Arteriosus may have to be kept patent in **'ductus dependent heart lesions'** like pulmonary atresia, tricuspid area with pulmonary stenosis, severe coarctation of aorta, hypoplastic left heart syndrome and TGA with intact ventricular septum. This is achieved in newborn babies by IV prostaglandin E1 0.05-0.2 mcg/kg/mt as infusion.

Differential Diagnosis of Continuous Murmur at the Base

1. *Venous hum:* Musical murmur at right upper sternal border due to kinking of large veins. It disappears while lying down or after occlusion of the vein.

2. *Aorto-pulmonary (AP) window:* Systolic murmur is more prominent. Colour Doppler will show the window defect. Left atrium and left ventricle will be enlarged.

3. *Pulmonary branch stenosis:* It is more common in congenital rubella syndrome. Pulse pressure is normal unlike in PDA, which is also more common in congenital rubella.

4. *VSD with AR/VSD with AR and MR:* VSD with AR can occur in supracristal VSD.

5. *Coronary arterio venous fistula:* It can be diagnosed by doppler/coronary angiography.

6. *Truncus arterious:* A single arterial trunk (truncus) supplies systemic, pulmonary and coronary circulations. The truncus gets blood from both ventricles through a VSD. There will be CHF and minimal cyanosis.

7. Aberrant left coronary artery with collateral circulation.

8. *Rupture of sinus of valsalva* aneurysm into right side of the heart.

CHAPTER 9

CARDIOVASCULAR SYSTEM

SECTION 9.3 A NEWBORN WITH CCF

Full term newborn delivered by vaginal route with poor feeding and respiratory distress was transferred to NICU.

On examination: Head sweats +, respiratory distress and tachypnea +, tachycardia +, cardiomegaly+, hepatomegaly +, pallor +, no cyanosis/clubbing. No cardiac murmur. Upper limb pulsations better felt than lower limb, Upper limb BP 68 mm systolic, lower limb BP 52 mm of Hg. The baby was normal on the day of delivery and became symptomatic on the second day.

DIAGNOSIS AND DISCUSSION

Coarctation of Aorta with CHF

A newborn baby with CHF without cardiac murmur manifesting after 15 hours of birth, when ductus closes should alert the possibility of coarctation of aorta. AV fistulas also cause CHF. So auscultation over the head and other parts of the body is indicated in such cases. Lower BP recorded in the lower limb is the clue to the diagnosis. Normally lower limb BP is more. Careful palpation will reveal radio femoral delay.

In preductal coarctation, reversal of flow through ductus leads to differential cyanosis in lower limbs. Juxta ductal and post ductal coarctation are more common. CoAs are more common in boys. It is important to look for radio femoral delay/weak pulse in lower limbs in a baby with unexplained CHF. Features of Turner syndrome like webbing of neck and peripheral edema should also be looked for, as CoA is the most common heart disease in Turner syndrome. Bicuspid Aortic Valve is the most common malformation in Turner. After the age of one year,

higher BP in upper limbs and lower BP in lower limbs become evident as against the normal pattern of higher BP in lower limbs. The BP difference may be more than 20 mm of Hg between the two limbs. Lower limbs may appear hypoplastic if there is no significant flow through PDA or collaterals. Systolic murmur may be heard in the base, especially when there is associated bicuspid aortic valve. Other left sided lesions like aortic stenosis or mitral stenosis may be associated with COA. **Shone complex** is CoA associated with left sided obstructive lesions like AS, MS, Subaortic stenosis etc.

ECG may show LVH and X-ray may show cardiomegaly, pulmonary congestion and left superior mediastinal shadow due to enlarged left subclavian artery. There may be notching of inferior border of ribs due to erosion caused by enlarged collaterals, but with sparing of the first 2-3 ribs. This becomes evident after infancy.

Complications are hypertension, intracranial hemorrhage, CHF, infective endocarditis/end-arteritis, aneurysm of descending aorta or collaterals and renal ischemia. Doppler studies and angiogram are diagnostic. Balloon angiopla-sty or surgical repair with anastomosis can be done. Re-stenosis may occur in some cases. Early detection and treatment of hypertension is essential.

Pulmonary valvular stenosis is the most common CHD in Noonan syndrome, which has a phenotype of Turner syndrome, but with normal karyotype.

This baby will benefit with fluid restriction, decongestives, prostaglandin infusion to keep PDA open and early surgery.

SECTION 9.4

A BLUE BABY WITH CRYING AND APNEIC BLUE SPELLS

A 10-month-old baby was admitted with several episodes of prolonged crying spell followed by apnea and intense blue-black discoloration:

On examination: Grade II PEM, 1° stunting. Developmental age corresponding to 6 months. No history of recurrent respiratory infection, central cyanosis +, clubbing +, polycythemic, no edema, RR 62/mt, HR 120/mt, CFT 2 seconds, no cardiomegaly, ejection systolic murmur +, pulmonary area with single pulmonary sound, no hepatosplenomegaly. The baby preferred to lie prone with pulled up legs.

DIAGNOSIS AND DISCUSSION

Cyanotic Congenital Heart Disease (CCHD) with decreased pulmonary flow, Tetralogy of Fallot with hypercyanotic blue spell

In TOF, cyanosis usually manifests 3-6 months after birth, when pulmonary stenosis becomes significant leading to right to left shunt. **Embryologically TOF is a monology with maldevelopment of conus/outflow tract of ventricle. Surgically, it is a dialogy with pulmonary stenosis and ventricular septal defect. Physiologically, it is a triology with PS, VSD and overriding of aorta, which facilitate right to left shunt into the aorta. Pathologically, it is a tetralogy with PS, VSD, overriding of aorta and RVH.**

In **Pink Fallot**, RV obstruction is mild and there is balanced shunt across VSD. VSD with acquired PS, and congenital PS with VSD without dextroposition of aorta are similar to pink TOF. TOF with ASD is called **Pentalogy of Fallot**.

PS may be infundibular, valvular or post valvular alone or in combinations. When PS is significant, blood flow to lungs is through PDA or **major aorto–pulmonary collateral arteries (MAPCAs)**. This may lead to the presence of a continuous murmur. Pulmonary atresia with VSD will manifest early in infancy unlike TOF.

The intensity of systolic murmur is inversely proportional to the severity of PS. The VSD is usually large and is situated at the root of the aorta and with overriding/dextroposition of aorta. Hence, ventricles pump into the aorta leading to mixing of blood and cyanosis. Cyanosis also get intensified depending on the degree of pulmonary outflow tract obstruction resulting in decreased oxygenation.

In the first few months of life, PS is mild, cyanosis is mild and increased left to right shunt through VSD may lead to recurrent respiratory infection and CCF. As the pulmonary stenosis increases, cyanosis increases and lung fields became oligemic. Failure to thrive may occur due to hypoxia. Polycythemia and consumption coagulopathy may lead to hemoptysis.

Squatting or squatting equivalents like 'prone frog like position, lying with pulled up legs' are resorted to by children for relief of hypoxia. Such procedures help to decrease shunt and oxygen debt and to improve pulmonary circulation by the following mechanisms. There will be shunting of relatively more oxygenated splanchnic blood into circulation. There will be compression of veins and reduced amount of hypoxic blood coming to the heart. There will be increase in systemic arterial resistance leading to deceased shunt to the aorta and therefore increase in pulmonary flow. Exertional dyspnoea may compel the child to rest in between activities. The child may rest in frog position.

Hypercyanotic blue spells or Tet spells occur in the first two years, in cases who are hemodynamically less adapted. It does not depend on the severity of the lesion. Hyperapnea leads to restlessness, gasping respiration and intensification of cyanosis. Syncope and convulsion may also occur. This is more common during morning hours, when the child cries or strain during defecation. The intensity of the murmur will decrease. Hypoxia, increased oxygen demand, supraventricular tachycardia, spasm of ventricular outflow tract and immaturity of the respiratory centre are the proposed causes. Spell may last for a few minutes or hours. It may be potentially fatal. Treatment includes oxygen, prone knee chest position or supine position with drawn up legs. Inj. morphine 0.2 mg/kg S/C will help to calm the child and the respiratory center and to decrease venous pressure. Propranolol 0.2 mg/kg IV will help to control tachycardia and sodabicarb to tackle acidosis. Prevention is by correction of anemia and oral propranolol 1mg/kg/Q6H. Propranolol may cause bronchospasm in asthmatics.

CCF may occur when there is anemia, infective endocarditis or complex lesions like associated AR, PR etc. CCF is rare in TOF except in infancy when L to R shunt is more.

Cerebral venous or arterial thrombosis may occur when there is vomiting, diarrhea or dehydration. This is more common below the age of 2 years. After the age of 2 years, brain abscess may occur usually without much focal neurological signs. The chance of systemic bacteremia bypassing the pulmonary vasculature through the direct shunt into the aorta and the presence of devitalized brain tissue following previous thrombosis are responsible for brain abscess.

X-ray will show 'boot shaped' normal sized heart with RV apex/upturned apex (coeur en sabot appearance). ECG will show RVH and RAD. Echocardiogram and catheterization help in delineating the anatomy prior to surgery. Palliative surgery includes various shunts to improve pulmonary circulation like Blalock-Taussig (BT) shunt producing a connection between subclavian to ipsilateral pulmonary artery, Waterston shunt between ascending aorta and Rt pulmonary artery and Potts shunt between descending aorta and Lt pulmonary artery.

Helen Taussig, is known as the mother of Pediatric cardiology, who advocated BT shunt resulting in the blue baby turning pink. Early total correction with infundibular/pulmonary valvuloplasty and patch closure of VSD is now preferred than the earlier two stage operation and initial shunt.

TOF is the cyanotic heart disease with better survival into childhood.

Hyperoxia test is useful to differentiate between Resp/Cardiac cases with cyanosis especially in the newborn. 100% oxygen for 10 mts followed by an ABG showing $PaO_2 < 70$ will confirm CCHD and > 150 mm of Hg will favour respiratory cause.

Differential Diagnosis: Other conditions with decreased pulmonary blood flow:

1. **Double outlet right ventricle with PS (DORV with PS):** Both great vessels arise from RV with mitral aortic discontinuity. Cardiomegaly may occur. Cyanosis is noted earlier than TOF. Surgery—Rastelli operation. There is more than 50% overriding of aorta unlike TOF with < 50%.

2. **Tricuspid atresia with PS:** Tricuspid valve is atretic and hence RA blood is shunted to LA through PFO. Pulmonary flow depends on shunt through VSD and the extent of PS. Cyanosis occurs at birth, ECG will show LAD. Surgical procedures—Rashkind balloon artery septostomy and bidirectional Glenn shunt between SVC and pulmonary artery and between IVC and pulmonary artery (Cavopulmonary anastomosis). Fontan operation is anastomosis between RA and pulmonary artery.

SECTION 9.5 A BLUE BABY WITH CCF

A two-day-old newborn baby was brought with tachypnea and cyanosis. Baby was normal at birth, weight of 3.5 kg. Next day, baby developed tachypnea and cyanosis.

On examination: Weight 3.8 kg, RR 70/mt, HR 160/mt, cardiomegaly +, ejection systolic murmur in the 2nd left intercostal space, hepato-splenomegaly and bilateral creps+. X-ray—cardiomegaly (CTR 65%), increased pulmonary markings with narrow pedicle (egg on end/egg on side appearance). ECG - RV dominance. Hyperoxia test - no improvement in PaO_2 with 100% oxygen administration.

DIAGNOSIS AND DISCUSSION

CCHD with increased pulmonary blood flow: Transposition of Great Arteries (D.TGA) with CHF

CHF is evident due to like tachypnea, tachy-cardia, cardiomegaly, hepatosplenomegaly, chest signs and increase in weight as against the usual 10% weight loss noticed soon after birth. Early CHF indicates increased pulmonary blood flow. Cardiomegaly with narrow pedicle (egg on end/egg on side appearance) and RV dominance and early symptoms starting on 2nd day (due to closure of PDA) suggests D.TGA. PDA usually closes within 15 hours after birth following oxygenation of the lungs. Ejection systolic murmur in the pulmonary area suggests flow through PFO. In D.TGA with VSD, pansystolic murmur in the 3rd and 4th space may be evident. Doppler ECHO

will confirm the diagnosis. Prostaglandin E_1 infusion to keep ductus arteriosus patent is the immediate step along with other measures like oxygen inhalation, fluid restriction and deconges-tives. **Rashkind balloon atrial septostomy** and **Jatene arterial switch** operation are the surgical interventions. In arterial switch, the great vessels are divided and reanastomosed at the correct sites. Coronary arteries will be reanastomosed to the neoaorta. Associated VSD should be closed in DTGA with VSD.

Other Cardiac Conditions

1. **L. TGA is corrected transposition:** The mitral valve is on right side and aorta arise from right side and vice versa. L. TGA is usually asymptomatic. There may be associated VSD/PS. Complete heart block also may be associated.

2. **D. TGA with DORV (Double Outlet Right Ventricle):** This is called Taussig Bing anomaly. There is supracristal VSD which allows double communication of RV to both aorta and pulmonary artery. This condition may require pulmonary artery banding followed by arterial switch operation.

3. **Tricuspid atresia without PS:** TA without PS manifests as TGA, but with LV dominence. TA with PS manifests as TOF, but with LV impulse and Left Axis Deviation in ECG. Pansystolic murmur of VSD is heard and pulmonary second sound will be single when associated

with PS. In TA, tricuspid valve is atretic and so RA blood gets shunted to LA though PFO or ASD. VSD supports pulmonary flow. In those without VSD/associated PS, PDA subserves pulmonary flow. Prostaglandin E_1 infusion/BT shunt are beneficial to keep PDA open. In those with increased pulmonary flow, pulmonary artery banding is useful. **Rashkind balloon septostomy** will increase flow in restrictive ASD/PFO. Another palliation is bidirectional **Glenn shunt** between SVC and pulmonary artery. In **modified Fontan operation,** RA is anastomosed to pulmonary artery. **Cavopulmonary anastomosis** between IVC and pulmonary artery is another procedure.

4. **Truncus arteriosus (Tr Ar):** Both ventricles pump into a common truncus and are exposed to systemic pressure. Pulmonary circulation may be maintained through MAPCAs. Initially cyanosis may be mild. When pulmonary pressure reduces and pulmonary flow increases, CCF will set in. Truncal valve will usually be atretic leading to regurgitation and high bounding pulse. Single pulmonary second sound, ejection click, ejection systolic murmur, apical mid diastolic murmur and basal early diastolic murmur due to truncal regurgitation are the other findings. X-ray will show cardiomegaly and increased pulmonary vascularity. There may be a right sided shadow due to right sided truncus and left sided shadow due to main pulmonary artery. Treatment is by **Rastelli repair** to establish continuity between RV and PA with closure of VSD.

5. **Single Ventricle (SV):** It is double inlet and double outlet ventricle with LV physiology which receives both vena caval and pulmonary venous flow and supports both systemic and pulmonary circulation. When there is significant PS, it will manifest like TOF. In SV, ECG will show normal, spiked or bifid 'p' wave. Palliative surgery includes aorto- pulmonary shunt in cases with PS or pulmonary artery banding in cases with increased pulmonary flow. Definitive surgery is **Glenn shunt followed by modified Fontan operation.**

6. **Hypoplastic left heart syndrome (HLHS):** The left sided structures like LA, mitral valve, LV, aortic valve and aorta are atretic. Systemic flow is maintained though PDA. There is associated ASD and VSD. Peripheral pulses are weak. There will be cardiomegaly, systolic murmur, tall 'p' wave and RVH. Treatment includes prostaglandin infusion to keep PDA open and balloon atrial septostomy. Norwood procedure and heart transplantation are the other options.

7. **Total anomalous pulmonary venous connection (TAPVC):** It is also called total anomalous pulmonary venous return (TAPVR). Here pulmonary veins drain into right side of the heart. In partial anomalous venous connection (PAPVC), there is no cyanosis. In 50% cases of TAPVC, PV drain into SVC **(supracardiac),** leading to **figure of 8 or snowman** appearance. RA to LA shunt is though PFO/ASD. In 25% cases, it is **'cardiac'** connection into coronary sinus or RA. In 20%, it is **'infracardiac'** into a common descending vein, IVC or portal vein. In the rest, it will be **'mixed type'.** Pulmonary congestion and pulmonary hypertension depends upon extent of obstruction of pulmonary veins. In infracardiac with severe obstruction, newborn presents like **RDS with perihilar pulmonary edema (washout lung), intense cyanosis and tachypnea without cardiomegaly or murmur.** Hyperoxia test will be negative indicating cardiac cause. This is the only true surgical emergency in newborn. The baby may not respond even to mechanical ventilation.

Those with moderate obstruction will manifest with cyanosis, CCF, PAH, gallop rhythm and systolic or continuous murmur. Those without obstruction will have mild or no cyanosis. **'Snowman appearance'** is due to supracardiac shadow due to dilated Rt SVC, Lt SVC and left innominate veins. ECG shows peaked P wave and RVH. Prostaglandin E_1 and balloon atrial septostomy are beneficial followed by surgical repair. Obstruction may occur in some post operative cases.

8. **Primary pulmonary hypertension (PPH):** Here pulmonary hypertension occurs without L to R shunt or corpulmonale. It usually presents in newborn period or as late as 2nd decade. Syncope, exertional dyspnea, Rt. heart failure, PR and TR occur. Sildenafil (Phospho-diesterase) inhibitor (Viagra) is tried in newborn babies in this condition.

9. **Eisenmenger physiology, Reversal of L-R shunt and pulmonary vascular disease (PVD):** PVD is a progressive condition. PVD is a complication of increased pulmonary flow. Initially venous pressure and then arterial pressure will increase. The clinical manifestations are cyanosis, dyspnea, arrhythmia, heart failure, pulmonary and tricuspid regurgitation and narrow split loud P_2. PR murmur is called **Graham Steel murmur.** X-ray will show prominent main pulmonary artery (MPA) and pulmonary pruning or oligemia beyond medial one third of lung field. ECG will show peaked

P wave and RVH. **Eisenmenger syndrome** is reversal through VSD and **Eisemenger complex** is reversal through ASD/PDA. PDA will lead to differential cyanosis manifesting only in the lower limbs.

Treatment is unsatisfactory. Oxygen, nitroprusside and prostaglandin infusion in venous hypertension are being tried. High altitude aggravates PVD. Heart and lung transplant is the other option.

Heath Edward's Classification of PVD

Type I: Medial thickening of pulmonary arteries.

Type II: Medial and intimal thickening.

Type III: Plexiform and aneurysmal dilatation of vessels.

CCHDs are approached as those with increased pulmonary blood flow/decreased pulmonary blood flow. Decreased pulmonary blood flow is TOF like physiology with less chance of recurrent respiratory infection and CCF. Increased pulmonary blood flow present with CCF. The differentiating features are given in Tables 9.5 and 9.6 as per pulmonary flow and ventricular hypertrophy.

SECTION 9.6
A BOY WITH ARTHRITIS AND CARDIAC FAILURE

A 9-year-old boy was admitted with fever, polyarthritis involving right knee, left elbow, left ankle, pedal oedema, dyspnea and cough. Initially he had arthritis involving one joint and later it subsided and another joint got involved.

On examination: Growth and development normal. PR 130/mt, RR 30mt, BP 90 mm systolic, pallor +, non tender pea sized subcutaneous nodules over spine and elbows +, polyarthritis +, JVP raised, cardiomeglay +, Heart sounds not well heard, pansystolic murmur mitral area conducted to other areas. Liver + 3 cm below costal margin, span 12 cm, lungs—bitateral creps +, other systems normal. He had 5 days of antibiotics 2 weeks back for fever and sore throat. Hb 9 gldl, TC 14,000/cu cm, P 78 L 20 E 2, ESR 50 mm/1st Hr. ASO 800 IU, X-ray chest-cardiomegaly+, diffuse bilateral haze +, ECG—PR interval 0.2 second.

DIAGNOSIS AND DISCUSSION

Acute Rheumatic Fever (ARF) with carditis and CCF

As per modified Jone's Criteria, he had 3 major + 2 minor criteria supported by essential criteria:

I. Major criteria

1.	Migratory polyarthritis	Present
2.	Carditis	Present
3.	Subcutaneous nodule	Present
4.	Erythema marginaturm	Absent
5.	Chorea	Absent

II. Minor criteria

1. Fever
2. Elevated acute phase reactants, leukocytosis. Elevated ESR (>30), and CRP (>6 mg/dl)
3. Arthralgia (When arthritis is not a major criteria)
4. Prolonged PR interval (When carditis is not a major criteria)
5. Previous history of rheumatic fever.

III. Essential criteria–evidence of recent Streptococcal infection: Positive throat swab/ASO titre >330 IU (definitive WHO cut off) > 250 may suggest streptococcal infection.

Rheumatic fever is a disease of molecular mimicry leading to cross reaction with one's own tissue. Age group is 2-15 years, 50% cases give a history of sore throat. Arthritis is migratory involving large joints. New joints get involved when the initial arthritis subsides. New joints getting involved before initial arthritis resolves is called 'Additive arthritis' seen in rheumatoid diseases. Small joints also may be affected rarely (Jaccods arthritis) in 23%. Monarthritis may occur in 5%. When Jone's criteria are not satisfied and with a positive ASO titre, the diagnosis is post streptococcal reactive arthritis (PSRA). PSRA is treated with Asprin/NSAID (Naproxen) for 6-8 weeks and penicillin prophylaxis is usually given for 6 months-1 year. The response will be poorer in PSRA than in ARF.

There will be no residual deformity in ARF **(ARF licks the joint, bites the heart and grips the basal ganglia—extrapyramidal system)**. Rheumatogenic strains of Beta hemolytic streptococci are M types 1, 3, 4, 5, 6, 18 and 24. HLA predisposition and B cell (non-T cell) Allo antigen mark genetic predisposition.

Carditis occurs in 40-60% cases and it is a pancarditis diagnosed by tachycardia out of proportion to fever (>10 beats/1°F), elevated sleeping pulse rate (SPR fall by <10 beats than wake), cardiomegaly, muffling of heart sounds, CCF, arrhythmia, cardiac murmurs, chest pain, pericarditis and Echocardiographic changes. Almost 50% of Rheumatic Heart Disease (RHD) give a history of RF. The initial murmurs of carditis include Carey Coombs diastolic murmur at apex due to valvulitis and Sea Gull's cooing pansystolic murmur at the apex due to valve ring dilatation and papillary muscle dysfunction. Early diastolic AR murmur also may rarely occur. The murmurs of carditis may resolve in 3-6 months. Chronic carditis persists for more than 6 months. It is very rare. Rheumatic heart disease (RHD) should be differentiated from carditis. Carey Coombs murmur and Sea Gull's murmur may disappear when carditis resolve. Persisting pansystolic murmur with loud P_2 indicates organic lesion, Rheumatic MR. Persisting AR murmur indicates Rheumatic AR. The AR murmur appearing initially usually does not disappear. Mitral MDM with presystolic accentuation suggest MS. MDM appearing 6 months to 2 years after carditis indicates Rheumatic MS. Pulmonary and Tricuspid valves are usually not involved. Rheumatic AS takes years to develop and hence, not seen in children. CCF occurring in a child with RHD is usually treated as Rheumatic Reactivation carditis. Mechanical CCF can also occur, but usually it is in adults and ESR will be normal in such cases.

ESR is very much raised upto 100 mm/1st hour in Rheumatic arthritis without carditis. In CCF, ESR tends to be lower. ECHO evidence of carditis may also be considered as a criterion for diagnosis as silent carditis is difficult to diagnose. However, ECHO evidence is not yet included as a diagnostic criteria.

Rheumatic chorea is called **Sydenham chorea or St Vitus dance**. It is more common in girls and usually occurs in 10-20 % cases of ARF. Chorea occurs several weeks or months after streptococcal infection and hence ASO titre may not be raised in such cases. It manifests as chorea, clumsiness, micrographia, hypotonia and emotional instability due to involvement of caudate nucleus. It may be unilateral in some cases (hemichorea) and may show recurrence even after treatment. S/C nodules and chorea are usually associated with carditis.

Treatment of RF involves oral or parenteral penicillin for 10 days followed by benzathine penicillin 12 lakh units deep IM every 3 weeks or oral penicillins twice daily for minimum 5 years/upto 21 years, whichever is later in cases with arthritis alone or for 10 years/upto 25 years in those with carditis. In RHD, it is given upto 35-40 years/preferably life long. In arthritis alone, aspirin is given for 4-8 weeks. In mild carditis, aspirin is given in full dose (100 mg/kg/day) for 2 weeks or till ESR becomes normal (<30 mm/1st hour) followed by 75 mg/kg/day for 8-12 weeks. In severe carditis with CCF, cardiomegaly or multivalvular involvement, full dose prednisolone (2 mg/kg/day) is given for 2 weeks followed tapering doses. Evening doses are tapered first to mimic physiological status and to prevent suppression of pituitary adrenal axis. Aspirin is added in a dose of 75 mg/kg/day when steroid is tapered. Antiinflammatory drugs are given for total 12 weeks in severe carditis. Haloperidol/diazepam is given in chorea. **Rebound arthritis** is a self limited condition with relapse of arthritis noticed while tapering or stopping antiinflammatory drugs.

Primary prevention of RF is by prompt treatment of all streptococcal infections. Skin infections do not usually cause ARF due to trapping of antigens in the fatty layer of subcutaneous tissue. The incidence of RF is 0.3/1000 in streptococcal sporadic infection and 3/100 in case of epidemic streptococcal infection.

Collagen vascular disease with multi system involvement including arthritis and carditis come in the differential diagnosis. But the course and prognosis are different. Viral fevers like chikungunya fever and other infections like brucellosis causes arthritis. Myocarditis may occur in certain viral fevers. Poncet's arthritis due to TB hypersensitivity may cause large joint arthritis.

SECTION 9.7

AN INFANT WITH TACHYCARDIA AND ACUTE CCF

A five-month-old baby was admitted with acute onset of tachycardia, tachypnoea, cardiomegaly and muffling of heart sounds.

On examination: Pallor, head sweats, cardiomegaly, hepatosplenomegaly, ejection systolic murmur, basal crepitation +, Hb 8 g/dl, TC 5000/cumm, P40, L55, E 5, ESR 20 mm/1st hour. ECG-HR. 150/mt, low voltage QRS complex with ST depression, ASO titre <200 IU.

DIAGNOSIS AND DISCUSSION

Viral Myocarditis with CCF

Absence of a history of congenital heart disease and young age group favor the diagnosis of myocarditis. ECHO will show poor ventricular function and sometimes pericardial effusion.

Diagnosis is based on clinical feature, raised CPK, viral markers and endomyocardial biopsy.

Treatment includes supportive care, fluid restriction, diuretics and dopamine with or without dobutamine. Digoxin is not usually given. Ribavirin, thiamine and carnitine are tried in some centers with variable results. Other treatment modalities include IV immunoglobulin, antivirals like pleconaril, acyclovir and steroid methyl prednisolone. Ionotropes are given in half dose with caution. Coxsackie A or B, adenovirus, HIV, ECHO virus, rubella, measles, varicella, influenza, EB virus etc. cause myocarditis. Fungi, rickettsiae, diphtheria, salmonella and leptospira also may cause myocarditis. Bradycardia as well as arrhythmia may occur in some cases. Myocarditis persisting beyond 6 weeks may persist as cardiomyopathy. ECMO (Extracorporeal membrane oxygenation) may be life saving in severe cases.

1. **DD: Endocardial fibroelastosis (EFE):** Primary EFE may occur with prenatal mumps infection in the mother or without any cause. Secondary EFE occurs in AS, COA, HLHS syndrome etc. Fibroelastic endocardial plaques and myxomatous degeneration of valves occur. ECHO will show poor LV function with bright echo shadows on endocardial surface. Treatment includes supportive care and heart transplantation in selected cases.

2. **Cardiomyopathy:** Dilated congestive cardiomyopathy, restrictive cardiomyopathy namely Endomyocardial fibrosis (EMF) and nutritional or metabolic cardiomyopathies have insidious onset and progressive course.

   Pompe's disease is glycogen storage disease with cardiomyopathy cardiotoxic drugs like adriamycin also cause cardiomyopathy.

   Type of Cardiomyopathies

   1. Dialated/congestive cardiomyopathy (DCM).

   2. Restrictive/obliterative cardiomyopathy (EMF).

   3. Hypertrophic obstructive cardiomyopathy (HOCM)—HOCM has a genetic predisposition (AD) and may cause sudden death. Digoxin is contraindicated in HOCM.

3. **Anomalous origin of left coronary artery from pulmonary artery (ALCAPA)**

   ALCAPA presents like DCM and angina may occur in young children. Rarely myocardial infarction may occur.

CHAPTER 9

CARDIOVASCULAR SYSTEM

SECTION 9.8 AN OLDER CHILD WITH FEVER AND CCF

A ten-year-old child was admitted with fever of 3 weeks duration. He was diagnosed to have a congenital heart disease in infancy, but was asymptomatic so far. He had pedal edema, exertional dyspnea and tachypnea.

On examination: Sweating +, fever +, clubbing +, pallor +, RR 40/mt, HR 130/mt, BP 90 systolic, JVP raised, CVS-mild cardiomegaly, pan systolic murmur-left lateral sternal border, P2 normal, Hepatosplenomegaly +, palmar erythema +; arthralgia +, Hb 8 g/dl, TC 18,000/cumm, P72, L26, E2, ESR 55 mm/1st, CRP 8 mg/dl, ASO 220 IU, Alb +, sugar nil, PC 5-8, RBC 5-10/HPF. Urine culture sterile. X-ray chest-cardiomegaly with slightly increased pulmonary vascularity.

DIAGNOSIS AND DISCUSSION

Infective Endocarditis (IE) with CHD, Probably VSD

Acute endocarditis can occur in normal heart especially in IV drug users, those with central lines and immunosuppression. Subacute endocarditis occurs in those with damaged heart like RHD, CHD, etc. Dental/oral procedures predispose to bacteremia. It presents with prolonged fever, chills, rigor, chest pain, arthralgia/arthritis, myalgia, tachycardia, splenomegaly, CCF, changing murmurs, arrhythmia, clubbing, stroke, petechiae/purpura, vasculitis and embolism. **Splinter hemorrhage** noted in nail beds, **Oslers nodes** in fingers and toes, **Janeway lesions** in

palms and soles, **Roth spots** in retina and hematuria are the other manifestations. ECHO will pick up vegetations > 2-3 mm size. Transesophageal ECHO is more useful. Absence of vegetations does not rule out IE. Refer Table 9.7 for diagnosis of IE.

The usual organisms are streptococcus viridans (mutans, sanguis, mitis) staph. aureus and epidermidis, enterococci (group D Streptococci), pneumococci, H. Influenza, Coxiella burnetti, Gonococci, Serratia, diphtheroids, Legionella, fungi and HACEK organisms (Hemophilus, Actinobacilli, cardiobacterium, Eikenella and Kingella). Aerobic, anaerobic and fungal cultures are needed to yield the various organisms. At least 2 cultures from 2 different sites should be taken. Empirical therapy includes supportive measures, decongestives and IV penicillin 3 lakh units/kg/day Q4H plus gentamicin 5-6 mg/kg/day Q8H. Aminoglycoside may be stopped after 2 weeks except in enterococci (Table 9.3). The treatment is usually given for 4-6 weeks. Amphotericin B is given in fungal endocarditis. In penicillin allergy and culture positive MRSA, vancomycin is given, 40-60 mg/kg/day Q8H. Ceftrixone IV OD may also be given after initial 2-4 weeks therapy if organism is sensitive to cephalosporin. IE is rare in infants. IE is an indication for early surgical correction of the underlying lesion, after control of the infection. For IE prophylaxis and therapy, refer Tables 9.2 and 9.3.

Culture Negative Endocarditis

This is diagnosed when patient has clinical and or ECHO evidence of IE with repeatedly negative blood culture. It is due to recent antibioic therapy or poorly growing fastidious organisms. The organism may be obtained after surgical excision of vegetation, thrombus or at autopsy. Filamentous fungal IE and IE caused by coxiella burnetii (Q fever), Brucella, Legionella, Bartonella and chlamydia are examples.

CHAPTER 9

CARDIOVASCULAR SYSTEM

A CHILD WITH CARDIAC TAMPONADE

A 9-year-old child was admitted with acute stabbing chest pain, fever and dyspnea. He was breathless and could not speak.

On examination: Cardiomegaly +, pulsus paradoxus > 20 mm of Hg +, Heart sounds muffled, pericardial rub +, Apex beat felt in the 5th space in the midclavicular line, but cardiac dullness was extending upto anterior axillary line. Liver +, 5 cm below costal margin. Neck veins distended. X-ray—cardiomegaly with globular contour. ECG–low voltage QRS with ST elevation and T inversion.

DIAGNOSIS AND DISCUSSION

Pericardial Effusion (PE) with Cardiac Tamponade

Globular heart with dullness outside the apex, muffled heart sounds, X-ray and ECG suggest PE. Cardiac tamponade is likely when pulsus paradoxus is >20 mm. ECHO showing anterior and posterior collection with reduced septal motion and collapse of RV outflow during diastole will confirm tamponade.

Treatment includes pericardial tap under ultrasound guidance or pericardiotomy along with appropriate antibiotics. Staphylococcal infection, TB, collagen vascular disease, malignancies, uremia etc. cause IE.

Constrictive Pericarditis

It may present similar to pericardial effusion with cardiac tamponade and may also mimic restrictive cardiomyopathy.

SECTION 9.10 — A NEWBORN WITH CCF AND EXTREME TACHYCARDIA

A twenty-day-old newborn was admitted with excessive crying, vomiting, tachypnea and mild fever.

On examination: Pallor +, RR 50/mt, HR 200/mt, CFT 3 seconds, liver + 3 cm, mild cardiomegaly, ejection systolic murmur +, ECG: Rate 200/mt, P wave absent, QRS narrow.

DIAGNOSIS AND DISCUSSION

Supraventricular Tachycardia (SVT) with CCF

SVT can occur with fever, exercise, anemia, thyrotoxicosis and beta agonists. In sinus arrhythmia, rate varies with respiration but, P wave is normal. In SVT, rate is usually > 200 and P wave will be absent or altered. The causes are increased automatically, reentry (>90% cases) or triggering by drugs like digoxin (Table 9.8). In **WPW syndrome**, short PR interval and slow upstroke of QRS (Delta wave) are seen.

Treatment includes vagal stimulation, keeping ice bag over face, Valsalva maneuver, drugs like digoxin, adenosine, and amiodarone and DC cardioversion.

24 hours Holter ECG monitoring may be needed in episodic SVT. Tachyarrhythmia may lead to recurrence. Such cases may need transcutaneous, intracardiac or oesophageal pacing/radiofrequency ablation (RFA). It may be fatal. It may also lead to cardiomyopathy (tachycardiomyopathy). Variants with long QT syndrome/Brugada syndrome may end up in sudden death.

In narrow QRS tachyarrythmias, adenosine is helpful in a dose of 100-250 mcg/kg/dose with N. Saline, given as a push. In wide QRS cases, amiodarone infusion in a dose of 5 mg/kg bolus followed by 5-15 mg/kg/mt is needed.

Table 9.1: Treatment of CHF

1. INOTROPES

1. Digoxin *	0.04-0.06 mg/kg loading dose, ½ stat and ¼ Q6H X 2 doses 12 hours later Maintenance 5/7 days, 0.01 mg/kg/day in 1-2 doses	IV 75% dose	SE: AV block, GI upset

2. DIURETICS

1. Frusemide	1-2 mg/kg/dose Q12H/Q6H	SE:Hypokalemia, alkalosis
2. Spirano-lactone	2-3 mg/kg/day Q12H/Q8H.	SE: Hyperkalemia

3. AFTER LOAD REDUCING AGENTS

1. Enalapril	0.1-0.2 mg/kg/day Q12 H	SE:Hyperkalemia cough, neutropenia
2. Captopril	1-3 mg/kg/day Q12H/Q8H	SE:Proteinuria, hypotension, neutropenia

* For slow digitalization, loading dose is skipped and only maintenance dose is given. Newborns and infants tolerate higher doses for digitalization.
Inodilators/Phosphodiesterase inhibitors like milrinone and amrinone may be tried in refractory cases.
SE—Side effect.

Table 9.2: Infective endocarditis prophylaxis

I. Standard Risk (Oral/Dental Procedure)

1. Ampicillin/Amoxycillin	– 50 mg/kg upto 2 g 1 hour before and 25 mg/kg upto 1 g 6 hours later
2. Penicillin allergy Erythromycin	– 20 mg/kg upto 1 g 2 hours before and 10 mg/kg upto 0.5 g 6 hours later
3. Clindamycin	– 10-20 mg/kg upto 600 mg 1hour before and 5 mg/kg 6 hours later

II. High Risk (Genitourinary/GIT procedures)

1. Ampicillin (IV) + Gentamicin (IV)	– Ampi as above + Genta 2 mg/kg upto 80 mg 30 mts before and 6 hours later
2. Penicillin allergy Vancomycin (IV) + Genta (IV)	– Vanco- 20 mg/kg upto 1 g as infusion 1 hour before and ½ dose after 8 hours + Genta as above

III. Special Risk (Cardiac surgery/Prosthetic valve)

1. Vancomycin (IV) + Genta (IV)	– 20 mg/kg upto 1 g as infusion starting with anesthesia and ½ dose Q8H X 3 doses and Q 12H X 2 doses more + genta
2. Cefazolin (IV)	– 30 mg/kg upto 2 g starting with anesthesia and ½ dose Q8H X 3 doses and Q 12H X 2 doses more

Table 9.3: Treatment of infective endocarditis

Agent	Drug	Dose	Duration
Strept. viridans	Penicillin and	2-3 lacs/kg/dQ4H	4-6 weeks
	Gentamicin	3-7.5 mg/kg/d Q8H upto 80 mg/dose	2 weeks
Enterococci	Ampicillin and	300 mg/kg/d Q 6 H upto 12 g/d	4-6 weeks
	Genta	as above	4-6 weeks
Strept viridans (Penicillin allergy)	Vancomycin Genta SOS	40-60 mg/kg/d Q8 H upto 2 g/d	4-6 weeks
Staph aureus	Cloxacillin	200 mg/kg/d Q6H upto 12 g/d	4-6 weeks
MRSA	Vancomycin Genta SOS	40-60 mg/kg/d Q8 H upto 2 g/d	6-8 weeks
Staph. epidermidis	Vancomycin	40-60 mg/kg/d Q8 H upto 2 g/d	6-8 weeks
	Rifampicin SOS	10-20 mg/kg/d Q 12 H upto 600 mg/d	6-8 weeks
Hemophilus	Ampi Genta SOS		
Unknown	Vanco,		6-8 weeks
	Genta		2-4 weeks
	Ampi SOS		6-8 weeks
Continuation phase:	Ceftrixone	100 mg/kg OD if sensitive (once a day therapy)	

Table 9.4: Syndromes and various conditions associated with CHD

I. Bone and Connective Tissue Disorder with Cardiac Defects
   1. Hurler syndrome — Valvular heart disease
   2. Marfan syndrome — Aortic dilatation
   3. Ellis-van Creveld syndrome — Septal defects
   4. SLE — Endocarditis

II. Teratogens/Environmental Agents Causing Cardiac Defects
   1. Congenital rubella syndrome — PDA, Pulmonary branch stenosis
   2. Fetal alcohol syndrome — Septal defects
   3. Fetal hydantoin syndrome — Septal defects

III. Miscellaneous Disorders with Cardiac Defects
   1. Holt Oram syndrome — Septal defects
   2. Noonan syndrome — PS
   3. William syndrome — Supravalvular AS
   4. Apert syndrome — Septal defects
   5. Carpenter syndrome — Septal defects
   6. Treacher Collins syndrome — Septal defects
   7. Goldenhar syndrome — Septal defects, PDA

IV. Chromosomal Anomalies with Cardiac Defects
   1. Trisomies 13, 18, 21 — Septal defects, AV canal defects
   2. Turner syndrome — Coarctation aorta, BAV
   3. Fragile X syndrome — PDA
   4. Penta X syndrome — PDA

Table 9.5: Differentiating features between CCHDs with increased pulmonary flow

Condition		Features
TGA	:	Cardiomegaly with narrow pedicle (Egg on end/side appearance)
TA without PS	:	LV impulse, LAD
Tr Ar	:	High bounding pulse, Rt sided and left side shadows in superior mediastinum due to truncus (Rt) and MPA (Lt)
HLHS	:	Low volume pulse

Table 9.6: Approach to CCHD

Increased Pulm Flow	Increased Pulm Flow	Decreased Pulm Flow	Decreased Pulm Flow	Decreased Pulm Flow
LVH/BVH	RVH	BVH	LVH	RVH
Truncus	TGA	TGA + PS	Tricuspid Atresia	TOF
Single ventricle	TAPVC	Single ventricle +PS	Pulm Atresia + hypoplastic RV	Ebstein anomaly
TGA + VSD	HLHS	Truncus + hypoplastic PA		

Table 9.7: Duke clinical criteria for diagnosis of IE

Major	Minor
1. Positive blood cultures (2) —typical organisms consistent with IE 2. Endocardial involvement —Vegetation (ECHO) —New valvular regurgitation	1. Predisposing heart lesion/IV drug use 2. Fever > 38°C 3. Vascular phenomenon 4. Immunologic phenomenon 5. Microbiological organism not consistent with IE 6. ECHO that do not meet major criterion

2 Major/1 Major+3 Minor or 5 Minor criteria→Definite IE.

Table 9.8: Classification of tachycardias

Narrow QRS (<120 ms/< 90 ms in young infants)	Wide QRS
Sinus tachycardia	Ventricular tachycardia
Ectopic/multifocal focus	SVT with aberrancy
Atrial tachycardia	SVT with bundle branch block
SA node reentry	Reentry tachycardia
WPW syndrome	WPW syndrome with fusion waves
Atrial flutter and fibrillation	Mahaim fiber disorder

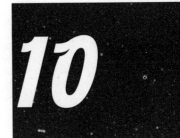

10

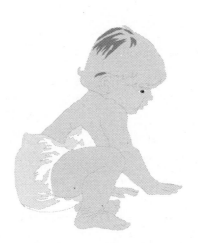

Genitourinary System

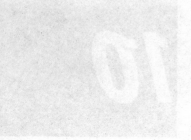

10

Genitourinary System

SECTION 10.1
A CHILD WITH ACUTE NEPHRITIS

A 3-year-old girl was admitted with puffiness of face, cola colored urine, dyspnea and oliguria. She had pyoderma treated with topical antibiotics 10 days back.

On examination: Growth and development normal. Afebrile, Pulse Rate 120/mt, RR 45/mt, BP 120 systolic, No chest indrawing, mild pedal edema +, Apex beat 5th space in the MCL, forceful, $S_1 S_2$ normal, no murmur, lungs B/L creps +, Abd- Liver + 3 cm, No Ascites, Hb 10 g/dl, TC 12000, P78, L20, E2, ESR 40, B urea 46 mg/dl S creatinine 1.1, S.Na 130 mEq/L, K 5.5 mEq/L, urine albumin +, pus cells (PC) 10-15/HPF, RBC- 5-10/HPF, RBC cast +.

DIAGNOSIS AND DISCUSSION

Acute Nephritic syndrome–Post Streptococcal Glomerulonephritis

Streptococcal etiology is evident by recent streptococcal impetigo. The common nephrogenic strains are serotype 49 (pyoderma) and serotype 12 (pharyngitis). It can be confirmed by positive ASO titre, Anti NADase, DNAase B, streptokinase, Hyaluronidase/Streptozyme test. ASO titre may not be positive following skin infection due to trapping of antigens in the S/C fat. In such condition, anti NADase may be positive. Other bacteria and viruses can cause nephritis and hence, may also be called **post infective glomerulonephritis.**

Acute glomerulonephritis/**Acute Nephritic syndrome** is suggested by the triad of oliguria,

hematuria and edema with or without uremia, acute renal failure (ARF) and hypertension. Oliguria is diagnosed when urine output is <400 ml/M^2 or <1ml/kg/hr. Hypertension is evident when systolic BP is above 95th centile for height (roughly > 90 + (Age x 2)). For e.g., in this child 90 + 6 = 96 mm of Hg. Uremia is evident by raised B urea, creatinine, and hyperkalemia. Fluid overload is evident by puffiness of face, edema, cardiomegaly, basal creps and dilutional hyponatremia. Cola colored urine and dysmorphic RBCs suggest glomerular disease. Fresh blood with eumorphic RBCs suggest lower tract disease. C_3 will be low in post infective glomerulonephritis and lupus nephritis, but will be normal in IgA nephropathy. USS will show poor corticomedullary differentiation (medical renal disease).

The complications are uremia, uremic encephalopathy, hypertension, hypertensive encephalopathy, seizures, hyperkalemia, hyperphosphatemia, hypocalcemia etc. The various causes of hematuria are given in Table 10.1.

Treatment of glomerulonephritis includes eradication of streptococci by penicillin/erythromycin x 10 days, fluid, salt and protein restriction, diuretics and prompt treatment of hyperkalemia. Fluid restriction = Insensible loss + last days output. Insensible loss is given as 10% Dextrose and output as N. saline + 10% Glucose (Table 10.2).

Thiazide diuretics and potassium citrate are beneficial to prevent nephrolithiasis. Calcium restriction is not undertaken in order to promote growth in idiopathic hypercalciuria. Nephralithiasis and calciurias are known causes of hematuria.

Hyperkalemia is treated with Soda Bicarb 1-2 mEq/kg/dose Q 12 H, Calcium gluconate 1ml/kg/dose Q 12H, Insulin–glucose regimen and K binding resins. Peritoneal dialysis is indicated in those refractory to medical therapy. Insulin-glucose promotes movement of K into the cells. Glucose is given in a dose of 1 g/kg/dose with 1 unit Insulin/3 g glucose. K binding Kayexalate is given 1 g/kg/d Q6-12H as oral or rectal.

Prognosis is usually good and recovery is complete in >90 % cases. <5% may develop complications. < 5% may develop chronic nephritis/Nephrotic Syndrome. AGN usually resolves in 2 months, but rarely urinary abnormality may persist upto 1 year.

Hypertension is treated by diuretics, Nifedipine/ACE inhibitors. The life threatening complications are ARF, CCF and hypertensive emergency including encephalopathy. The dose of nifedipine is 0.25-0.5 mg/kg/dose.

SECTION 10.2 CHILD WITH GROSS HEMATURIA

A 10-year-old boy was admitted with gross hematuria. He had fever, but no dysuria. He had similar episodes 6 months back, which was treated in a local hospital.

On examination: Growth and development—Normal. Tachycardia +, BP normal. All systems within normal limits. B urea 56 mg/dl, S.Creatinine 1.1, C3 Normal, S.Na, S.K.& S. cholesterol normal. USS Abdomen–medical renal disease. Urine alb +, RBC plenty, WBC 1-3/HPF.

DIAGNOSIS AND DISCUSSION

IgA Nephropathy/Berger Disease

It is a cause of recurrent hematuria, often para infectious. In IgA nephropathy, C_3 is normal unlike other glomerulonephritis. IgA mesangial deposits, in the absence of SLE and HSP, is seen in biopsy. In 30%, disease may be progressive.

Differential Diagnosis: Other causes of hematuria (Table 10.1). Glomerular diseases cause cola colored/altered blood with dysmorphic RBCs and bladder and urethral conditions cause fresh blood with eumorphic RBCs. Hematuria may be benign, familial and recurrent. It is usually due to thin basement membrane disease, loin pain hematuria syndrome, urolithiasis, tumors, idiopathic hypercalciuria etc. In Alport's, it is familial with hearing loss.

IgA nephropathy is parainfectious unlike post infectious glomerulonephritis. It is a chronic glomerular disease, more common in males, with mild to moderate proteinuria < 1 g/24 hours. S. IgA has no diagnostic value. The poor prognostic indicators are altered renal function, persistent hypertension and prolonged proteinuria. Diagnosis is confirmed by biopsy. ACE inhibitors, losarten (Angiotensin Receptor Blocker), methyl prednisolone and omega 3 fatty acids are also tried in refractory cases.

CHAPTER 10

GENITOURINARY SYSTEM

SECTION 10.3

A CHILD WITH ACUTE UREMIA, PALLOR AND BLEEDING

A 2-year-old child, who was under treatment for diarrhea and respiratory infection in a local hospital for the last 10 days, was referred with rapid onset of pallor, irritability, lethargy, oliguria, hematuria and skin bleeds.

On examination: Anemic, BP 130 systolic, hepatosplenomegaly +, petechiae +, Hb 7 g/dl, Peripheral Smear–evidence of hemolysis with helmet cells, burr cells, fragmented RBCs+, Retic count 3%, platelet count 32,000/cmm PT, APTT Normal, B urea 100 mg/dl, S. creatinine 1.2, S.Na 135, S.K.5 mEq/l.

DIAGNOSIS AND DISCUSSION

Hemolytic Uremic Syndrome (HUS)

Differential Diagnosis: Acute diarrhea with sepsis and DIC, Acute diarrhea with prerenal uremia/renal—Acute tubular necrosis.

HUS usually occurs below 4 years of age and may follow ADD/ARI. Post ARI HUS tends to be more severe. Enteropathogenic E. coli (EPEC) elaborates verotoxin, that lead to glomerular thrombus formation and occlusion, hemolytic anemia, thrombocytopenia and uremia. DIC is unlikely in this case as evidenced by normal PT and APTT. Other bacteria and viruses can also cause HUS.

Treatment includes supportive care, antibiotics, FFP, platelet transfusion, packed cells and early peritoneal dialysis. Some may have fatal outcome and some may rarely develop chronic disease with CRF.

Post diarrheal case is designated D+ and post respiratory D—.

The poor prognostic indicators are post respiratory (D—), Severe azotemia and anuria. In HUS, hyperkalemia may be mild compared to other types of ARF.

Prerenal uremia is due to dehydration and reduced kidney perfusion. It will promptly respond to fluid correction and serum creatinine will remain normal unlike in renal and post renal uremia.

Acute tubular necrosis (ATN) may occur in prolonged dehydration and insufficient perfusion. Urine sodium will be> 40 mEq/L in this condition. Recovery will take more time in this compared to prerenal uremia. Post renal is due to obstructive uropathy, posterior urethral valve etc.

SECTION 10.4   A CHILD WITH RECURRENT EDEMA

An eight-year-old girl was admitted with massive edema and loose stools, no hematuria/oliguria. She had similar episode of edema 2 months back, treated in a local hospital.

On examination: Pallor +, pitting edema and facial edema +, Rt sided pleural effusion +, Ascites +, abdominal tenderness +, BP 110 mm of Hg, Temp 99° F, HR 90/mt, RR 30/mt. CFT 2 seconds, B urea 32 mg/dl, S.Creatinine 0.7, S Na 130/mEq/l S.K.4 mEq/l, S.cholesterol 412 mg/dl, urine Ab +++, PC 3-4/HPF. RBC Nil, granular cast +, urine PC ratio 3.5, 24 hours urine protein 2 g.

DIAGNOSIS AND DISCUSSION

Nephrotic Syndrome–Minimal Change(MCNS) with ADD and Probably Peritonitis

Minimal change NS is the most common type of NS. Being a girl, SLE should be ruled out. Similarly, other histologic types may occur in children > 8 years of age. Loose stools and abdominal tenderness may indicate bacterial especially pneumococcal peritonitis in a case of NS.

NS is diagnosed by massive edema, massive proteinuria > 2 g/day (> 40 mg/m^2/hour or 1g/m^2/day or 50 mg/kg/day), Protein Creatinine (PC) Ratio >2, hypoalbuminemia <2.5 g/dl and hyercholesterolemia > 200 mg/dl and absence of nephritic features like oliguria, hematuria and hypertension. C$_3$ levels will be normal in MCNS, but low in SLE. It is important to screen the child for TB (Mantoux, X-ray chest) and HBsAg before starting treatment. Urine culture and sensitivity should be done to rule out associated UTI. USS Abdomen may reveal edematous kidneys, bowel wall edema and ascites. Other significant kidney changes may be absent.

Treatment includes supportive care, control of infection and steroids. Ascitic tap will reveal presence of peritonitis. Spontaneous pneumococcal or E. coli peritonitis should be treated with CP and ceftriaxone for 10-14 days. Single donor plasma (SDP) should be administered for intravascular volume expansion and hypoalbuminemia. Diuretics can be given after SDP/IV albumin. Potassium sparing diuretics like spironolactone 3-5 mg/kg/day can be given when there is massive edema/ascites. Prednisolone 2 mg/kg/day upto 60 mg/day is started in divided doses after preliminary investigations. Full dose steroid is given for 6 weeks followed by 1.5 mg/kg alternate day as single dose in the morning for another 6 weeks. Onset in infancy and age > 8 years usually indicate significant change NS. NS associated with hepatitis B is treated with lamivudine and not steroids. CMV, Malaria, Syphilis etc., are other causes of NS.

Remission, relapse, steroid dependence and resistance are all defined:

1. **Remission:** Proteinuria < 40 mg/m^2/hour or <1g/kg/day or urine protein nil/trace.

2. **Relapse:** Proteinuria > 40 mg/m^2/hour or urine protein 3+/4+ with edema after attaining remission.

3. **Frequent relapse:** 2 or more relapses within 6 months of remission/3 or more in any 12 months period.

4. **Steroid dependence:** 2 relapses during steroid therapy or within 2 weeks of stopping steroid.

5. **Steroid resistance:** Failure to achieve remission after 6-8 weeks of steroid therapy or after 1 month steroid therapy + 3 doses of pulse methyl prednisolone.

Other Types of Nephrotic Syndrome

a. **Membranous glomerulopathy (MGN):** Age group usually above 8 years. Nephritic presentation with microscopic hematuria may occur. C_3 normal. Renal vein thrombosis may occur in MGN. Cyclophosphamide orally or as IV pulses may be beneficial. Biopsy will show thickening of glomerular basement membrane.

b. **Membrano–proliferative glomerulonephritis (MPGN):** MPGN occurs in older children and young adults. Biopsy is diagnostic.

c. **Rapidly progressive glomerulonephritis (RPGN):** RPGN presents with crescents in Bowman capsule. RPGN may also be post streptococcal. It may present as A/c nephritic or nephrotic syndrome. IV Methyl prednisolone or oral prednisolone, cyclophosphamide and azathioprine are tried along with supportive measures. PD may be needed in some cases.

d. **Congenital nephrosis:** Onset is in infancy. It may be part of Denys Drash syndrome (NS, Wilim's tumor and genital anomalies), Finnish type Congenital nephrosis or secondary to CMV/Syphilis.

e. **NS associated with HBV infection/Malaria - pl. malariae.**

f. **Toxin/Drug induced NS:** Penicillamine, heavy metals, captopril, ethosuximide, lithium, phenytoin etc.

g. **Other DD:** Focal segmental glomerulo- sclerosis (FSGS), IgA nephropathy, IgM nephropathy.

Frequent relapser is treated with full dose steroid × 1 month followed by Alternate Day steroid (1.5 mg/kg/dose) × 1 month, which is stepped down by 0.5 mg/kg/dose once a month. **Infrequent relapser** is treated with full dose steroid till remission of albuminuria (trace/nil) for 3 days and then A/D steroid (1.5 mg/kg/dose) for month. **Steroid resistance** is treated with Methyl prednisolone pulse doses (30 mg/kg/day) for 3-5 days followed by steroid (0.5 mg/kg/dose). Cyclophosphamide/alternate drugs may be added as per renal biopsy result. **Steroid dependent** cases may benefit with levamisole 2-3 mg/kg/ dose OD/AD with steroids for 2 months. The dose of cyclophosphamide is IV/Oral 2-3 mg/kg/d titrated to response in NS. In SLE, the dose is IV/ Oral 15-25 mg/kg once a month.

MCNS shows normal histology on light microscopy. There is retraction of capillary epithelial foot process leading to increased permeability and loss of negative charge of membrane, preventing repulsion of albumin leading to selective proteinuria and filtering of other low molecular weight substances.

Prognosis is good in MCNS. Remission and exacerbations may occur upto young adulthood/ adolescence. Infections are the usual precipitating agents for relapse. Cerebrovascular accidents (CVA) due to thrombosis, renal vein thrombosis etc. may occur due to the hypercoagulable state. Hypercholesterolemia usually resolves with dietary restriction and correction of hypoalbuminemia. The use of statins is restricted in initial episode, but may be needed in long standing cases. Dietary restriction of salt and fluid are mandatory when there is massive edema and oliguria. Protein food and fruits can be given unlike in AGN. Fat restriction is essential. In long standing cases, calcium supplements, phosphate restriction and vitamin D supplement may be needed. **Hydrotherapy** is also advisable, i.e., making the child stand in a drum with warm water. It induces diuresis and fluid exchange by osmosis.

SECTION 10.5 A CHILD WITH STUNTING OF GROWTH AND ANEMIA

A 3-year-old child was brought with stunting of growth and pallor of insidious onset. She had no other specific complaints.

On examination: Pallor +, no edema, Growth retardation +, Wt 8 kg, Height 75 cm, BP 120/70 mm of Hg, Hb 6 g/dl, TC 5000/cumm, P62, L32, E6, ESR 80 mm/1st hour, PS—Normochoric RBCs, WBC–normal, no evidence of hemolysis, Retic count 1%, B urea 68 mg/dl, S creatinine 4.2, S.Na 130 mEq/l, S.K.4.8 mEq/l, S Ca 6 mg/dl, S.P 6.5g/dl, SAP 880 IU/l. S HCO3 12 mEq/l, USS abdomen—small kidneys, No other abnormalities, GBR 20.

DIAGNOSIS AND DISCUSSION

Chronic Kidney Disease (CKD) with Chronic Renal Failure (CRF) Secondary to Contracted/hypoplastic Kidneys with Growth Retardation and Anemia

The most common cause of CRF< 5 years is hypoplasia, malformation or obstruction of kidneys and >5 years is hereditary disorders, polycystic kidneys, Alport syndrome, RPGN/glomerulonephritis, chronic UTI etc. Growth retardation sets in when GFR falls <50% and CRF became evident when GFR falls < 20%.

Diet: Low salt, low protein, low phosphate diet. Liberal carbohydrate and salt free fat (coconut oil/salt free butter) can be given. High biological value protein can be given (upto 1 g/kg/day) to promote growth as per GFR. Calories for the height age may be initially started rather than for the chronological age. Fluid may be restricted to two third of the requirement if edema is present.

Hypertension is treated with diuretics, fluid restriction and nifedipine or ACE inhibitors. Enalapril is preferred than captopril due to high B. urea. ACE inhibitors are contraindicated in bilateral renal artery stenosis. The angiotensin receptor blocker (ARB), Losartan potassium, is a well tolerated antihypertensive (Dose 25-50 mg OD or BD). Hyponatremia may be dilutional and is treated with fluid restriction in cases with edema. Hyperkalemia >5 mEq/l is treated with dietary restriction, 10% Calcium gluconate 0.5-1ml/kg/dose Q12H slowly IV, Soda bicarb 2 ml/kg/dose diluted with equal volume distilled water, Kayexelate (Potassium binding resin) and insulin glucose regimen. Salbutamol nebulization is also beneficial. Acidosis is managed by giving soda bicarb. The dose of soda bicarb is calculated as follows:

HCO_3 (mEq) = 0.3 x weight (kg) x (desired value (20)—observed value) 0.3 is the multiplication factor as only ½ correction is attempted with soda bicarb. For other constituents like sodium, potassium etc., 0.6 is the correction factor. Blood volume is around 60% of the body weight.

Rickets should be anticipated/prevented/treated with 1,25 Di OH Cholecalciferol (0.25 mcg/day) plus calcium carbonate 50-200 mg/kg/day to prevent hypocalcemia. Hyperphosphatemia is the rule in renal rickets. It is ideal to keep the 'Cadman product' around 40 to ensure optimum minerali-

CHAPTER 10

GENITOURINARY SYSTEM

zation (S. Ca x S.P = 40). When the product is > 55, phosphate binders like calcium acetate (Hypophos) may be given and when it is > 65, all supplements may be stopped temporarily. SIMILAC is a low phosphate formula. Anemia is treated with packed cells transfusion and Erythropoietin S/C weekly. Nephrotoxic drugs should be avoided.

Peritoneal dialysis (PD) may be done to tide over acute crisis and to support life till transplantation or other definitive therapy is available. PD is usually done using Type I Fluid (1.5%). Type II (8.7%) may be used in overhydrated patients. Higher strengths may be preparedly by adding 25% glucose to Type I solution. Usually 20-40 cycles are planned with 20-50 ml/kg fluid/cycle. 4 mEq/l of 7.5% K Cl is added from 4th cycle onwards. While on PD, fluid and diet restriction may be lifted as per clinical judgement.

Chronic ambulatory PD is undertaken in ambulant patients. Hemodialysis is rarely undertaken in children. The prognosis of CRF is variable, depending on the etiology and available treatment options.

Calculation of GFR (ml/min/1.73 m^2)

* $\dfrac{K \times Ht \text{ (cm)}}{S. \text{ creatinine (mg/dl)}}$

* **K Preterm—0.35 × length divided by S creatinine**

   K Infant—0.45 × length divided by S creatinine

   K Adolescent girl and child—0.55 × height divided by S creatinine

   K Adolescent boy—0.70 × height divided by S. creatinine.

Protein allowance as per GFR in renal failure

Stage	0-1 year	1-5 years	5-10 years
Mild (GFR 20-40)	1.8 g/kg/d	1.4 g/kg/d	1.0 g/kg/d
Moderate (GFR 5-20)	1.4 g/kg/d	1.0 g/kg/d	0.8 g/kg/d
Severe (GFR <5)	1 g/kg/d	0.8 g/kg/d	0.6 g/kg/d

SECTION 10.6 A CHILD WITH RECURRENT UTI

A 2-year-old boy was brought with history of recurrent urinary tract infection (UTI), dysuria and fever with chills and vomiting.

On examination: Growth and development normal. No edema, vitals stable, physical examination normal, Urine—Alb. +, sugar nil, PC plenty, RBC 5-8/HPF, pus cast +, urine culture—Klebsiella sensitive to 3rd generation cephalosporin, USS abdomen B/L Hydronephrosis –Rt ><Lt.

DIAGNOSIS AND DISCUSSION

Febrile UTI—Culture Positive with Hydronephrosis Probably due to Vesoureteric Reflux (VUR)

UTI may be classified into simple/complicated. Complicated UTI is usually recurrent/associated with anatomic anomalies/due to unusual organisms other than E coli like klebsiella, proteus, pseudomonas etc. The chances for kidney scarring is more in children below 4 years of age and those with anatomic defects and in boys especially infants. DMSA scan using Technetium labelled 2-3 dimercapto succinic acid will confirm scarring of kidneys. Flow can be assessed using DTPA scan. Micturating/voiding cystourethrography (MCU/VCU) will delineate reflux, which is usually warranted in those below 2 years and in those with USS abnormalities or scarring.

Grade I: VUR–reflux into distal ureter without dilatation

Grade II: reflux upto collecting system

Grade III: reflux into dilated ureters and blunting of calyceal fornices

Grade IV: reflux into grossly dilated urters

Grade V: massive reflux with tortuous ureters and hydronephrosis.

Prompt treatment for 10-14 days with appropriate dose of antibiotics preferably parenteral, is advised followed by uro prophylaxis in young children upto 4-5 years (with one third dose as single dose till VU reflux subsides (usually for 6 months to 2 years) or till documenting no VUR in MCU). Monthly urine culture may be done in the initial follow up period to look for breakthrough infection.

MCU is advocated in recurrent, complicated UTI and those with USS abnormalities or poor stream to look for obstructions/reflux. This is preferably done 2-3 weeks after control of infection. The complications are septicemia and bladder perforation. Perforation may be silent during overfilling of the bladder. It may also occur due to mechanical pushing of the catheter. MCU should be done under full dose of antibiotic cover, even in those on prophylaxis.

It is controversial, to undertake MCU for every child with a single episode of UTI. VU reflux may be present congenitally in some families and siblings of those with UTI, without even a single episode of UTI. And scarring has been reported in those without reflux. So, subjecting the genital organs to high radiation will have to be weighed with the benefit from the procedure. When reflux is detected, uroprophylaxis will have to be continued. As per current recommendation, MCU should be repeated to look for resolution later. However, it may be done at least in all infants with culture positive UTI and those with USS abnormalities.

Fever with chills and loin pain and plenty of pus cells with pus casts suggest pyelonephritis and need parenteral antibiotics like 3rd generation cephalosporin initially. Lower UTI and cystitis may be afebrile and treated with oral antibiotics. Surgical repair of VUR is recommended in those with breakthrough infection while on prophylaxis and those with severe grades IV and V reflux.

Asymptomatic bacteriuria is seen in many children especially adolescent girls. This may be the forerunner of a reproductive tract infection (RTI) later in life.

| SECTION 10.7 | # A CHILD WITH URETERIC COLIC AND HEMATURIA |

A 10-year-old boy was brought with hematuria and severe colicky pain radiating from loin to groin. He had similar episodes with hematuria during the episodes.

On examination: Growth and development normal, vitals stable, no pallor, Alb trace, PC 5-8/HPF, RBC plenty, oxalate crystals+.

DIAGNOSIS AND DISCUSSION

Urolithiasis with Ureteric Colic Probably Calcium Oxalate Stones

Differential Diagnosis: Loin pain hematuria syndrome without stones

Calcium oxalate stones are radio opaque and are visible in X-rays, cystine and struvite stones are mildly radio opaque and uric acid stones are non opaque, but are seen in USS. Struvite stones follow infection and are triple phosphates of magnesium, ammonium and calcium. Cystinuria and hyperoxaluria may run in families and are in born errors of metabolism. Hyperuricemia and hypercalciuria are other causes of stone. Urine calcium creatinine ratio > 0.2 (in infants it may be upto 0.8) or urine calcium > 4 mg/kg/day are diagnostic of hypercalciuria. It may be idiopathic or part of hypercalcemias. Idiopathic hypercalciuria is treated with thiazide and citrates to inhibit

stone formation. Dietary restriction of calcium is not usually undertaken in growing children. Potassium citrate can be given as it is an inhibitor of stone formation.

Oxalate crystals are of 2 types, envelope type and needle type. The envelope type crystals may be seen in standing urine. So, fresh urine sample should be repeated for confirmation. Estimation of urine oxalate and uric acid, serum uric acid and oxalate and urine calcium are beneficial.

Treatment includes dietary restriction, plenty of oral fluids and specific drugs like Allopurinol in uric acid stones and B_6 in oxalate stones. Stones may be removed surgically, endoscopically or by extracorporeal shock wave lithotripsy (ESWL). The latter is possible when stone can be crushed in a fluid medium like in the collecting system or bladder.

The diagnostic tools for urolithiasis are abdominal X-ray (KUB), USS abdomen, and spiral CT with or without contrast. Dietary restriction and adequate hydration are the keys for management (Table 10.3). Analysis of the stones, that are obtained after passing or surgery, can give valuable information about the type of stone.

CHAPTER 10

GENITOURINARY SYSTEM

SECTION 10.8 A BABY WITH FAILURE TO THRIVE AND ACIDOSIS

A 5-month-old baby was brought with severe failure to thrive and tachypnea.

On examination: Growth <3rd centile, development delayed with partial head control only. Hb 9 g/dl, TC 10,000/cumm, P62, L38, E 0, ESR 43 mm/1st Hr. ABG—Metabolic Acidosis—HCO_3 8 mEq/l. Urine PH. 5.8, B urea 35 mg/dl, S. Na 132 mEq/l., S.K 3 mEq/l. USS Abdomen—Nephrocalcinosis, Anion gap 15 mEq/l.

DIAGNOSIS AND DISCUSSION

FTT, Renal Tubular Acidosis Probably Distal RTA (Type I) with Nephrocalcinosis

The defect is lack of acidification in distal tubule. FTT, normal Anion gap acidosis with relatively higher urinary PH compared to serum acidosis hyperchloremia and hypokalemia are the features. Nephrocalcinosis/nephrolithiases is more common in Distal RTA. Type I Distal RTA may occur as Autosomal dominant/Recessive condition or a sporadic condition/secondary to SLE, obstructive uropathy, pyelonephritis and Medullary sponge kidney (MSK).

Type II Proximal RTA: Defect is reduced bicarb absorption in proximal tubule. Acidosis is more and urinary PH may be less than 5.5 due to distal acidification. It is either autosomal dominant/sporadic/secondary to hyperparathyroidism, interstitial nephritis or due to drugs/toxins and medullary cystic kidney (MCK). There may be Fanconi syndrome with glycosuria, phosphaturia, aminoaciduria, creatininuria etc. Proximal RTA is severe initially, but may resolve later.

Type III RTA is a variant of type I.

Type IV RTA is hyperchloremic acidosis with hyperkalemia and mineralocorticoid deficiency.

MSK is a sporadic condition associated with dilatation of terminal collecting ducts, associated with pyelonephritis, hypercalciuria, nephrocalcinosis and distal RTA. Life span and renal function remain normal.

MCK is associated with dilatation of distal tubules and collecting ducts (AD/AR inheritance), with proximal RTA. Red blonde hair and renal insufficiency are seen.

Shohl solution that supplies 1 mEq/ml of bicarbonate is supplemented in young children and soda bicarb tabs in older children to tackle acidosis. In those with hypokalemia and acidosis, polycitra is given that supplies 1 mEq/ml of sodium, potassium and 2 mEq/ml of bicarb.

Dose: Distal RTA–3 mEq/kg/day Q4H of Bicarb.

Proximal RTA: 15 mEq/kg/day QH of Bicarb. Potassium binding resins are useful in Type IV RTA.

Shohl solution/Litre	Polycitra solution/Litre
Citric Acid–140 g	Potassium citrate–110 g
Sod Citrate–90 g	Sodium citrate–100 g
Water upto I L	Citric acid–66.8 g
	Water–1 Litre

Bartter Syndrome is a rare condition with hypochloremic metabolic alkalosis with hypokalemia and increased renin aldosterone levels. It may be AR/Sporadic. It presents with FTT, polyuria, dehydration, muscle weakness, cramps and constipation. Increased Prostaglandin E2 leads to platelet function defects. Urine chloride is increased. Treatment - K. supplements upto 250 mEq/day with liberal sodium chloride. Indomethacin 3-5 mg/kg/day Q8H is beneficial as anti prostaglandin agent. K sparing diuretic, spirano-lactone is also beneficial. 1 ml of 7.5% KCl gives 2 mEq/ml of K and 1.5 ml of oral potassium chloride gives 2 mEq of K.

'**Anion gap**' represents unmeasured anions. Normal-12 (8-16) mEq/l. Anion gap=(S. Na+S.K.)-(S.cl+S. HCO$_3$). High Anion gap acidosis is seen in lactic/Ketoacidosis and Normal Anion gap is seen in RTA and diarrhea.

Table 10.1: Various causes of hematuria

Conditions	Remarks
I. Glomerular Conditions	
1. Post infective glomerulonephritis	C3 low
2. IgA nephropathy	C3 normal
3. Alport syndrome	Familial, deafness+
4. Rapidly progressive glomerulonephritis (RPGN)	Fatal progression
5. Hemolytic Uremic Syndrome	Bleeding, Hemolytic anemia, thrombocytopenia
6. SLE	ANA, DsDNA +ve
7. Nephritic Onset Nephrotic Syndrome	Massive proteinuria, High S.cholesterol
8. Henoch-Schönlein purpura/ anaphylactoid purpura	Skin vasculitis
9. Good Pasture disease	Lung involvement, C3 normal
II. Hematologic Conditions	
1. Coagulopathies	Generalized bleeding, prolonged PT/APTT
2. Thrombocytopenia	Low platelet count with normal PT/APTT
3. Renal vein thrombosis	Palpable kidneys (Doppler USS of renal veins show occlusion)
III. Urolithiasis and Related Conditions	
1. Calcium oxalate/Uric acid stones— radiologic/sonologic evidence, ureteric colic	
2. Hypercalcemias/idiopathic hypercalciuria without hypercalcemia (> 4 mg/kg/day or calcium–creatinine ratio > 0.2), in infants calcium excretion is more and the ratio may be up to 0.8	
IV. Anatomic Conditions	
1. Polycystic kidneys	
2. Vascular malformations	
V. Others	
1. Drugs—cyclophosphamide	
2. Strenuous exercise	
3. Tumors	
4. Loin Pain Hematuria syndrome – similar to urolithiasis, but no stones	
5. Thin Basement Membrane Disease – benign familial hematuria	
6. Cystitis/UTIs	

Table 10.2: Insensible water loss (400 ml/M^2)	
Age group	*ml/kg/day*
Newborn	30
Infant	25
Underfive child	20
Older children	15
Adult	10

Table 10.3: Dietary items rich in oxalate, uric acid and calcium		
Oxalate rich items	*Uric acid rich items*	*Calcium rich items*
1. Gingley seeds	1. Chicken, beef, pork	1. Crab, prawn
2. Tea and coffee	2. Sardine	2. Gingly seeds
3. Spinach	3. Liver	3. Amaranth, spinach
4. Almond, cashew	4. Spinach	4. Mackerel, sardine, shark
5. Amla, Plantain flower	5. Cauliflower	5. Mutton
6. Drum stick and coriander leaves	6. Chocolate, cocoa	6. Milk
7. Horse gram, kesari dhal		7. Ragi

CHAPTER 10

GENITOURINARY SYSTEM

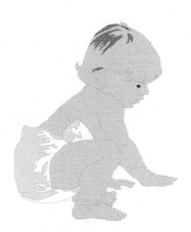

Hemato Oncology

11

Hemato Oncology

SECTION 11.1   AN INFANT WITH SEVERE ANEMIA

A 4-month-old boy was admitted with insidious onset of pallor noticed around two months of age. No bleeding manifestations.

On examination: Growth and Development Normal. Liver and spleen not palpable. TC—6000/cumm, P 20, L 78, E 2, platelet 4.5 lakhs/cumm, ESR 40, Hb 6 g/dl, Retic Count < 1%, PS—RBC—No evidence of Hemolysis. WBC—Relative Neutropenia and thrombocytosis, HbF 4%, Bone marrow—Cellular marrow with reduced RBC precursors.

DIAGNOSIS AND DISCUSSION

Pure Red Cell Aplasia (PRCA)/Congenital Hypoplastic Anemia or Diamond Blackfan Anemia

Reduced RBC precursors with normal WBC and platelet precursors is the hallmark of the disease. It may be familial in 20% cases. Chromosomal study will be normal unlike Fanconi's pancytopenia. Dysmorphism and triphalangeal thumb may be seen in 1/3 cases. Raised 'i' antigen levels are seen. Hepatosplenomegaly is usually absent. It manifests usually by 2-6 months of age. Reticulocytopenia and high HbF are noticed. Erythropoietin will be elevated in these cases. Parvovirus B_{19} infection may cause aplastic crisis with involvement of other blood elements as well.

Treatment includes repeated packed RBCs with diuretics and deferoxamine to chelate extra iron. Chelation is undertaken when S. ferritin is >1500 mg/dl. The oral chelating agent is deferiprone (L1). Chelating agents may affect growth and hence should be undertaken with caution in underfives. Prednisolone is given 1-2 mg/kg/day in divided doses initially and may be maintained on a daily or alternate day basis to stimulate bone marrow. Pulse methyl predniso-lone 30 mg/kg/day × 3-5 days may be tried in refactory cases followed by 0.5 mg/kg/day oral prednisolone or minimum dose to keep up Hb on a long term basis. IV immunoglobulins, Anti thymocyte globulin, cyclosporine, cyclophospha-mide, androgens, interleukin –3 and BM stem cell transplantation are the other modalities tried in congenital and acquired cases. Splenectomy may be needed in those who develop spenomegaly and hypersplenism especially in children >6 years of age.

Differential Diagnosis:

1. **Transient Erythroblastopenia of Childhood (TEC)**

   TEC is transient and recovers in a few months. It is seen between 6 months to 3 years of age. It may follow viral infections. It may also be immune mediated transient suppression of BM. Hb F is normal. It may be severe anemia (normocytic) and may need packed RBC transfusion. RBC Adenosine Deaminase (ADA) will be normal in TEC, but elevated in PRCA. Steroids are not beneficial.

2. **Physiological Anemia of Infancy (PAI)**

   In newborn, Hb is 16 g/dl, it falls to 9-10 g/dl by

2-3 months and may remain low for a few weeks and gradually rise to 11 g/dl by 6 months of age. PAI is more exaggerated and rapid in preterm babies. In them, it may fall to 7-9 g/dl by 1-2 months of age. Erythropoietin will be low.

The causes of PAI are the following:

1. Reduced erythropoietin (EPO)—due to hepatic to renal switchover of production.

2. Reduced erythropoiesis with increase in O_2 saturation to > 95%.

3. Short RBC life span upto 90 days compared to normal 120 days.

4. Hemodilution due to increase in plasma volume.

5. Reduced hematopoietic factors like iron, folic acid, B_{12}.

Treatment includes packed RBCs and Erythropoietin (EPO). Prophylactic iron 2-3 mg/kg/day from 2-4 weeks onwards in preterms and 4 months onwards or earlier in term babies may be beneficial. Folic acid is given in a dose of 100-500 mcg/day. EPO is given in a dose of 200-250 IU/kg/dose S/C thrice weekly.

3. **Vitamin E deficiency related hemolytic anemia of prematurity can also cause anemia. There will be evidence of hemolysis.**

4. **Fanconi's pancytopenia**–All 3 blood elements will be reduced.

5. **Aplastic crisis in hemolytic anemias** due to Parvovirus B_{19} infection.

6. **Sideroblastic Anemia/Hypoplastic anemia associated with Pearson–Marrow Pancreas Syndrome**

Here, FTT, neutropenia and thrombocytopenia may be associated. Exocrine pancreatic dysfunction and Diabetes mellitus are usually associated disorders. Lactic acidosis, renal Fanconi syndrome and neurological impairment are the other features associated with this. It is a mitochondrial DNA deletion syndrome.

Sideroblastic anemia presents with hypochromic microcytic anemia with sideroblasts in bone marrow and perinuclear collar of hemosiderin granules in nucleated RBCs. It may be a X-linked recessive condition or may be associated with Pearson marrow pancreas syndrome/malignancies. It may respond to high doses of pyridoxine—200-300 mg/day. G-CSF (Filgastim) is useful in neutropenia.

7. **Acquired Pure Red Cell Anemia**

This is seen in conditions like thymoma, chloramphenicol administration, Parvovirus B_{19} infection, intrauterine infections, HIV etc.

SECTION 11.2

A CHILD WITH NUTRITIONAL ANEMIA

A 4-year-old girl was brought with pallor and exertional dyspnea. She was malnourished and coming from a poor socio-economic status. She also had worm infestation and pica.

On examination: Grade III PEM and 2 degree stunting and 3 degree wasting present. Pallor, leukonychia, knuckle pigmentation, angular stomatitis and glossitis +, Blood Hb 5 g/dL. TC 4500/cu mm, P36, L40, E 24. ESR 34 mm/1st hour. Retic count 1%, PS: Dimorphic anemia, RDW 25% (increased). Eosinophilia present, platelets adequate. CVS ejection systolic murmur +.

Diagnosis and Discussion

Malnutrition with Nutritional Anemia, Eosinophilia and Worm Infestation, Probably Iron and Folic Acid Deficiency

Malnutrition and poor SE status point to nutritional anemia. History also suggests worm infestation, supported by presence of eosinophilia. Knuckle pigmentation suggests folic acid and B_{12} deficiency. B_{12} stores are said to be adequate for a decade. B_{12} deficiency may present alone or as part of pernicious anemia. Iron deficiency is the most common deficiency among women and children. It is usually associated with poor dietary intake, increased demand or blood loss in the form of bleeding P/R, menorrhagia, pregnancy, lactation or HW/WW infestation.

Iron store is only 0.5 g in newborn compared to 5 g in adults. Bioavailability of iron is more from breast milk and from heme iron and non vegetarian diet than from vegetarian diet or non heme iron. Iron absorption will be reduced with concurrent intake of tea and coffee. Iron is absorbed from proximal jejunum with the help of the duodenal protein 'mobilferrin'. Lactoferrin in breast milk, vitamin C and the reduced form, ferrous iron promote absorption. Co fortification of iron with vitamin C is a novel approach. Iron fortification of cereals and double fortification of salt with iodine and iron are already in use. Elemental iron powders and iron fumarate microencapsulated sprinkles are newer interventions in place of oral iron tablets.

Inherited disorders of iron homeostasis is another area under current research. Mutations in DMT 1, Ireg 1 genes play a role in iron transport across brush border and basolateral membranes of enterocytes respectively. Hepcidin expression in hepatocytes play a key role in intestinal iron absorption, Hepcidin expression is inappropriately decreased in hemochromatosis and is increased in anemia of chronic infection. Other hepatic proteins are also essential for normal homeostasis, including HFE, transferrin receptor 2 (TfR2). Homojuvelin function is for modulating expression of hepcidin. Hepcidin is now identified as an iron regulating hormone.

In infants, iron stores get depleted by 4-5 months when birth weight doubles. In LBW and preterm babies, this may occur earlier. Among adolescents, anemia is common due to very high iron requirement for growth spurt and relatively poor intake due to food fads, dieting etc. Menstrual loss is also significant in girls.

Pica is eating of unedible substances. It may be due to craving for iron. But, it may also aggravate anemia due to worm infestation and may also result in lead poisoning. Microcytic hypochromia anemia with basophilic stippling occurs in lead poisoning. Eating mud is geophagia, eating raw rice is amylophagia and eating ice is pagophagia. These picas are seen in various socio-economic sections.

Irritability, cardiomegaly, tachycardia, hemic murmur and CCF occur when Hb falls <5-6 g/dL. In 15% cases, there may be splenomegaly. Iron deficiency also leads to reduced work efficiency, learning ability, cognitive functions and attention span. Iron depletion leads to lack of iron in the bone marrow and tissues. Iron status can be determined by serum iron, transferrin, ferritin and bone marrow iron. Transferrin is measured as iron saturation/iron binding capacity. It is inversely proportional to serum iron. Iron stores is reflected in ferritin level. Bone marrow staining for iron with Prussian blue is confirmatory for iron stores. Iron deficiency leads to reduction in iron dependent enzymes like Monoamine Oxidase (MAO), cytochromes, catalases and peroxidases. It also results in reduction in dopaminergic receptors in the brain. Low Dopaminergic receptors will lead to unopposed opiate receptor activity and reduced learning ability. Learning ability is a balance between dopaminergic and opiate receptors.

Iron Deficiency Anemia (IDA) is the final stage of iron deficiency. The three stages are iron depletion, iron deficiency and iron deficiency anemia. IDA may also lead to rigid RBCs and increased chance of thrombosis as in cases of polycythemia. Another cause for thrombosis may be associated thrombocytosis.

In iron deficiency, serum iron will be low (normal 50-150 mcg/dL) and iron binding capacity will be increased. Bone marrow will not show hemosiderin on staining with Prussian blue. Serum ferritin will be low in IDA, ferritin is also an acute phase reactant and so it may not be very reliable in the context of infections or inflammations (normal ferritin—Newborn 25-200 ng/mL, 1 mo- 200-600 and 15-200 in adults). To make 1 mg iron bioavailable, roughly 10 mg elemental iron should be taken. The usual iron requirement is 10-20 mg/day. It increases to 30-40 mg/day during increased demands like pregnancy and lactation. The highest iron requirement is for adolescent boys, upto 50 mg/day. During adolescent period, lot of iron and calcium are trapped in the body and hence administration of weekly iron (100 mg) on Saturdays during teenage/adolescent clinics is considered an effective intervention. Boys need iron due to high requirement and girls need more iron due to menstrual loss and rapid growth. This will prevent anemia and reduce maternal and infant mortality by preventing anemia during pregnancy and delivery and by ensuring iron transfer to the baby. Similarly, 250 mg calcium also can be given on a weekly basis.

Therapeutic dose of iron is 3-6 mg/kg/day and prophylactic dose is 2 mg/kg/day. Iron should be given for at least 3 months to replenish stores. Parenteral iron preparations like iron dextran (Imferon 1 ml= 50 mg) or Iron sucrose (Orofer S-1 ml = 20 mg) also may be given. Iron sucrose is associated with less reactions. It is given as infusion, 2.5 ml diluted in 100 ml of N. saline, upto 100 mg/day.

Parenteral iron dose (mg) = weight X (Target Hb – Actual Hb) x 2.5. 25% extra may be given to replenish stores in children. During pregnancy, 500 mg extra iron is usually given.

Packed RBC is given in a dose of 5-10 ml/kg/dose when Hb is < 5 g/dL or when there is hemodynamic instability. Chronic anemia is often better tolerated than acute anemia. Iron rich food items are meat, 3 Gs (green leafy vegetables, grams and grains), dates, watermelon etc. Cooking in iron vessels is said to increase iron intake. The response to iron is given in Table 11.1.

Dimorphic anemia is seen when there are multiple deficiencies like iron plus folic acid (FA)/B_{12}. Both microcytes and macrocytes will be seen. In isolated folic acid/B_{12} deficiency, there will be megaloblastic or macrocytic anemia. In megaloblastic anemia, there may be associated hypersegmented neutrophils, neutropenia, giant platelets or thrombocytopenia. Clinically there may be periungual/knuckle pigmentation. Chronic diarrhea may also be seen in FA deficiency. Tropical sprue, short bowel syndrome, malnutrition, malabsorption, anticonvulsant and antimalignant drugs and goat's milk/powdered milk consumption are the causes of FA deficiency. S folic acid will be low, < 3 ng/ml (Normal 15-20 ng/ml). Serum LDH will be elevated. Treatment includes FA 1-5 mg/day for 4 weeks or more. In congenital folate malabsorption, inj folic acid may be beneficial. FA rich items are green leafy vegetable, fruits, organ meat like liver, kidneys etc. Bioavailability of FA from leafy vegetables is variable. FA is absorbed through out the intestine. Pterroylpolyglutamate in cabbage, lettuce are less well absorbed than pteroylmonoglutamate (folic acid). Pteroypolylglutamate is not biologically active. FA is reduced by dihydrfolate reductase to tetrahydrofolate, which is polyglutamated in the tissue. The requirement is 100 mcg/day.

Vitamin B_{12} deficiency is usually an Autosomal Recessive genetic disorder called pernicious anemia (PA). It is also called 'Addisonian anemia'. It may also occur in short bowel syndrome, ileal resection/atresia, blind loop syndrome or fish tapeworm (Diphyllobothrium latum) infestation. In PA, there is deficiency of intrinsic factor and achlorhydria, especially in the adult. Juvenile type PA manifests after 1-10 years due to exhaustion of B_{12} stores. The manifesta-tions are glossitis, irritability, ataxia, paresthesia, hyperreflexia, clonus, extensor plantar reflex and coma. Serum B_{12} will be less than 100 mg/ml. It may also present early with skin pigmentation, regression of milestones etc. Treatment is by Inj. B_{12} 1 mg/day × 2 weeks followed by 1mg/month. Strict vegetarians are liable to develop B_{12} deficiency. High dose oral therapy may be effective due to mucosal diffusion.

In Schilling test, Inj B_{12} 1 mg is given IM to saturate the stores followed by administration of radiolabelled B_{12}. A 24 hours urinary excretion < 5% of the given dose indicate ileal malabsorption. This test is usually done to identify ileal or distal malabsorption. Urinary excretion of Methy malonic acid is suggestive of B_{12} deficiency. Serum LDH will be elevated in deficiency.

Red Cell Distribution Width (RDW) is normally 12-15%. It is increased in aniso-poikilocytosis like IDA. It is narrow in thalassemia trait. The various causes of hypochromic microcytic anemia are given in Table 11.2. The classification based on RDW and MCV is given in Table 11.3. It is useful in identifying thalassemia trait from IDA.

CHAPTER 11

HEMATO ONCOLOGY

SECTION 11.3

A CHILD WITH SEVERE ANEMIA REQUIRING FREQUENT BLOOD TRANSFUSIONS

A 3-year-old child was brought for blood transfusion due to severe anemia. He had several previous transfusions for anemia since infancy. He was born out of consanguinous marriage.

On examination: His growth was retarded. Development normal. He had an apparently large head, severe pallor with no bleeding manifestations, hepatosplenomegaly and hemic murmur +. There was mild jaundice also. Hb 4 g/dL, TC 10400, P56, L3 E7 M1, platelet 2 lakhs, retic count 12%, RBC hypochromic, microcytic with poikilocytosis and target cells, nucleated RBCs +. HbF 6 %, X-ray skull showed widening of medullary space with 'hair on end appearance' and X-ray chest showed cardiomegaly, S. Bilirubin 3 mg/dL, Liver enzymes normal, Hbs Ag negative, HCV antibody negative.

DIAGNOSIS AND DISCUSSION

Thalassemia Major/Beta Thalassemia/ Cooley's Anemia

It is an Autosomal Recessive condition, with severe hemolytic anemia manifesting in the second half of infancy, when HbF starts falling. The presence of jaundice and pallor points to hemolysis. It warrants frequent blood transfusions. Extra medullary erythropoiesis is evident by hepatosplenomegaly and increased medullary erythropoiesis by widening of marrow spaces evident in the skull. Extreme cases may have 'Chipmunk facies'.

The long term complications include hemosiderosis affecting heart leading to arrhythmia, hemosiderosis of pancreas leading to diabetes and that of liver leading to liver dysfunction. This is the rule when iron chelation is not routinely undertaken.

It is a hemoglobinopathy due to failure of synthesis of beta chains. The chromosome for Alpha chain is on chromosome 16 and that for Beta, Gamma and Delta chains on chromosome 11. There are 4 genes for Alpha and 2 genes for Beta chains.

Hb A→2 Alpha chains +2 Beta chains

Hb A2→2 Alpha + 2 Delta chains

Hb F→2 Alpha + 2 Gama (resistant to alkali)

Hb B (Barts)→ 4 Gamma (seen in Alpha Thalassemia)

Hb H→4 Beta (seen in Alpha Thalassemia).

Hb F is 90% at 6 months of gestation and 70% at birth and < 2% by 1 year of age. Hb A is 10% at 6 months of gestation and 30% at birth. Normal Hb A: Hb A2 ratio is 30:1.

These patients need protection against blood borne disease like HBV, HCV, CMV, malaria, syphilis, HIV and so on. Parvovirus B_{19} infection may lead to aplastic crisis. Blood borne diseases can be avoided by vaccinations and proper screening of blood before transfusion. Normally, retic count is 1% as RBC destruction is 1%/day.

It may increase to 3-8% in maximum marrow activity.

$$\frac{\text{Corrected}}{\text{Retic Count}} = \frac{\text{Observed PCV}}{\text{Normal PCV}} \times \text{Retic count}$$

Hemolytic Anemias are mainly of 4 types:

1. Due to membrane defect—e.g., Hereditary spherocytosis

2. Due to Hb defect—e.g., Sickle cell disease, thalassemia

3. Due to enzyme defect—e.g., G6PD deficiency

4. Extrinsic defects—e.g., immune → autoimmune hemolytic anemia and non immune → snake venom/toxin mediated.

1. **RBC membrane defects**

Membrane defects affect the shape of RBCs leading to hemolysis, e.g., Hereditary spherocytosis (HS), elliptocytosis, stomatocytosis, acanthocytosis and paroxysmal nocturnal hemoglobinuria (PNH).

HS is usually AD. AR inheritance is also described. In dominant type (AD HS), there is defect in **Beta spectrin**, the protein that maintains the RBC shape. In Recessive type (ARHS), there is defect in **Alpha spectrin**. In HS, the RBCs lose the dump bell shape/concave shape and become spherical and get destroyed in the spleen. It may manifest with mild to severe hemolysis at any time from newborn to adulthood. It may also remain dormant without clinical manifestations. One of the parents is usually affected with variable severity of expression. Spherocytes are smaller in size than normal RBCs and do not have central pallor. Spherocytes will be >15-20% of the total RBCs. USS will show splenomegaly and gall stones, beyond usually 4 years of age due to increased calcium bilirubinate. BM will show erythroid hyperplasia and all other elements will be normal. Osmotic fragility will be increased. Spherocytes are also seen in conditions like ABO incompatibility, burns, Wilson disease, Clostridium sepsis,

auto immune hemolytic anemia etc. and other conditions with rapid bone marrow regeneration. Hypersplenism may lead to pancytopenia in some cases.

Treatment of HS includes packed RBC transfusion with iron chelation. The goal is to keep Hb >10 g/dL and splenectomy may be done in those above 6 years of age, requiring frequent transfusion. They also need vaccinations to prevent infections by microbes with capsular antigens namely HIB, pnemovax and meningovax prior to splenectomy and oral penicillin prophylaxis after splenectomy. The vaccination should be given at least 2 weeks prior to surgery. Thrombocytosis may occur after splenectomy and also sepsis by encapsulated organisms.

Paroxysmal nocturnal Hemoglobinuria (PNH) is an acquired defect, which makes the RBCs liable to destruction by activation of serum complement. There may also be associated thrombocytopenia and leucopenia. It may progress to aplastic anemia or AML. Treatment includes prednisolone, antithymocyte globulin (ATG), androgen like danazole and BM transplantation in resistant cases. Hemoglobinuria is more in the night and early morning and hence the name.

2. **Hb defects/Hemoglobinopathies**

There are 3 types of Hemoglobinopathies: (1) Single amino acid substitution—e.g., (HbS) – Sickle Cell Anemia (2) Amino acid deletion or insertion and (3) Absent or defective synthesis of one or more Hb chains.

Sickle cell anemia (SCA) is an AR condition, seen more commonly among tribes. It is due to substitution of valine in the six position instead of glutamic acid in Beta chain of HbA leading to abnormal HbS. The RBCs become rigid and lead to sickling. The heterozygote carrier state offers protection against malaria. HbS can be detected by electrophoresis and HbF is elevated. **Sickle cell crisis** is due to ischemia and vascular occlusion by masses of sickled RBCs in any internal organs. The manifestations start by 2-4 months of age when most of the HbF get replaced by HbS instead of HbA. **Hand Foot syndrome** is due to acute symmetric dactylitis. Other manifestations like autosplenectomy, leg ulcers and priapism are extremely painful conditions. There will be huge splenomegaly with hypersplenism leading to leukopenia and thrombocytopenia. Blood smear will show sickled cells, Howel Jolly bodies due to remnants of hemolysed RBCs and retculocytosis. There may be neutrophilia and thrombocytosis with low ESR. Osmotic fragility will be increased. HbS may be upto 35 to 45% and HbF upto 2-20%. Sickling may be demonstrated by **Sickling test** in deoxygenated state. Treatment is symptomatic and includes anti-inflammatory drugs and corticosteroids in painful crisis, frequent blood transfusions and splenectomy. BM stem cell transplantation is beneficial. Carriers are asymptomatic, but in high altitude, heterozygous cases also may develop ischemia. HbC is substitution of lysine in the 6th position instead of glutamic acid. HBE is substitution of lysine in the 26th position.

In hemoglobinopathies, Hb electrophoresis will confirm the diagnosis. The patients should be protected from blood borne disease. Parvo virus B$_{19}$ infection may lead to aplastic crisis in those with hemolytic anemias. Transfusion requirements vary from disease to disease and case to case.

Hypertransfusion refers to packed RBC transfusion to keep Hb > 10 g/dL, to ensure proper growth of the child. **Supertransfusion** refers to keeping Hb > 12 g/dL to prevent change in facies by increased medullary erythropoiesis. 500 ml blood delivers around 200 mg iron and hence Desferrioxamine 50 mg/kg/dose may be given as IV infusion or as subcutaneous injection after each transfusion. It may also be given using infusion pumps. This is essential especially when serum ferritin exceeds 1500-2000 ng/mL. Chelated iron in urine will show **'vinrose color'**.

Packed cell requirement more than 240 ml/kg/year and hypersplenism are indications for splenectomy especially after 6 years of age. **Neocyte transfusion** using young RBCs (neocytes) with more life span is also advisable.

Alpha thalassemia is due to deletion of all the 4 alpha globin genes. It leads to hydrops fetalis. Deletion of 3 genes lead to **thalassemia intermedia syndrome** and two lead to alpha thalassemia trait and deletion of one is asymptomatic leading to silent carrier. In alpha thalassemia, HbF, HbA and A2 cannot be synthesized and Hb Barts (4 Gamma) is synthesized. HbB has increased affinity for oxygen. In Beta thalassemia, deletion of one gene leads to trait and two leads to thalassemia major.

RBC Enzyme Defects

G6PD (Glucose 6 Phosphatase dehydrogenase) deficiency is X-linked recessive, that manifest in males. It usually leads to episodic anemia precipitated by oxidant drugs like aspirin, sulpha and antimalarials. Exposure to naphthalene balls may cause hemolysis. It offers protection against P. falciparum malaria even in heterozygous females. It manifests in boys with acute hemolysis, hemoglobinuria and jaundice. Newborns may present with hemolysis following transfer of oxidant drugs through placenta or breast milk. There will be Heinz bodies or precipitated Hb in RBCs with polychromasia and reticulocytosis. G6PD level less than 10% of normal is diagnostic. After a blood transfusion, 3-4 months period should be allowed before the test. It is better to do the test before blood transfusion.

Pyruvate kinase deficiency (PKD) is an AR condition and hence can occur in both genders. The defect is on chromosome 21q.

There are other less common **congenital non spherocytic hemolytic anemias** due to deficiency of enzymes of glycolysis and RBC nucleotide metabolism. **Pyrimidine 5' nucleosidase deficiency** (P5'ND) manifests with mild chronic hemolysis with basophilic stippling.

Basophilic stippling is the hallmark of lead poisoning, but serum lead level will help to differentiate between the two conditions. P5'ND is usually autosomal recessive. If the deficiency is also there in the brain, there may the mental retardation. Reticulocyte maturation requires disposition of intraerythrocytic RNA, which is no longer needed for protein synthesis when it matures to RBC. Pyrimidine nucleotide formed by action of ribonuclease on ribosomal RNA is hydrolysed by P5'N enzyme. In its deficiency, substrates accumulate leading to hemolysis and anemia. MRI or UV spectroscopy for cellular extracts in RBCs and enzyme assay are confirmatory. There is no specific therapy. Folic acid is beneficial in all hemolytic anemias with rapid RBC regeneration.

The various causes of hypochromic anemias are given in Table 11.2.

Hemolysis due to Extrinsic Factor

1. Immune anemia–blood group incompatibility–Coomb's test positive.
2. Autoimmune–autoimmune hemolytic anemia (AHA)–Coomb's test +, Evans syndrome with anemia and thrombocytopenia–Coomb's +, SLE.
3. Hemolysis in malignancies.
4. Hemolytic anemia due to microbes, EBV,CMV, mycoplasma.

5. HA due to drugs/toxins–immune—methyldopa, levodopa and non-immune-penicillin, cephalosporins, snake venom etc.

AHA-Warm Antibodies

AHA may be due to warm antibodies as in SLE, lymphoproliferative disorders, immunodeficiency or due to unknown causes. The warm antibodies are active between 35-40°C upto 260-500 IgM molecules are needed for Coomb's positivity. So, there may also be Coomb's negative AHA. Repeat testing may be done periodically. Treatment includes IVIG, steroids and androgens.

AHA—Cold Antibodies

Cold antibodies are active <37°C. In EBV, CMV, mycoplasma etc., cold antibodies mediate hemolysis. In lymphoproliferation and paroxysmal cold Hbinuria, it may be seen. Paroxysmal Cold Hbinuria (PCH) is a cold agglutinin mediated HA. In these conditions, exposure to cold should be avoided.

Cold Agglutinin Test: This test is positive in cold antibodies and mycoplasma infection. Equal volume RBC fluid and blood is mixed on a glass slide and is kept in the refrigerator for 30 seconds. This will lead to 'chilly powder' like agglutination in positive cases.

SECTION 11.4 A 3-YEAR-OLD CHILD WITH PANCYTOPENIA

A 3-year-old child was brought with pallor and bleeding from gums. He had these symptoms from infancy and had previous blood transfusions. He was born out of consanguinous marriage and his brother had died of similar illness. His sister is apparently normal.

On examination: Growth < 3rd centile. He had pigmentation around mouth, multiple café au lait spots and hypoplastic thumb. Hb 3/dL, TC 3000/cu mm, platelets 28,000/cu mm, HBF 5%, RBCs macrocytic with anisopoikilocytosis, BM dry tap, Trephine biopsy—Hypocellular marrow with decreased RBC, WBC and megakaryocyte precursor. No blast proliferation.

DIAGNOSIS AND DISCUSSION

Fanconi's Pancytopenia

Congenital and hereditary pancytopenia are constitutional (Fanconi's pancytopenias). Acquired pancytopenias are due to radiation, drugs, chemicals, viruses, immune disease like SLE, paroxysmal nocturnal hemoglobinuria (PNH) and preleukemic conditions. HIV may rarely manifest with hypergammaglobulinemia, antinuclear antibodies and pancytopenias. Chloramphenicol, NSAIDs, antiepileptic drugs and gold salts produce idiosyncratic type of pancytopenia whereas cytotoxic agents and benzene cause dose related pancytopenia. EBV, CMV, HBV, parvovirus B_{19} and HIV are the viruses that lead to pancytopenias. Chromosomal breaks in karyotype and raised HbF point to constitutional type and rule out acquired types. The asymptomatic sister also should be evaluated for chromosomal breaks before recommending her as a bone marrow donor for BM stem cell transplantation.

Severe pancytopenia is characterized by ANC< 500/cu mm, platelet count < 20,000 and Retic count < 1% with hypocellular BM. Febrile neutropenics need special care and they should be initiated on higher antibiotics like ceftazidime, vancomycin and amikacin. Astreonam is preferred in renal insufficiency, compared to aminoglycoside.

Fanconi's pancytopenia is an AR condition with chromosomal breaks, abnormal cytokine network, reduced GM CSF stem cell factor and IL 6. It may manifest around 1 year of age, usually as a single cytopenia like thrombocytopenia and progress to pancytopenia. Radial defects include absent radius, hypoplastic thumb etc. **TAR syndrome** is thrombocytopenia absent radius syndrome. In **Amegakaryocytic thrombocytopenia**, initially there is only thrombocytopenia. It has a fatal course and pancytopenia evolve later on. In **dyskeratosis congenita**, there is hyperpigmentation, nail dystrophy, leukoplakia, cataract etc., with pancytopenia. 10% of cases may have chromosomal breaks. The variant of pancytopenia without physical stigma of Fanconi's is called **'Estren Damashek syndrome'**.

Treatment includes steroids, androgens like inj testosterones 100 mg once a month, dinabol (menabol) 15-25 mg/day and stanazolol 0.5-1mg/

kg/day. IL 3 and IL 6 are also being tried. Some especially acquired cases may response to anti lymphocyte globulin (ALG), anti thymocyte globulin (ATG), granulocyte colony stimulating factor (G CSF-Nupogen) and granulocyte macrophage colony stimulating Factor (GM CSF-Leucomax). Some aplastic anemias may evolve into leukemias and G CSF may unmask such proliferation. This issue should be discussed with the parents before starting treatment. Irradiated blood products should be given to those on immunosuppressive therapy or those who are planning BMT. Similarly androgen therapy may be withheld in those going for BMT. BMT donor should be selected carefully as asymptomatic siblings may have chromosomal breaks.

SECTION 11.5 A WELL CHILD WITH ECHYMOSIS

A 5-year-old child otherwise healthy was admitted with ecchymosis of one week duration.

On examination: Growth, development, general and systemic examination within normal limits. Blood counts normal except platelet count—38000/cu mm.

DIAGNOSIS AND DISCUSSION

Immune Thrombocytopenic Purpura/Idiopathic Thrombocytopenic Purpura (ITP)

The term 'immune' is preferred than idiopathic in this condition.

Cause of Thrombocytopenia

1. Congenital: TAR syndrome, Amegakaryocytic thrombocytopenia, Fanconi's pancytoenia
2. Thrombopoietin deficiency
3. Kasalbach Merrit syndrome (MS) with cavernous hemangiomas
4. Wiskott Aldrich syndrome (WAS)—X-linked recessive with immunodeficiency, CSOM, eczema and decreased release of platelets in boys
5. Thrombocytopenia associated with thrombasthenia–Bernad Soulier syndrome
6. Immune thrombocytopenic purpura—ITP with peripheral destruction of platelets
7. Hypersplenism
8. Thrombotic thrombocytopenic purpura, HUS, DIC due to increased consumption
9. Auto immune conditions like Evan syndrome, SLE
10. Bone marrow infiltrations like leukemias
11. Aplastic anemias with reduced precursors
12. Drugs/toxins, infection induced thrombocytopenia
13. Neonatal thrombocytopenia due to intra uterine infections or maternal antibodies.

Neonatal thrombocytopenia may be due antibodies transferred from mothers with SLE or ITP. Rarely, it may be Allo immune when mothers platelet count is normal due to transplacental alloantibodies.

In ITP and conditions with peripheral destruction of platelets, BM will show increased proliferation of megakaocytes. Thrombocytopenia is always an indication to do BM aspiration to differentiate between aplasia, leukaemia and ITP before starting treatment.

Platelet count <20,000/cu mm and overt bleeding are definite indications to give platelet transfusion (around 1bag/10 kg body weight). Count < 40-50,000 may be associated with bleeding. Spontaneous bleeds occur with < 20000 count. In DHF and other hemorrhagic fevers, platelet transfusions are usually not warranted, unless there is severe bleeding or count <10,000/cu mm.

In ITP, 2 mg/kg prednisolone is given for 2-3 weeks or till count comes up to normal. ITP may be self limited in many cases. So, if the count is showing upward trend or if there is no further bleeding, it may be left alone with close monitoring. In refractory cases, IVIG, methylprednisolone pulses, Anti D etc. are tried. Anti D antibody is given to Rh +ve cases only. The dose is 50 mcg/kg × 2 days. It acts by combining with macrophage Fc receptors and preventing destruction.

Thrombocytopenia persisting for more than 6 months is called **chronic ITP** and need IVIG/ methylprednisolone pulsing, vincristine and even splenectomy. Retinal bleeds herald IC bleed. Tranexamic acid may be tried in minor bleeds.

In **thrombasthenia**, count may be normal or slightly reduced. In Glazmann's, count is normal with absent platelet aggregation and absent clot

retraction. Hence, platelets are seen singly in blood smear. In Bernard Soulier, count may be low with Ristocetin induced agglutination defects. Such patients may benefit with platelet transfusion during overt bleeding. Platelet function tests and clot retraction test should be done in them. Usually clot retracts with clean sera in 2 hours time.

Skin and mucosal bleeds are usually seen in capillary fragility and platelet disorders whereas deep bleeding into joint and muscle occur in coagulation defects. BT is prolonged in bleeding disorders and CT in coagulation defects. PT is prolonged in liver disorders and vitamin K deficiency. APTT is prolonged in Hemophilias. In DIC, both PT and APTT are prolonged. An approach to bleeding diathesis is given in Figure 11.1.

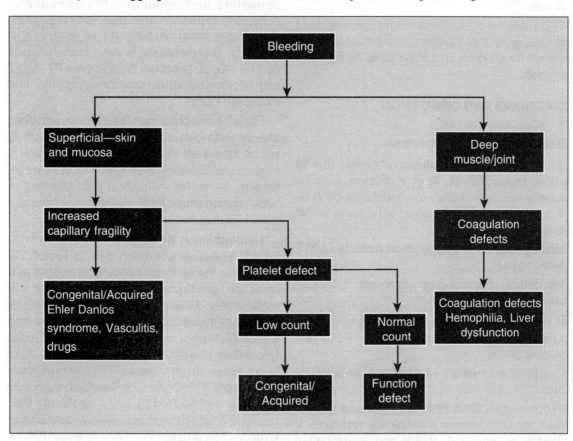

Fig 11.1: An approach to bleeding diathesis

SECTION 11.6 · A 6-YEAR-OLD CHILD WITH REPEATED HEMARTHROSIS

A 6-year-old boy was admitted with hemarthrosis right knee. He had several previous episodes earlier and had history of increased bleeding following injury. His maternal uncle had similar illness.

On examination: Growth and development normal, general and systemic examination normal except for effusion right knee joint. APTT >100 seconds.

DIAGNOSIS AND DISCUSSION

Hemophilia with Hemarthrosis

Hemophilia is a coagulation disorder due to either factor VIII, IX, XI or V defects. Specific assays are confirmatory in coagulation defects. But, mixing studies can give useful clues in this respect.

Mixing studies in coagulation defects (APTT prolonged)

VIII defect—Corrected by aluminium hydroxide absorbed plasma

IX defect—Corrected by aged serum

XI deficiency—Corrected by both adsorbed plasma and serum

Coagulation inhibitors—Defect not corrected by both.

Prothrombin time (PT) is prolonged in liver disorder, DIC, Vitamin K deficiency and factor V deficiency. Factor II, V, VII and X are called prothrombin complex and all except Factor V

need vitamin K for synthesis. **Coagulation inhibitors** are antithrombin III, protein C & S and their deficiency may lead to thrombosis. The **fibrinolytic system** consists of plasminogen activators and inhibitors. Plasminogen is converted to plasmin, that lyse fibrin to produce fibrin degradation products (FDP) or fibrin split products. D Dimer assay is very sensitive to pick up this. This state occurs in DIC where PT, APTT are prolonged with thrombocytopenia and increased FDP.

Classic hemophilia manifests in boys with deep bleeding into joint/muscle. The coagulant activity will be as low as 1% in severe cases to 30% in mild cases. Bleeding may manifest at any age, for e.g., in newborn umbilical cord bleeding or later—during injury, tooth extraction or circumcision. ICH may rarely occur.

Hemophilia A or classic hemophilia is X-linked recessive condition due to factor VIII deficiency. Hemarthrosis should be treated with local ice, pressure bandage and factor VIII replacement. 1 unit plasma contains 1 unit factor VIII and 20-40 unts/kg is usually given for arresting bleed. Factor VIII is available as 250-500 units lyophilised powder. The shelf life is only 8-12 hours. Fresh frozen plasma (FFP) is less effective in Hemophilia A. Cryoprecipitate is cheaper and one bag yields 75-125 units of Factor VIII. Epsilone amino caproic acid (EACA) 50-100 mg/kg dose Q 6H is useful in minor injuries and dental procedures. It delays lysis of formed clost.

Desmopressin nasal spray may raise factor VIII activity and may be useful in nasal and other minor bleeds. Tranexamic acid is also useful in minor bleeds. It is antifibrinolytic agent given in a dose 500-1000 mg Q8-12 H. In those with factor VIII antibodies, factor IX concentrate and porcine factor VIII may help.

Hemophila B is **Christmas disease** due to factor IX deficiency. It is also X-linked recessive condition. It is similar to Hemophilia A, but responds to FFP, Factor IX and not to Factor VIII. Specific factor IX assay will confirm it. Half life of factor IX is 24 hours. One unit will rise coagulant activity by 1-1.2%. 1 ml FFP contains 1 unit of factor IX.

Hemophilia C is due to factor XI deficiency. It is rare. 2-3% of hemophilics have this and it is AR. It can manifest in females also. Half life of

factor XI is 40-80 hours. Bleeding is corrected by FFP and not by VIII or IX.

Parahemophilia or Owren's disease is Factor V deficiency. It is AR condition. Occurring in both genders.

Von Willebrand's disease is AD/AR condition. VW protein includes platelet adhesive component, VW factor and factor VIII carrier protein. Parameters like BT, APTT and platelet aggregation are usually prolonged. They respond to FFP, Factor VIII and Desmopressin nasal spray.

Among the coagulation factors, Factor XII deficiency, does not produce bleeding, but thrombosis. Hemophilia is a chronic disabling disease. Poor response to treatment may be due to inhibitors. It is also called 'Royal disease' as it was present in the pedigree of Queen Victoria.

CHAPTER 11

HEMATO ONCOLOGY

SECTION 11.7

A 4-YEAR-OLD CHILD WITH RAPIDLY DEVELOPING ANEMIA AND BLEEDING GUM

A 4-year-old boy was admitted with general weakness, pallor, bleeding gums of 2 weeks duration.

On examination: Sick looking child, growth and development normal, pallor +, bleeding gum +, ecchymosis +, cervical and axillary lymph nodes +, hepatosplenomegaly +, sternal tenderness +, Hb 5 g/dL, platelet 30,000/cu mm, WBC 100,000/cu mm with 80% lymphocytes, 10% neutrophils and 10% immature cells, X-ray chest—no mediastinal mass. S. Uric acid 10 mg/dL, B urea 44 mg/dL, S. P 8 mg/dL, S.Ca 7 mg/dL, S.Na 130 mEq/L, S.K.5 mEq/L.

DIAGNOSIS AND DISCUSSION

Acute Lymphatic Lymphoblastic Leukemia with Tumor Lysis Syndrome

Acute onset of pallor, bleeding, lymphadenopathy and organomegaly suggest acute leukemia. There may be associated infection, parotid swelling, bone and joint involvement, cranial nerve palsies, **mediastinal/superior vena caval compression** by mediastinal nodes and tumor lysis syndrome. **Tumor lysis syndrome** is characterised by hyperuricemia, hyperphosphatemia, hyperkalemia with or without hypocalcemia and hypo/hypernatremia. Lymphocyte predominance and blasts confirm ALL. It is the most common malignancy in children followed by CNS tumors. In AML, thrombocytopenia may be less marked and there may be features of DIC in M3 type.

Treatment and prognosis depend on the type and cytogenetic characteristics. On the whole, pre B cell ALL (75%), has better prognosis than mature B cell (5%) and mature T cell (1%) types. AML accounts for 15-20% of all leukemias. AML has poorer outcome. Common ALL antigen (CALLA) positivity and polyploidy in leukemic cells indicate better outcome.

Treatment of leukemia includes supportive care and specific chemotherapy as per accepted protocols. 5-year 'Event Free Survival (EFS)' is the rule in most of the cases with good prognosis. Mediastinal compression including vena caval and tracheal compression is rare, but may occur in T cell ALL or lymphomas. Tumor lysis syndrome occurs with abnormally high counts around 2 lakhs/cu mm in AML and 3 lakhs/cu mm in ALL. Under the microscope, ALL blasts have 'convent school girl appearance due to uniform size and shape of cells and AML blasts have 'college girl's appearance'. Diagnosis is confirmed by bone marrow aspiration/Biopsy. CSF study may be necessary in some cases.

All—Good Prognostic Factors

1. Age 1-10 years.
2. Gender–Female, due to high testicular relapse among boys.
3. WBC Count—<1 lakh/cu mm and > 2 lakhs/cu mm.
4. Pre B cell/B progenitor cell Type and CD 10—CALLA Positive cells.
5. Absence of mediastinal/CNS involvement.

Types of ALL and AML (French American British—FAB Classification)

ALL	AML
L1–Small Homogeneous	Mo and M1–Myeloblastic with no maturation
L2–Large Heterogeneous	M2 with some maturation
L3–Large Homogeneous	M3 Promyelocytic
	M4 Myelo–monocytic
	M5 Monocytic
	M6 Erythro leukemia
	M7 Megakaryocytic leukemia

Treatment regimen in given in Table 11.4.

Total duration is 36 months in boys and 30 months in girls

Radiotherapy is usually reserved for local relapse; e.g. CNS/testicular relapse. Remission is usually achieved by 4-6 weeks and boys are treated for longer period, 36 months (in view of testicular relapse) and girls for 30 months. Leukemia cases may come in clusters or during certain seasons.

Radiation, viruses, carcinogens, oncogenes and underlying conditions like Down Syndrome, immunodeficiency states and chromosomal breakages may evoke neoplasmic proliferations.

AML is more resistant to treatment and may be associated with Fanconi's pancytopenia, Diamond Blackfan syndrome, Bloom syndrome, previously treated malignancies etc. Pancytopenias and myelodysplastic syndromes usually evolve into AML. AML is treated with multi drug chemotherapy. Daunomycin and cytosine arabinoside are the common drugs.

Pneumocystis carinii pneumonia (PCP) treatment and prophylaxis with co-trimoxazole is usually given during treatment (10 mg/kg/dose Q12H is given for treatment and half the dose for prophylaxis). Pneumocystis jerovecci is the current name for PCP.

Chronic Myeloid Leukemia (CML) is rare in children, but juvenile CML may occur. There are 2 types of CML—Philadelphia chromosome Ph +ve (2) Ph -ve. Ph+ve has better prognosis. Drug of choice in CML is busulfan (myeleran). Ph chromosome is a specific 22 deletion with 9-22 balanced translocation.

CHAPTER 11

HEMATO ONCOLOGY

CHAPTER 11

HEMATO ONCOLOGY

A 9-YEAR-OLD GIRL WITH MEDIASTINAL COMPRESSION SYNDROME

A 9-year-old child was admitted with hoarseness of voice, tachypnea, cough, venous congestion in eyes and neck and prominent chest. She became acutely ill and had pallor and fever of 2 weeks of duration.

On examination: Pale, sick looking, evidence of tracheal and superior vena caval compression+, cervical lymphadenopathy and hepatosplenomegaly, reduced air entry right with dullness and mediastinal shift to the left. X-ray chest showed pleural effusion right with mediastinal shift,. Hb 8 g/dl, TC 15,000/cu mm, P 40, L60. ESR110/mm/1st hour, platelet 1.2 lakhs/cu mm. Pleural tap yielded hemorrhagic fluid and cytology slowed malignant cells. BM: No malignant infiltration or increased blast cells.

DIAGNOSIS AND DISCUSSION

Non Hodgkin's Lymphoma (NHL) with Hemorrhagic pleural effusion and Mediastinal Compression Syndrome

NHL is a rapidly progressive disease and sometimes there may be BM infiltration leading to leukemic phase of lymphoma. Lymphoma cells may replace 25% of marrow in contrast to total replacement in ALL and there is less severe thrombocytopenia in NHL as compared to ALL.

Classification of NHL

1. B cell Vs. T cell. Cell lymphoma*

2. Large cell (anaplastic) Vs. Small cell and Mixed cell lymphoma

3. Follicular (indolent) Vs. Diffuse (Aggressive)

4. High grade Vs. Intermediate Vs. Low grade lymphoma.

*T cell lymphoma may be associated with gluten sensitive enteropathy.

Staging of NHL

Stage I: Single site/nodal or extra nodal.

Stage II: Two or more nodal/single site + single node/single site—GIT.

Stage III: Nodal/extranodal on either side of diaphragm/extensive—GIT.

Stage IV: Any of the above + CNS/BM involvement.

Hodgkin's lymphoma: It is rare in children compared to NHL; Cell of origin is B cell/T cell/ monocyte. Reed Strenberg cell is pathognomonic of Hodgkin's disease.

Histology Types

1. Nodular sclerosing

2. Mixed cellularity

3. Lymphocyte predominant

4. Lymphocyte depletion type.

A subset has no constitutional symptoms

B subset has constitutional symptoms

Staging of Hodgkin's Lymphoma (Ann Arbor Classification)

Stage I: Single node/Extranodal.

Stage II: 2 or more nodal/extra nodal on same side of diaphragm.

Stage III: Nodal/Extra nodal on either side of diaphragm or splenic involvement.

Stage IV: Diffuse disseminated disease.

Treatment includes radiotherapy; chemotherapy as per standard regimen and surgical excision.

MOPP regimen for HL includes: Mustard Nitrogen, Oncovin (Vincristine), Procarbazine and Prednisolone.

ABVD regimen for BM involvement: Adriamycin (doxorubicin) Bleomycin, Vinblastine and dacarbazine.

CHOPP regimen for NHL: Cyclophosphamide, Hydroxy adriamycin (Doxorubicin), Oncovin, Prednisolone.

Prognosis is not good due to rapid dissemination in NHL compared to HL.

EB virus is related to Burkitt's lymphoma and nasopharyngeal carcinoma. It is an oncogenic virus.

SECTION 11.9

A 1½-YEAR-OLD CHILD WITH PROPTOSIS, ATAXIA AND ABDOMINAL MASS

A one-and-half-year-old child was brought with unsteady gait pain lower limbs and proptosis.

On examination: Child pale, BP 130/90, hepatomegaly and irregular mass left side of abdomen +, Proptosis and ecchymosis in both eyes, bilateral nystagmus +, Hb 8 g/dL. TC 12,000/cu mm, P 70, L28, E2, Platelet 1.5 lakhs, X-ray chest–No mediastinal mass or pleural effusion, USS abdomen—solid mass in left suprarenal region with calcification. X-ray of lower limbs show mottled and moth eaten pattern in tibia.

DIAGNOSIS AND DISCUSSION

Neuroblastoma—Hutchison's Type with Opsoclonus Myoclonus Cerebellar Syndrome

Neuroblastoma is the 2nd most common solid tumor in children second to brain tumor. It originates in neural crest of sympathetic nervous chain any where from posterior fossa to coccyx and in adrenals. Metastasis occurs into bone, bone marrow, liver, lung and brain. Biopsy will show round cell with Homer-Wright rosettes, areas of hemorrhage and calcification. It usually presets as a mass lesion in the neck, thorax or abdomen. Horner syndrome and paraplegia may occur. Ataxia and Opso–myoclonus are usually primary non-metastatic manifestations. Primary tumor may be undetectable in some cases. There may be hypertension in a few cases unlike all cases of pheochromocytoma. In pheochromocytoma, there is very slow inactivation of

catecholamines to VMA and HVA leading to hypertension.

Neuroblastoma may occur in families and there may be associated deletion of chromosome 1 and 17 and n-myc oncogene. **Pepper type** has primary and secondary lesions on right side of body with liver metastasis. **Hutchison type** has primary on right side with raccoon eyes and skull deposits. Raccoon eyes denote proptosis and ecchymosis due to orbital deposits. Intravenous pyelography (IVP) will show 'drooping lily appearance' with lateral and downward displacement of renal pelvis.

Staging of neuroblastoma

Pediatric oncology group	Evan's staging
• Stage A: Resectable tumor	• Stage I: Localized to organ of origin
• Stage B: Unresectable tumor	• Stage II: Extension beyond organ of origin, but not crossing midline
• Stage C: Tumor with node lymph metastasis	• Stage III: Extension beyond midline and bilateral lymph node
• Stage D: Metastasis beyond lymph node	• Stage IV: Remote disease in skeleton/soft tissue/distant node

Contd.

Contd.

- **Stage DS:** Small adrenal primary with metastasis to skin, liver/BM
- **Stage V:** S or Stage V with localized tumor with metastasis to skin, liver/BM

Stage S—denotes systemic involvement.

Urine VMA and monoclonal antibodies are elevated in neuroblastoma. Spontaneous remission may occur in some cases. Surgery, chemotherapy and radiotherapy are useful. Radiotherapy and excision are done for localized tumor. Chemotherapy is given for large tumors followed by surgery. Chemotherapy includes cyclophosphamide, doxorubicin, cisplastin, etoposide, melphalan, vincristine and carboplatin in various combinations.

CHAPTER 11

HEMATO ONCOLOGY

A 10-MONTH-OLD BABY WITH HEMATURIA AND RIGHT LUMBAR MASS

A 10-month-old baby with normal growth and development came with a bout of hematuria. The local doctor detected a palpable right lumbar mass probably renal. BP 110/80, other general and systemic examinations unremarkable.

DIAGNOSIS AND DISCUSSION

Wilms' Tumor/Nephroblastoma

Wilms' tumor is the most common renal neoplasm in children. It presents as an accidentally detected mass or with hematuria and hypertension in some cases. USS or X-ray will show curvilinear calcification and IVP will show medial displacement of renal pelvis unlike in neuroblasoma with lateral displacement. The tumor is smooth with firm consistency and may cross the midline. CT/MRI may show extension to IVC.

Wilms' tumor may occur in isolation or in association with chromosomal anomaly, 11p deletion with hemi hypertrophy, aniridia, genitourinary anomalies. Others are **WAGR syndrome** (Wilms' tumor, aniridia, genitourinary anomalies and retardation of mentation) and **Denys Drash syndrome** (Wilms' tumor, nephropathy and genitourinary anomalies).

In resectable tumor, immediate resection should be done followed by chemotherapy/radiotherapy. In large tumors, chemotherapy is beneficial using oncovin, dactinomycin and adriamycin. Prognosis is usually good in early cases.

Staging of Wilms' Tumor (Wilms' Tumor Study Group)

- Stage I: Completely resectable tumor with intact capsule
- Stage II: Completely respectable, but with local spread
- Stage III: Intra abdominal extension
- Stage IV: Hematogenous metastasis
- Stage V: Bilateral renal tumor.

SECTION 11.11 A 6-YEAR-OLD CHILD WITH ICSOL

A 6-year-old child presented with headache of one month duration, more in the morning and projectile vomiting. She had incoordination and intention tremor on right side of body. There was lateral rectus palsy right side. The child had head tilt to right side and neck rigidity. There was papilledema and bilateral up going plantar and brisk DTR. Growth and development were normal. CT scan showed a posterior fossa mass in the right cerebellum with solid and cystic areas and hydrocephalus.

DIAGNOSIS AND DISCUSSION

Posterior Fossa ICSOL—Cebellar Astrocytoma

CNS tumors are the 2nd most common malignancy in children, second to leukemia and the most common solid tumor in children, the second being neuroblastoma. CNS tumors arise from **neuroectodermal cells** (medulloblastoma/pineoblastoma), **glial cells** (astrocytoma, ependymoma, glioma), **embryonic remnants** (craniopharyngioma, dermoid, epidermoid tumors, neurofibromas, choroid plexus papilloma and teratomas).

Supratentorial and infratentorial tumors vary in clinical presentation. Infratentorial tumors obstruct CSF flow early in the course and manifest early with papilledema and is more common in children <12 years, but supratentorial tumors may remain obscure till late phase or present with focal signs. Both supra and infratentorial tumors occur with equal frequency in older age group. Chromosomal defects and defects in epidermal growth factors (EGF) may be seen in CNS tumors. Increased ICT will lead to sutural separation and positive crack pot sign or Macewen sign. Optic atrophy may occur in long standing ICT. In brainstem glioma, onset may be acute. Multiple cranial nerve plasies and pyramidal signs occur. Cerebellar astrocytoma is the most common posterior fossa tumor followed by medulloblastoma and brainstem glioma. Ispilateral cerebellar signs occur in astrocytoma whereas truncal ataxia and metastasis along CSF axis occur in medulloblastoma.

Craniopharyngioma is the most common supratentorial tumor in children. It produces calcification, compression of 3rd ventricle, hydrocephalus and visual defect—bitemporal hemianopsia due to compression of optic chiasma. Growth retardation, hypopituitarism, diabetes insipidus, hypothyroidism. Addison disease etc are the other manifestations of craniopharyngioma.

Choroid plexus papilloma leads to slowly progressive hydrocephalus. Choroid plexus carcinoma is malignant.

Diencephalic syndrome is due to lesion of hypothalamus with FTT, emaciation, but normal linear growth.

Metastasis/Secondary brain tumors are rare in children like leukemia or lymphoma. Facial nerve, sciatic or peroneal nerve palcies may occur in some cases with metastasis.

Treatment of CNS tumors include modalities like surgery, radiotherapy and chemotherapy. Stereotaxic biopsy and excision are now possible without conventional surgery. Similarly focal and focused radiotherapy and brachytherapy by implantation of radiation seeds are also possible.

The clinical triad for diagnosis includes headache, projectile vomiting and papilledema in posterior fossa tumors. In some cases, the tumor may be slow growing (pituitary adenoma) or may be isodense with brain tissue (brainstem glioma). Repeated imaging and follow up may be needed.

Pituitary or hypothalamic tumors may present with precocious puberty, galactorrhea etc. Gelastic seizures are seen in hypothalamic hamartoma. Surrogate markers of tumors include beta HCG, alpha feto protein etc. Meningeoma is a benign tumor.

Table 11.1: Response to iron therapy	
Day 1	Subjective improvement
Day 2	Erythrocyte hyperplasia
Day 3	Reticulocytosis
Day 4-30	Rise in Hb
1-3 months	Restoration of stores

Table 11.2: Conditions that lead to hypochromic microcytic anemia		
	Condition	Clinical features
1.	Iron deficiency anemia	- RDW increased, Low retic count
2.	Thalassemia	- Hemolytic anemia, High retic count
3.	Sideroblastic anemia	- Sideroblasts in BM, perinuclear collar of hemosiderin in nucleated RBCs
4.	Lead poisoning	- Basophilic stippling with high S lead
5.	Congenital non spherocytic hemolytic anemia	- Basophilic stippling with low S lead hemolytic anemia (Pyrimidine 5'Nucleotidase deficiency)

Table 11.3: Classification of Anemia based on RDW and MCV

Microcytic Homogeneous RDW-N	Microcytic Heterogeneous RDW-I	Normocytic Homogeneous RDW-N	Normocytic Heterogeneous RDW-I	Macrocytic Homogeneous RDW-N	Macrocytic Heterogeneous RDW-I
Heterozygous thalassemia	Iron deficiency anemia, HbS-Beta thalassemia	Normal, Chronic diseases, CML, HS	Mixed deficiency, Myelofibrosis, Sideroblastic	Aplastic anemia	B_{12}, Folate deficiency, Immune hemolytic anemia

Table 11.4: Treatment of acute leukemias

Phase I: Induction of Remission (4-6 weeks)

1. Vincristine – 1.5 mg/M^2/IV/week (up to 2 mg/dose)

2. Prednisolone – 40 mg/M^2/day/PO Q 8H (upto 60 mg/day)

3. L. Asparaginase – 10,000 U/M^2/IM/dose biweekly

Phase II: CNS Prophylaxis * (Triple intrathecal—Triple IT)

Weekly x 6 followed by 2 monthly for next 2 years.

Age	Methotrexate (mg)	Hydrocortisone (mg)	Cytosine Arabinoside (mg)
0-2 years	10	10	20
2-8 years	12.5	12.5	25
>8 years	15	16	30

* Cranial irradiation is not undertaken in initial therapy, it is done in CNS relapse

Phase III: Maintenance phase

1. 6 mercaptopurine (6 MP)—50 mg/M^2/PO/day

2. Methotrexate—20 mg/M^2/week/PO/IV/1M

Phase IV: Reinforcement Therapy

1. Vincristine—monthly once IV through out the course.

2. Prednisolone—PO for 1 week every month.

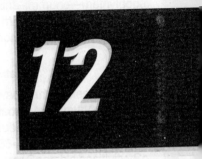

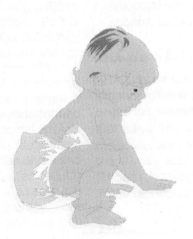

Nervous System

12

Nervous System

A 10-MONTH-OLD BABY WITH AN ABNORMALLY SMALL HEAD

A 10-month-old baby was brought with delayed development and abnormally small head. Baby's birth weight was 2.4 kg. No history of vomiting or seizures, baby could roll over, no sitting balance, no pincer grasp, social smile +. Mother had febrile illness in the first trimester.

On examination: Weight 8 kg, Length 70 cm, OFC 39 cm, AF just open, sutures palpable with step formation, large ears +, receding forehead +, No hypertonia/spasticity, DTR brisk, plantars both upgoing. Other systems examination unremarkable. Head circumference of both parents normal.

DIAGNOSIS AND DISCUSSION

1. **Primary microcephaly with developmental retardation.**
2. **Intrauterine infection with microcephaly.**

A diagnosis of cerebral palsy is not made in this case because there is no demonstrable central motor deficit like pyramidal or extrapyramidal signs. Receding forehead and large bat ears suggest primary microcephaly. Intrauterine infection is also possible due to 1st trimester pyrexia. But, there are no other features like hepatosplenomegaly.

Microcephaly is divided into primary or genetic microcephaly and secondary or non-genetic. In craniosynostosis/craniostenosis, brain growth is normal and so there will be features of increased ICT. Sutures will be prematurely closed with abnormal shape of head and sharp suture lines that are palpable like 'the keel of the ship'. In microcephaly, due to defective brain growth, there will be no features of ICT and the sutures will be felt 'overriding with step formation'.

Primary autosomal recessive (AR) microcephaly presents with severe MR, slanting forehead, prominent 'bat ears' and seizures. Primary autosomal dominant (AD) microcephaly presents with mild MR, slanting forehead, upward slant of eyes and seizures. Linear growth is usually normal. Microcephaly is <3SD and macrocephaly is >2SD compared to the normal.

In microcephaly, treatment is usually unsatisfactory Neuro developmental patterning (NDP) and seizure control are beneficial. In craniostenosis, craniotomy and craniofacial reconstructive surgery may benefit the child.

The different causes of microcephaly are given in Table 12.1.

CHAPTER 12

NERVOUS SYSTEM

SECTION 12.2 A 6-MONTH-OLD BABY WITH LARGE HEAD

A 6-month-old baby was brought with excessive crying and mild fever. He had a large head.

On examination: Growth-weight and height <5th centile, OFC-47 cm and development—social smile +, cooing sounds +, head control +, could not roll over or reach out for objects, vitals stable, sun setting sign +, AF bulging, swelling noted at lumbar spine region, hypertonia and pyramidal signs in both lower limbs. Baby had treatment for fever in a local hospital for 2 weeks prior to admission.

DIAGNOSIS AND DISCUSSION

Hydrocephalus, meningomyelocele with paraplegia probably Arnold Chiari Malformation Type II and meningitis.

Differential Diagnosis

1. **Hydrocephalus—post meningitic sequelae.**
2. **Intrauterine infection with hydrocephalus** in view of growth retardation and development delay.

In any baby with excessive crying and mild fever, meningitis should be ruled out. In infants, paradoxical irritability may be seen due to stretching of nerves in meningitis while handling. Generally, baby will get consoled while handling. In infants with open AF and relatively small spinal cord and relatively large foramen magnum, neck rigidity may not occur unlike in older children where spinal cord fills up the foramen magnum

and the skull is a closed box. It is always desirable to do repeat LP and document CSF clearance on completion of antibiotics as ongoing meningitis and partially treated meningitis may lead to more sequelae in young infants. Ongoing ventriculitis may also occur in some cases.

Large head may also occur in hydranencephaly, thick cranium as in rickets, osteopetrosis, skeletal dyplasias, widening of marrow spaces as in hemolytic anemias. Megalencephaly is due to storage disorders like Tay Sachs, Canavans disease etc.

X-ray skull may show silver beaten appearance due to increased ICT. Calcifications occur in periventricular region in CMV and diffuse calcification in toxoplasmosis. Imaging like cranial ultrasound is useful in infants with open AF. CT or MRI will show ventricular dilatation and any other associated defects.

Medical treatment includes antiedema measures and acetazolamide to decrease CSF production. Ventriculo-peritoneal or ventriculo-atrial shunt are useful in large collections. Treatment of underlying cause and physiotherapy are other management options. CSF study should be done to rule out ongoing infection before shunt operations. Bowel and bladder care are important in meningomyelocele. Folic acid supplement periconceptionally should be advised to prevent neural tube defect in subsequent pregnancy.

The different causes of hydrocephalus are summarised in Table 12.2.

SECTION 12.3

ONE YEAR OLD BOY WITH FEVER AND SEIZURE

A one-year-old boy was admitted with high fever and one episode of generalized seizure lasting for 10 minutes. There was no previous history of seizures, but had positive family history of febrile seizure in the father.

On examination: He was febrile and crying, but was feeding. Vitals stable except Temp 101° F, AF closed, throat was congested. There were no other positive findings. Growth and development normal.

DIAGNOSIS AND DISCUSSION

Febrile Convulsion

DD Meningitis

Meningitis should be ruled out in view of fever and increased crying. CSF study is usually done in first episode of febrile fit or when clinical suspicion of meningitis is there. It is worth eliciting a history of seizure disorder in the family, afebrile fits before and looking for neuro cutaneous markers, head trauma and perinatal insults or development delay. In normal children and those with seizure disorder, fever may lower seizure threshold. Even in epileptics, the first fit may be a febrile fit.

Febrile fit is divided into simple and complex or atypical. Simple febrile fit is a brief fit lasting for less than 10-15 minutes with normal sensorium before and after the fit. It is associated with rapid rise of temperature above 39°C in the age group 6 months to 6 years. It may also occur from 3 months of age and upto 8 years of age. **Atypical febrile fit** is diagnosed when fit lasts for > 15 minutes, focal fit, frequent fits in single episode of fever, with evidence of brain damage or EEG abnormalities persisting after 2 weeks of the fit. There is 9% increased chance for epilepsy in them compared to 1% in others. Mesial temporal sclerosis may be seen on imaging in some cases.

Seizure should be controlled with diazepam/ lorazepam along with control of fever by antipyretics and tepid sponging using lukewarm water. Ice sponging is not desirable due to unpleasant feel, shivering that may evoke further thermogenesis and vasoconstriction of skin blood vessels leading to increase in core temperature. Warm sponging will be pleasant and will lead to skin vasodilatation and heat loss and also subsequent faster evaporation of moisture leading to cooling of skin.

The chance for recurrence of febrile seizure is more especially in boys and when the first fit occurs below 1 year of age.

Prophylaxis includes hydrotherapy, antipyretics (oral or rectal) and oral or rectal diazepam for 2-3 days of fever in a dose of 0.2 mg-0.3 mg/kg/ dose. Clobazam is also beneficial instead of diazepam, which causes less drowsiness compared to diazepam. The dose is 0.25—0.5 mg/kg/dose 12 hourly. Long-term anticonvulsant are given in selected cases of atypical febrile fit for 1½ -3 years using phenobarbitone or valparin.

Other anti-epileptic drugs (AEDs) are not useful. Iron supplementation is also said to benefit those with breath holding spells and febrile fit. These two conditions have a temporal association with iron deficiency.

In focal/psychomotor/temporal lobe epilepsy, carbamazepine is given. Valparin in a broad spectrum AED. Myoclonic epilepsy has poor outcome and treatment includes nitrazepam, ACTH and ketogenic diet.

SECTION 12.4 — A 12-YEAR-OLD GIRL WITH PERSISTENT HEADACHE

A 12-year-old girl was brought with persistent headache for 2 months. She had headache in one of the frontal region associated with lacrimation and rhinorrhoea and often relieved by sleep or vomiting. Her mother had treatment for migraine in childhood. The girl also had psychological stress due to poor school performance.

On examination: Growth, development, vitals and physical examination within normal limits.

DIAGNOSIS AND DISCUSSION

Migraine—Cluster Headache

Differential Diagnosis:

1. Sinusitis.
2. Other extra cranial causes.
3. Refractory error.
4. Dental causes.
5. Psycho-somatic illness.
6. Tension headache—muscular/myogenic.
7. Abdominal epilepsy.
8. Trigeminal neuralgia.
9. ICSOL.

The term **'cephalalgia or cephalgia'** is used to denote headache due to any cause. Brain is insensitive to pain. Meninges and blood vessels are sensitive to pain.

Migraine is the most likely diagnosis in this girl. It is the most common type of vascular headache (Refer Table 12.3).

It is diagnosed by recurrent symptoms with symptoms free intervals and at least 3 out of the following 6 criteria:

1. GI disturbances.
2. Throbbing nature of headache.
3. Unilateral location of headache.
4. Relief with sleep.
5. Visual/sensory/motor aura.
6. Positive family history.

She has 1, 3, 4 and 6 features. The precipitating factors are anxiety, stress, hormonal changes, food allergies, exposure to bright light and loud notice, smell of certain perfumes, personality trait with high achievement. The chemical mediators are high serotonin and a vasodilation 'P' polypeptide. The other types of vascular headache are fever associated toxic headache and headache due to high BP.

Headache due to ICSOL and increased ICT are associated with morning headache and projectile vomiting and neurological localization.

Tension headache is dull or tight constant generalized headache and is associated with anxiety provoking circumstances. In sinusitis, purulent or blood stained discharge from nose and worsening during day time may be seen. There will be sinus tenderness and collections visible in X-ray of para nasal sinuses (PNS).

Refractory errors lead to eye strain. The child will be holding books closer to the face than elbow level. Moving closer to TV while watching will be observed.

Abdominal epilepsy presents with cyclical vomiting and butterfly sensation in abdomen and headache. EEG will be abnormal.

Migraine responds to antiemetics and analgesics. Cyproheptadine (serotonin antagonist) is useful in vascular headache, flunarizine in migraine, mefenamic acid in clutter headache and propranolol in tension headache. ENT, ophthalmic and psychological evaluation should be done before starting long term medications. Avoidance of offending light, sound, performs and other strong smell and food items like Chinese food, aginomoto, beef, chocolate, may be beneficial in some cases. Very rarely 'Alice in wonderland syndrome' may be associated with migraine.

SECTION 12.5
AN INFANT WITH ACUTE HEMIPLEGIA

A 10-month-old baby was admitted with weakness of right side of body. He had no fever and was well when he went to bed in the night.

On examination: Growth normal, developmental history normal. No anemia or polycythemia. Vitals stable. Dense facio-brachio-cural hemiplegia right involving face upper limb and lower limb with loss of conjunctival, abdominal, cremasteric reflexes. Other systems within normal limits.

DIAGNOSIS AND DISCUSSION

Acute infantile/young stroke or acute infantile hemiplegia (right), probably cerebral thrombosis involving left internal capulse due to Middle Cerebral Artery (MCA) thrombosis

Hemiplegia evolving overnight is usually due to thrombosis. Absence of alteration in sensorium and seizures exclude hemorrhage. Embolism is unlikely due to absence of predisposing factors like right to left shunt, infective endocarditis, cardiac arrhythmia, atrial myxoma etc. Embolism is more common into the left hemisphere due to the straight origin of left common carotid and internal carotid arteries compared to the right side, where it arises from the common brachiocephalic artery. Internal carotid artery thrombosis may follow injury to pharynx during fall with a pencil or lollypop stick in the mouth or following retropharyngeal abscess. Middle cerebral artery (MCA) thrombosis and venous thrombosis are more common in CCHDs with polycythemia.

Vasculitis syndrome may cause venous/arterial thrombosis. **'Moya Moya disease or puff of smoke disease'** is more common in girls and is characterised by basal artery occlusion and telangiectasia/collaterals that are picked up in angiogram as the puff of smoke. MR angiogram or Digital subtraction angiography will show it clearly. It presents with headache, bilateral motor paralysis and chorea. Left hemispherical lesions may lead to aphasia by affecting speech centre.

Superficial or deep vein thrombosis may occur in meningitis, otitis, mastoiditis, dehydration, polycythemia, malaria and vasculitis syndromes like SLE. Presence of anti-phospholipid antibody (APLA syndrome) is a risk factor for thrombosis. The 3 Ps associated with venous sinus thrombosis are pregnancy, puerperium and use of oral pill. Anemia in addition to polycythemia also may cause thrombosis due to rigid RBCs with decreased oxygen delivery. Hypercoagulable states may occur in deficiency of Anti-thrombin III. Protein S and C, presence of anti-cardiolipin antibodies, lupus anticoagulants and anti-phospholipid antibodies (APLA).

Intracranial hemorrhage (ICH) usually occurs in AV malformations. It follows severe unilateral headache always confined to the same side of the head. Associated bruit may be heard on auscultation on the affected side of head. ICH can also occur in hemophilia, ITP and collagen vascular diseases/vasculitis syndromes. The other causes of infantile/young stroke include hyperlipidemia, metabolic conditions like homocystinuria, infections like herpes encephalitis, cerebral tumors and complicated migraine.

Treatment aims at early re-perfusion of affected area, neuroprotection, nootropics and rehabilitation by physiotherapy.

1. **Early re-perfusion:** Adequate hydration should be achieved. Thrombolytic agents like urokinase, streptokinase and recombinant tissue plasminogen activator (r TPA) may be beneficial for reperfusion within 6 hours of onset. These agents are contraindicated in hemorrhage. Among anticoagulants, heparin is not safe. Low molecular weight (LMW) heparin may be used during first 48 hours. Antiplatelet drugs like aspirin (5 mg/kg/day), dipyridamole and ticlopidine are useful.

Vasodilators like pentoxyfiline may help to improve collateral circulation.

2. **Neuroprotective agents:** Calcium channel blockers like nimodipine if started with 12 hours of onset and N Methyl D Aspartate Receptor blockers (NMDA) may be useful in some cases. Inhibitors of excitatory neurotransmitters like glutamate and glycine antagonists are also tried. Antioxidants and nitric oxide donors are other agents that are used.

3. **Nootropics:** These are agents that improve brain function. Piracetam (100 mg/kg/day) IV for 4 days from day 1 of onset followed by oral medicine for 1 month may improve aphasia and neurological function. **Surgical intervention** may be essential in arterial malformation and for creating anastomosis in thrombosis.

SECTION 12.6

A CHILD WITH BIRTH ASPHYXIA AND NEUROLOGICAL DISABILITY AND SEIZURES

A 2½-year-old girl was brought with development delay and toe walking. She was a term LBW baby with BW 2.2 kg and had special care for birth asphyxia and neonatal seizure.

On examination: Growth < 3 centile including OFC. Development: social smile +, vocalises and combines mono syllables, she can sit and walk with support, has toe walking with stiff tendo achillis. Difficulty in swallowing +, dysarthria +, concomitant squint +, All 4 limbs showed clasp knife hypertonia with exaggerated DTR, clonus +, tendo achillis contracture +, abdominal reflexes–retained, bilateral up going plantars. Muscle power grade III plus. Seizures were controlled with valproate. Vision and hearing grossly normal.

DIAGNOSIS AND DISCUSSION

Cerebral palsy with spastic quadriplegia, seizure disorder, developmental delay and malnutrition

Cerebral palsy (CP) is non progressive central motor deficit of posture and movement due to defect in the developing brain, often associated with MR, special sense organ defects and epilepsy. It was first described by Little as 'Little' diplegia' in premature babies. It may be the sequelae of perinatal asphyxia, perinatal infection, metabolic disorders, neonatal jaundice, neonatal seizures or developmental malformation of the brain. The incidence of CP 2/1000 noticed in olden days is remaining same even now with the best

possible obstetric and neonatal care. Hence, the role of developmental malformation/vulnerability to asphyxia is postulated as an important cause of CP rather than iatrogenic causes.

Around 10% of asphyxiated babies develop CP and 10% of CPs give a definite history of asphyxia. In those with low APGAR score persisting at 10 mts, the incidence of CP in 60%.

Spastic monoplegia is usually seen in preterm babies with mild disability and usually not associated with seizure/MR/special sense organ defects. Spastic diplegia is the usual type in preterm babies with lower limb affection more than upper limb and usually not associated with other disabilities. In preterm babies, periventricular lower limb fibres are more affected during hypoxia as deeper blood vessels are less and superficial cortical vessels are more before maturity. Whereas in term babies, the insult occurs in the superficial cortex due to end arteries superficially, with little collaterals (circle of Willis), but with more deeper vessels.

Spastic hemiplegia is due to an insult occurring in one hemispheric cortex and upper limb is more affected than lower limb. Due to cortical involvement, there may be seizures and MR. There may be shortening of the affected side and associated focal or generalised seizures. The affected hemisphere i.e., opposite to the clinical disability will show atrophy or porencephalic cyst. Spastic triplegia may also occur, with 3 limbs affected. Spastic quadriplegia usually occur in full term babies with asphyxia. It is usually associated with seizure and mental retardation. In FT babies, deeper penetrating vessels are more compared to the superficial cortical end arteries without mutual communication. Pseudobulbar palsy is spastic (UMN) with increased jaw jerk and bulbar palsy is flaccid (LMN).

In dystonia/chorio athetoid CP, there is cogwheel rigidity and extra pyramidal signs. There may be associated deafness. It is usually associated with bilirubin encephalopathy/kernicterus leading to 'status marmoratus' and gliosis of basal ganglia.

Atonic/hypotonic CP usually evolves into spasticity with age and there is more severe MR. In double hemiplegia, both upper limbs are more affected than lower limbs. In mixed type, there is spasticity and choreo-athetoid movements.

In CP, there is no progressive deterioration of functions, but, there will be slow attainment of milestones. Antigravity muscles are more weak leading to postural abnormality, foot drop, tendoachillis contracture etc. CNS Imaging, EEG, vision and hearing evaluation are mandatory. Thyroid function test, TORCH Screen, Karyotyping etc. may be done in selected cases.

Differential diagnosis of CP is slowly progressive neuro degenerative disorders. Some of these manifest in infancy and childhood and others only in adulthood.

Treatment includes multi-disciplinary team approach with physiotherapy and occupational therapy. Seizure control, special schooling and appliances are beneficial. Tendon lengthening operation, Rhizotomy for reducing severe in hypertonia in spastic diplegia and botox (botulinium toxin) or phenol injections into affected spastic limb are also being tried. Benzodizepines or baclofen for spasticity, carbamazepine for dystonia and levodopa for athetosis are also beneficial.

'Spastic society' is a support group comprising of patients, their parents and well wishers. Community based rehabilitation (CBR) and Home based rehabilitation (HBR) are breakthrough in this field as centre based rehabilitation cannot be made available to all and at the doorstep (Also Refer Chapter 16.5).

The various classifications of CP are given in Table 12.4. The various levels of retardation and guidelines for rehabilitation are given in Table 12.5. The common neuro-degenerative disorders are given in Table 12.6.

In spasticity, there is hypertonia in certain groups like anti-gravity muscles, but in rigidity both agonists and antagonists have increased tone. Abdominal reflexes are retained in congenital hemiplegia, but are lost in acquired hemiplegia.

CNS localisation an art add on to science (Refer Table 12.7). The various cranial nerves are shown in Figure 12.1.

CHAPTER 12

NERVOUS SYSTEM

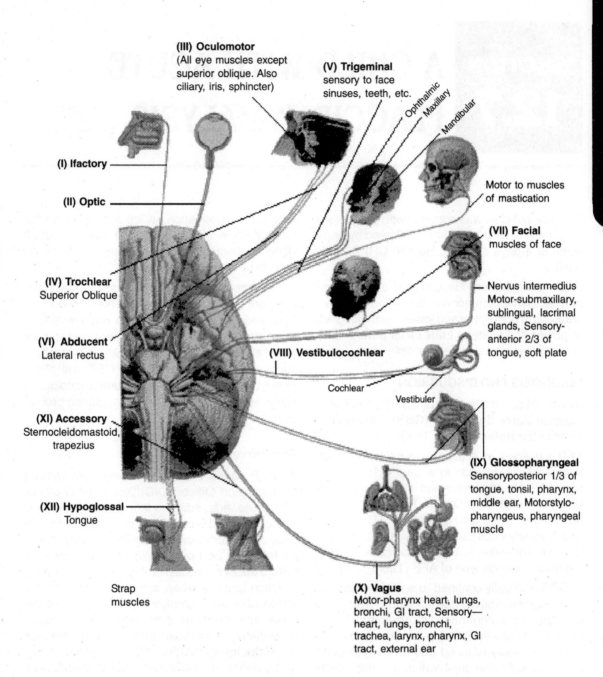

(III) Oculomotor
(All eye muscles except superior oblique. Also ciliary, iris, sphincter)

(V) Trigeminal
sensory to face sinuses, teeth, etc.

Ophthalmic

Maxillary

Mandibular

(I) Ifactory

(II) Optic

Motor to muscles of mastication

(VII) Facial
muscles of face

(IV) Trochlear
Superior Oblique

Nervus intermedius
Motor-submaxillary, sublingual, lacrimal glands, Sensory-anterior 2/3 of tongue, soft plate

(VI) Abducent
Lateral rectus

(VIII) Vestibulocochlear

Cochlear

Vestibuler

(XI) Accessory
Sternocleidomastoid, trapezius

(IX) Glossopharyngeal
Sensoryposterior 1/3 of tongue, tonsil, pharynx, middle ear, Motorstylo-pharyngeus, pharyngeal muscle

(XII) Hypoglossal
Tongue

Strap muscles

(X) Vagus
Motor-pharynx heart, lungs, bronchi, GI tract, Sensory—heart, lungs, bronchi, trachea, larynx, pharynx, GI tract, external ear

Fig. 12.1: The cranial nerves

Fig. No. 49 (Plate 12)

CHAPTER 12

NERVOUS SYSTEM

SECTION 12.7   A CHILD WITH ACUTE FLACCID PARALYSIS (AFP)

A 7-year-old child was admitted with progressive weakness of both lower limbs followed by upper limbs of 4 days duration. He had URI 2 weeks back.

On examination: Growth and development normal, Sensorium normal, B/L symmetric LMN paralysis of both upper and lower limbs with grade III power and bilateral LMN facial paralysis, no sensory involvement, bladder distended.

DIAGNOSIS AND DISCUSSION

Acute Flaccid Paralysis (AFP) Probably Guillain-Barré Syndrome (GBS)—Ascending Type (Also Refer Section 16.8)

AFP is defined as acute flaccid paralysis of less than 4 weeks duration in a child < 15 years of age. AFP should be informed immediately to the District RCH/Medical Officer. The target for AFP reporting is 1/one lakh population <15 years of age. Recently it has been increased to 2. In places where poliomyelitis is almost eradicated, GBS is the most common type of AFP (Table 12.8).

GBS is usually confined to spinal nerves, but may progress to bulbar palsy or lead to diaphragm paralysis or autonomic disturbances. Nerve conduction velocity (NCV) in the affected nerves will be markedly reduced due to demyelination and EMG will show denervation patterns. Distal muscles show more weakness than proximal, unlike in myopathies with more affected proximal muscles. Post infectious demyelination is often less severe compared to the rare type of parain-fectious demyelination, which occurs during the viral infection without the usual latent period. It denotes altered immune response, which usually tend to be more severe.

Treatment includes physiotherapy and supportive care. Plasmapheresis and methyl prednisolone and IVIG may be tried to remove/reduce demyelinating antibodies. Bowel and bladder care are of extreme importance. Nursing in 'water bed' will help to avoid bed sore. CSF will show pleocytosis in first week and albumino cytological dissociation in 2nd week, i.e., increased protein with few cells.

AFP Surveillance

All AFP cases should be reported to District Immunisation Officer (DIO)/District RCH officer with name, age, address etc. This is called 'line listing'. An EPID no: should be obtained for the case and 2 stool samples (8 g/thumb size) should be taken at 24 hours apart and sent for viral culture under cold chain facility. The yield for virus isolation is more when sample is sent within 2 weeks of onset of paralysis. DIO should visit the case and confirm it as AFP. DIO should immediately undertake **'ring immunization or outbreak immunization (OBI)'** in the locality by giving minimum 500 doses of OPV to underfive children residing in a 5 km radius area in a rural setting or among 3000-5000 population in an urban setting. The stool culture report should be obtained and if positive the case will be confirmed as polio. If negative, the case can be discarded as negative. If stool sample is insufficient, the case should be referred for expert review before discarding the case. In doubtful cases, CSF study, nerve conduction studies etc. may be done to differentiate between GBS, transverse myelitis and polio. All AFP cases should be followed up on 60th day to look for residual paralysis. This can be achieved through the surveillance network even if the child shifts residence or move out to another area or country by contacting the regional health team or WHO surveillance team.

In case of a confirmed case of polio, it should be treated as a medical emergency and **Mop Up Immunization (MUI)** should be undertaken by giving 2 doses of OPV to underfive children at one month interval in that region and the neighbouring states.

Pulse Polio Immunization (PPI) is undertaken on National Immunization Days (NIDs) by giving 2 extra doses at 1 month interval on a national/continental basis to eliminate wild virus and flood the vaccine virus in the community. For polio eradication, routine immunization should also be strengthened. Out of the P_1, P_2 and P_3 viruses, P_2 is eradicated in India.

Vaccine Associated Polio (VAP) is rare. Suspected cases should be confirmed by viral culture, isolation and serotyping. It is about 1/> one million doses and usually by P_2 virus.

Spinal Cord Tumors: Bladder involvement usually occurs in spinal cord tumors and nerve root involvement as in GBS. In spinal cord **intramedullary tumors** like astrocytoma, ependymoma etc. bladder involvement is early. In **extramedullary tumors** like extradural lesions due to deposit from neuroblastoma or lymphoma or intradural due to neurofibroma or meningioma, bladder involvement may be late. MRI scan is ideal for confirmation of such lesions. Extramedullary tumors may present with **Brown Sequard syndrome** with ipsilateral spasticity and contralateral loss of pain and temp.

Bladder Involvement: Cortical lesions lead to uninhibited contractile bladder with frequent voiding (Refer Fig. 12.2).

UMN lesions between pons and sacral micturition centre leads to UMN spastic bladder and sphincter and lesions at the sacral micturition centre leads to two types of neurogenic bladder:

i. Type A: Hyporeflexive detrusor with spastic sphincter with enormous distension and over flow incontinence; and

II. Type B: Hyperreflexive detrusor and flaccid sphincter with urinary incontinence.

In conus-cauda lesions and peripheral neuropathy, there will be flaccid (UMN) autonomous bladder Fig. 12.2.

Bladder innervation is given is Table 12.9.

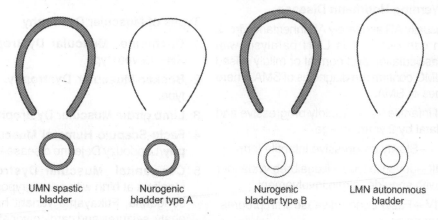

| UMN spastic bladder | Nurogenic bladder type A | Nurogenic bladder type B | LMN autonomous bladder |

Fig. 12.2: Types of bladder

CHAPTER 12

NERVOUS SYSTEM

SECTION 12.8 A 5-MONTH-OLD FLOPPY INFANT

A 5-month-old baby with generalised muscle weakness was brought with tachypnea. He was born of consanguinous marriage. He had no milestones except social smile. First child died in infancy due to similar illness.

On examination: Severe hypotonia with ragged doll appearance/pitched frog appearance. Generalised muscle wasting, face bright with normal eye movements. Tachypnea noted with paradoxical movement of chest wall and abdomen. Tongue showed fasciculation. CPK 200 IU/L (N <160), Fundus normal, no hepatosplenomegaly, DTR absent. ENMG (Electro-neuro myogram): Nerve conduction normal, fibrillation potential and denervation pattern.

DIAGNOSIS AND DISCUSSION

Spinal Muscular Atrophy–Infantile Form— Type I Werding Hoffmann Disease

SMA is usually AR and rarely AD inheritance/fresh mutation can occur. It is LMN paralysis with tongue fasciculation and normal or mildly raised CPK. ENMG confirm the diagnosis of SMA. There are 4 types of SMA.

Type I infantile form—rapidly progressive and severe, fatal by 2 years of age.

Type II—Slowly progressive infantile form.

Type III—Juvenile type—Kugelbreg Welander disease with shoulder girdle involvement.

Type IV—Fazio Londe disease with progressive bulbar palsy.

Juvenile Amyotropic Lateral sclerosis is degeneration of anterior horn cells and corticospinal tract with onset in late adolescence.

Treatment is unsatisfactory and includes supportive care and physiotherapy to prevent contractures. Many children may handle computer keyboard, but writing with pencil may be difficult. The genetic defect of SMA is on chromosome 5. It is the second most common neuromuscular disease following Duchenne muscular dystrophy. SMA may occur in non consanguinous parents due to the clustering of the mutant gene in many families.

In **muscular dystrophies**, CPK is markedly increased and there may be cardiomyopathy, NCV normal. EMG—Myopathic pattern. There may be pseudohypertrophy of calf muscles in DMD.

Types of Muscular Dystrophy

1. **Duchenne Muscular Dystrophy (DMD).** XR—Severe type.

2. **Becker Muscular Dystrophy.** XR—Milder type.

3. **Limb girdle Muscular Dystrophy**—AR.

4. **Facio-Scapulo Humeral Muscular Dystrophy**/Landouzy Dejerine disease—AD.

5. **Congenital Muscular Dystrophy**–AR— Manifest at birth with arthrogryposis multiplex congenita, Fukayama variant has microcephaly, seizures and cardiomyopathy.

6. **Myotonic Muscular Dystrophy**/Steinert Disease—AD—myotonia manifest by 3-5 years, EMG—'Diver Bomb discharges', Myotonia is usually elicited by a shake hand.

7. **Myotonia Congenita**/Thomsen Disease.

   AD/AR, Myotonia manifest by 2-3 years and there may be pseudohypertrophy of calf muscles.

   Paramyotonia–Myotonia in cold temperature only.

8. **Metabolic and Endocrine myopathies:**

   Glycogen storage disease—Pompes, lipid myopathies (muscle carnitine deficiency) hypo/hyperkalemic periodic paralysis, Vit E deficiency.

Hypothyroidism with pseudo hypertrophy of calf muscle is called Kocher Debre Semelaigne syndrome.

9. **Mitochondrial myopathies**—exclusively inherited from mother.

   a. Kerns Sayre syndrome.

   b. Chronic progressive ophthalmoplegia.

   c. MERRF—Myoclonic Epilepsy and Ragged Red Fibre syndrome.

   d. MELAS–Mitochondrial myopathy, encephalopathy, lactic acidosis stroke like episodes syndrome.

   The various causes of floppy infant are given in Table 12.10.

SECTION 12.9 A GIRL WITH FEVER AND ALTERED SENSORIUM

A 12-year-old girl was admitted with fever, altered sensorium, convulsions of 1 day duration. She was well previously.

On examination: No meningeal signs. Growth and development normal. She was febrile, Tachycardia +, tachypnea +, BP–normal and she was unresponsive. No papilloedema, Brisk DTR—both lower limbs with upgoing plantars.

DIAGNOSIS AND DISCUSSION

Acute Encephalitis Syndrome

Differential Diagnosis: ADEM

1. Acute Disseminated Encephalomyelitis (ADEM)—in view of the clinical picture with brisk DTR suggestive of spinal cord demyelination.

2. Encephalitis may be specific or non-specific. JE may lead to personality and behavioral changes and Herpes Encephalitis may lead to focal seizures and focal neurological signs and EEG will show PLEDs (periodic lateralizing electrical discharges). Entero viruses, measles etc are the others.

3. Encephalopathy: Reye Encephalopathy may follow viral infection with repeated vomiting, hypoketotic hypoglycemia, ICT raised without focal deficits.

Imaging–MRI will pick up demyelination. CSF study may be normal or may show mild pleocytosis without hypoglycorrhachia and normal or raised protein.

ADEM or acute disseminated encephalomyelitis is a demyelinating disorder involving brain and spinal cord. There may be altered sensorium, convulsion and features of spinal cord white matter demyelination leading to brisk reflexes. Differential diagnosis of ADEM is **Acute encephalitis syndrome**. MRI can pick up the demyelinating lesions. It may run a relapsing course with myelination occurring again at the same site unlike **multiple sclerosis** involving demyelinating plaques occurring at different sites at different point of time. In ADEM, IV gamma-globulin, plasmapheresis and supportive care may be beneficial. Acyclovir and ceftriaxone are also usually given in view of associated viral/pyogenic infection.

Table 12.1: Differential diagnosis of small head

I. **Primary microcephaly**
- AD microcephaly
- Chromosomal anomalies
- Cornelia de Lange (limb anomalies and synophrys)
- AR microcephaly
- Dysmorphic syndromes
- Rubinstein Taybi (broad thumb + beaked nose)
- Smith Lemli Optiz (dolicocephaly+ ptosis)

II. **Secondary microcephaly**
- Radiation embryopathy
- Fetal hydantoin syndrome
- HIE/Cerebral palsy
- Maternal PKU
- IU infections
- Fetal alcohol syndrome
- Sequel of meningoencephalitis
- CNS malformation

III. **Conditions associated with craniostenosis**

Craniostenosis lead to abnormal shape of head.
1. **Scaphocephaly**—fusion of sagittal suture.
2. **Plagiocephaly**—abnormal shape in certain areas.
   (1) Frontal plagiocephaly—fusion of coronal and sphenofrontal suture.
   (2) Occipital plagiocephaly—fusion of lambdoid suture.
3. **Trigonocephaly**—fusion of metopic suture.
4. **Turricephaly**—fusion of coronal, sphenofrontal and sphenoethmoid sutures.
5. **Brachycephaly**—fusion of bilateral coronal sutures.
6. **Oxycephaly/Acrocephaly**—high skull due to fusion of coronal suture.
7. **Clover leaf skull/deformity**—prominent frontal bones with or without hydrocephalus.
8. **Lacunar skull**—bony ridging and multiple bony depressions similar to silver beaten appearance of increased ICT.
9. **Cranio-facial dysostosis**/Genetic/Sporadic syndromes with craniostenosis.
   i. **Crouzon syndrome**—AD inheritance with brachycephaly and proptosis.
   ii. **Apert syndrome**—AD/sporadic with Crouzon facies and syndactyly with or without cleft palate.
   iii. **Carpenter syndrome**—AR inheritance with clover leaf skull, post axial polysyndactyly, corneal opacity, CHD and coxa/genu valgus.
   iv. **Chotzen syndrome**—AR with plagiocephaly, brachysyndactyly and ptosis.
   v. **Pfeiffer syndrome**—AD/sporadic with turricephaly, brachysyndactyly and hypertension.

Table 12.2: Causes of hydrocephalus

1. Aqueductal stenosis—4th ventricle not dilated.
2. 4th ventricle outflow obstruction—4th ventricle also dilated.
3. Intrauterine infection especially Toxoplasmosis/CMV.
4. Arnold Chiari Malformation (ACM) type I—late presentation with headache, neck pain, diplegia and urinary frequency and cerebellar tonsil herniation.
5. ACM type II—early presentation with meningomyelocele and paraplegia.
6. Dandy Walker malformation—cystic expansion of 4th ventricle with or without agenesis of posterior cerebellar vermis and corpus callosum.
7. Post meningitic sequela with obstructive hydrocephalus due to obstruction within ventricular spaces.
8. Post meningitic sequela with communicating hydrocephalus—communicating with cisterns and subarachnoid space due to scarring of absorptive subarachnoid villi.
9. Increased CSF production—Choroid plexus papilloma.
10. Tumors especially posterior fossa tumors leading to CSF blockage.

Table 12.3: Types of migraine
1. **Common migraine**—no aura.
2. **Classic migraine**—with aura.
3. **Migraine variants**—cyclical vomiting.
4. **Complicated migraine**—with vertebro basilar insufficiency, ophthalmoplegia, hemiplegia.
5. **Cluster headache**—with unilateral lacrimation and rhinorrhoea.

Table 12.4: Various classifications of CP

Physiologic	Topographic	Etiologic	Functional
Spastic	Monoplegia	Prenatal	Class I- No disability
Hypo/Atonic	Diplegia	Natal	Class II - Mild limitation
Dystonic	Hemiplegia	Postnatal	Class III - Significant limitation
Choreo-Athetoid	Triplegia	Perinatal	Class IV - No useful activity
Ataxic	Quadriplegia		
Mixed	Double hemiplegia		

Table 12.5: Levels of retardation and functional rehabilitation

Mild retardation	Mainstreaming as per developmental age or special schooling
Moderate retardation	Special schooling/stereotyped workshop activities
Severe retardation	Training for Activation of daily Living (ADL)
Profound retardation	Custodian care preferably at home by the mother rather than in a common facility

Table 12.6: Common neuro degenerative diseases

1. Storage disorders–Tay Sachs, Sandhoff's, Neiman Pick, sialidosis (cherry red spot and metabolic screen).
2. Leukodystrophies—Alexander's disease with macrocephaly, Canavan with macrocephaly and increased urinary N. Acetyl aspartic acid, MLD with metachromatic granules in urine and diagnostic sural nerve biopsy, Krabbe Disease with hypertonia and delayed nerve conduction and globoid histiocytes in white matter.
3. Spino cerebellar ataxias–Ataxia telengiectasia, Friedreich's ataxia.
4. Extrapyramidal degenerations—Huntington's chorea.
5. Mineral metabolism—Copper-Wilson disease and Menkes kinky hair disease, Iron-Hallervorden Spatz disease.
6. Others—Rett syndrome with acquired microcephaly and hand washing movement and ataxia (Female), Heller's (Male counterpart to Rett).
7. Multiple sclerosis.
8. Slow virus–SSPE (Measles virus), Rubella, CMV, HIV. Subacute spongiform encephalopathies—Kuru, Creutzfeldt-Jakob disease (CJD/ mad cow disease).
9. Leighs encephalopathy.
10. Peroxisomal disorder.

Table 12. 7: Localisation of CNS Pathology

1. **Cortex**—Contralateral paralysis with or without loss of cortical sensations like touch localisation, two-point discrimination, stereognosis and graphesthesia, presence of altered sensorium and convulsion and also aphasia when dominant hemisphere is affected.

2. **Subcortical areas**—Less dense contralateral hemiplegia with variable sensory loss, Convulsion may occur due to cortical edema.

3. **Internal capsule**—Contralateral dense facio-brachiocrural hemiplegia with or without sensory loss.

4. **Midbrain—Weber syndrome**—Ipsilateral LMN 3rd nerve palsy with contralateral hemiplegia.

5. **Pons—Milard Gubler**—Ipsilateral LMN 7th nerve palsy with contralateral hemiplegia (6th N plays has no localizing value, it may be affected in any increased ICT), **Pontine hemorrhage** presents with pyrexia, pinpoint pupil and paralysis (3Ps).

6. **Medulla**—Ipsilateral LMN bulbar palsy of IX-X cranial nerves and contralateral hemiplegia with pooling of secretion and dysphagia (Similar pooling of secretion and dysphagia may occur in bilateral UMN bulbar palsy as in cerebral palsy. This is called 'pseudobulbar palsy', but there will be exaggerated jaw jerk and preserved gag reflex).

7. **Spinal cord**—Ipsilateral motor paralysis with loss of posterior column sensation and contralateral loss of pain and temp. Spinal cord lesions are localized by **sensory level** according to dermatomes, **motor level** according to muscles involved and **reflex level** according to DTR and superficial reflexes like anal, cremasteric, planter, abdominal etc.

   a. **Sensory level**—Xiphisternum—T6

      Subcostal—T8

      Umbilicus—T10

      Groin—T12

   b. **Motor level**—Biceps C5, C6

      Triceps—C6,C7

      Quadriceps—L2,L3, L4

      Gastrocnemius—S1,S2

   c. **Reflex level**—Conjunctival Afferent Vth nerve and Efferent VIIth, Abdominal T6—T12

      Plantar—L5, S1

      Cremasteric—L1-L2

      Anal—S3-S4.

8. **Position of eyes**

   Doll's eye present—intact brainstem connections.

   Persistent upward gaze—pineal lesion.

   Persistent gaze to opposite side of lesion—irritation lesions like hemorrhage.

   Persistent gaze to same side of lesion—irritating brainstem lesions.

9. **Nystagmus**

   Cerebellar lesions—Pendular nystagmus with slow component to midline especially intentional nystagmus.

   Labyrinthine lesions—Rotary nystagmus with vertigo.

   Congenital eye lesions—Roving nystagmus due to lack of visual fixation.

CHAPTER 12

NERVOUS SYSTEM

Table 12.8: Differential diagnosis of AFP

1. **Poliomyelitis:** It is viral infection with destruction of anterior horn cells. It presents with fever, myalgia, asymmetric motor paralysis and post polio muscular atrophy. There may be pleocytosis in the CSF with normal or raised protein during acute phase. Nerve conduction will be normal.

2. **GBS:** It is a post viral demyelination of nerve roots. It presents with symmetric ascending or descending paralysis with or without sensory numbness/paraesthesia and autonomic disturbances leading to hypertension. Albumino cytological dissociation may be seen in 2nd week of illness with increase in protein more than the increase in the cells in the CSF. There may be complete recovery in most cases and residual paralysis may occur in some cases. Nerve conduction will be very much delayed.

3. **Transverse myelitis:** It may be due to viral inflammation or immune mediated demyelination of a spinal cord segment with a definite sensory motor and reflex level. Flaccid paralysis will soon evolve into UMN/spastic paralysis below the level of the lesion. Initially DTR may be absent due to spinal shock, but plantars may be upgoing. CSF may be normal or may show slightly elevated protein and cells. It may lead to complete recovery or residual paraplegia.

4. **Traumatic neuritis:** It follows an IM injection to sciatic nerve leading to local paralysis and it presents with foot drop, absent ankle jerk and preserved knee jerk and delayed nerve conduction only in the sciatic nerve.

Table 12.9: ABCS of bladder innervation

A. **Alpha adrenergic**—Sympathetic T11-L2, through Hypogastric nerve → Sphincter contraction.

B. **Beta adrenergic**—Sympathetic—T11-L2 through Hypogastric nerve →Detrusor relaxation.

C. **Cholinergic**—Parasympathic S2-S4, through Pelvic Nerve→Detrusor contraction.

S. **Somatic**–Motor S2-S4, through Pudendal nerve→Sphincter relaxation.

Table 12.10: Causes of floppy infant and LMN paralysis

1. **Cortex**–Hypotonic CP-Brisk reflexes, central motor deficit with or without mental retardation.
2. **Anterior horn cell**—SMA, poliomyelitis, progressive motor neuron degenerations like Pena Shokeir and Marden Walker syndromes.
3. **Nerve root**—Guillain Barré syndrome.
4. **Peripheral nerve**—HSMN—Hereditary sensory motor neuropathy, post diphtheretic paralysis, Refsum's disease, toxic neuropathies, polyarteritis nodosa, Hansen's disease.
   Types of HSMN:
   Type I: Peroneal Muscular Atrophy–AD–Stork leg foot drop, pes cavus.
   Type II: Peroneal Muscular Atrophy—Axonal type— AD—Slowly progressive.
   Type III: Dijerine Sottas disease—AD with nerve thickening.
   In HSMN, CPK is normal and EMG—Myopathic pattern.
5. **Autonomic Neuropathies**—Riley Day—Familial Dysautonomia
6. **Myoneural Junction**—Myasthenia Gravis.
   Botulinum toxin, organo-phosphorous poison.
7. **Muscle**—Myositis, Dermatomyositis.
   Myopathies, Muscular Dystrophies (CPK raised in dystrophies).
   Benign Congenital Hypotonia—improves in later life, AD.
   In congenital myopathies, CPK is normal and NCV is normal.
   Types of myopathies:
   1. Myotubular.
   2. Nemaline rod.
   3. Central core

Fig. Nos. 35 to 45 (Plates 8 to 11) for various CNS and related conditions.

13

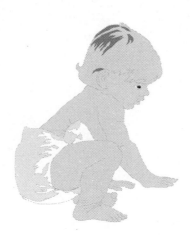

Endocrinology

A CHILD WITH SEVERE SHORT STATURE AND NORMAL INTELLIGENCE

A 6-year-old child was brought for evaluation of short stature. He was normal at birth (BW 3.2 kg) and growth retardation was noticed around one year of age. Dietary intake was normal.

On examination: Height 86 cm, Weight 11 kg and OFC 48 cm. Development–Normal. He was a good student studying in Std I. Vital signs normal. Blood counts, urine. RE, RFT, LFT–within normal limits. X-ray wrist: two carpals only. General and systemic examination within normal limits except growth retardation. No dysmorphism. There was no family history of similar short stature in childhood or adulthood among parents or close relatives.

DIAGNOSIS AND DISCUSSION
Hypopituitarism

Differential Diagnosis: Other Causes of Short Stature

1. Laron syndrome (End organ defect—GH normal)
2. Somatomedin/IGF/IGF Binding protein (IGFBP) deficiency
3. Constitutional/Maturational Growth Delay (MGD)
4. Syndromic dwarfing: Seckel syndrome, Russel Silver syndrome
5. Nutritional dwarfing
6. Emotional deprivation
7. Chronic systemic diseases
8. Primordial dwarfing
9. Genetic/Racial/Familial Short Stature
10. Others: Skeletal/Metabolic/Chromosomal/ Endocrine defects.

Growth Assessment (Also Refer Section 2.1)

Expected Weight = 20 kg, Height = 116 cm and OFC – 51 cm

Weight for age–11/20 × 100 = 55% (Grade IV PEM-IAP)

Height for age–86/116 ×100 = 74% (3rd Degree stunting–Waterlow)

Weight for Height–11/12 × 100 = 91.6% (No wasting–Waterlow).

OFC–3 cm less than expected, but development and intelligence normal. Chronological Age (CA) = 6 years, Height Age (HA) = 2 years, Mental Age (MA) = 6 years and Bone Age (BA) = around 1 year only. At 6 years–5-6 carpals and epiphysis of lower end of radius are expected. Here, CA = MA > HA > BA. This points to an endocrine cause without mental retardation as BA is the most severely affected and MA is least affected. In Hypothyroidism, MA will also be affected. Dietary history and clinical features do not suggest malnutrition and on examination wasting is absent. In malnutrition, CA > HA = BA, MA will be variable. In MGD, CA > HA = BA and MA = CA. Syndromic malformation and primordial dwarfing are unlikely due to absence of clinical features and absence of growth retardation at birth.

Retarded height age without significant wasting point to endocrine cause supported by retarded bone age. In hypothyroidism, mental age is retarded and in hypopituitarism, mental age is normal. Normal growth at birth and growth failure becoming evident later and a growth velocity less than 4-5 cm per year is suggestive of hypopituitarism. Some cases of hypopituitarism may have hypoglycemia/associated panhypopituitary with TSH, ACTH and GNRH deficiency and micropenis. Those with destructive lesions of pituitary may show visual defect, enlargement or destruction of sella and calcification or ICSOL on imaging as in craniopharyngeoma. Confirmation of GH deficiency is by 'stimulation test'; early morning growth hormone estimation (Basal value) 20 minutes after vigorous exercise or basal and 30 minutes and 60 minutes after L Dopa, insulin, glucagone, arginine or clonidine. Insulin should be given with caution as hypoglycemia may already be there in some cases with hypopituitarism. Clonidine stimulation test is usually safe. Around 4-5 mcg/kg/dose is given with BP monitoring. In Hypopituitarism, GH values < 7 mcg/dL is diagnostic of GH deficiency. Normally, the values will be above 10 mcg/dL.

Laron syndrome is end organ defect with GH insensitivity–GH level will be normal or high in the presence of typical clinical features of GH deficiency and normal IGF levels, unlike IGF deficiency. IGFBP deficiency occurs in malnutrition.

Syndromic dwarfing is usually present at birth. Seckel syndrome is bird headed dwarfism with small head and sharp nose. There may be associated GH deficiency in some cases of Seckel's. Russel Silver syndrome presents with LBW, triangular face, frontal bossing, hemihypertrophy/hemiatrophy and clinodactyly.

Constitutional/Maturational delay (MGD) and nutritional dwarfing are discussed in Section 2.1.

GH Replacement Therapy (GHRT) is very expensive (6 mg = 18 units costing nearly 7000 Indian Rupees). It is given in a dose of 0.3 mg/ kg or l unit/kg/week S/C in 6-7 divided doses on a daily basis. It should be started as early as possible and may be continued till growth stops. GH therapy is also beneficial in other forms of short stature like Turner syndrome, syndromic dwarfing, idiopathic short stature etc. In conditions like Pickwickian syndrome, Prader Willi syndrome etc., it is given to tackle central obesity. In such cases, sleep apnoea or fall in oxygen saturation noted by pulse oximeter during sleep is a contraindication to GH therapy, as it may be associated with increased mortality in them.

In panhypopituitarism, other supplements also may be needed like Thyroxine in TSH deficiency, hydrocortisone in ACTH deficiency and cyclical hormones in females and Testosterone enanthate 100 mg IM in males on a monthly basis for 3 months or more for GnRH deficiency. This is usually started from the age of 13 in girls and 14 in boys. Testosterone treatment is also beneficial in those with micropenis and MGD.

Somatomedin/IGF deficiency is rare with usually increased GH. This may be a primary defect or secondary to emotional deprivation. IGF binding proteins may be low in some cases as a primary defect or secondary to malnutrition.

Hyperpituitarism occurs as **overgrowth syndrome**, may occur due to hyperplasia or tumor. There may be increased TSH, ACTH and GnRH in some cases. Increased TSH and other thyroid stimulating hormones like Long Acting Thyroid Stimulator (LATS) may mediate hyperfunction of thyroid. Increased ACTH may lead to **Cushing's Disease** with adrenal hyperfunction and hyperpigmentation as ACTH is one of the chief pigmentary hormones (Central cause). **Cushing's syndrome** is due to adrenal cause for hyperfunction. **Cushingoid syndrome** is due to exogenous steroids.

Increased GnRH may lead to precious puberty. Excess GH will produce **gigantism** in those with open epiphysis and **acromegaly** in those with closed epiphysis. Height age and bone age will be advanced, but sexual maturation may be normal. In tumors, there may be features of increased ICT. Mc Cune Albright syndrome and GnRH producing pancreatic tumors may produce similar picture.

Cerebral gigantism (Sotos syndrome) is overgrowth syndrome probably due to hypothalamic defect. But bone age may not be advanced unlike in pituitary gigantism. Other features are familial incidence, associated mental retardation and increased risk for malignancy.

GH therapy is also thought to increase ICT and risk of leukemia. GH can be suppressed by somatostatin or its analog, Octreotide.

CHAPTER 13

ENDOCRINOLOGY

SECTION 13.2 A CHILD WITH POLYURIA AND POLYDIPSIA

A 3-year-old child was brought with polyuria and polydipsia. No history of polyphagia or weight loss. Urine output 5 L/24 hours with excessive drinking at night also. Urine Sp. gravity was 1005. On water deprivation, it increased to 1010. Urine sugar-Nil. Her skin was dry without sweating.

DIAGNOSIS AND DISCUSSION

Diabetes Insipidus—Neurogenic (DI)

Differential Diagnosis:

1. Diabetes Mellitus–Polydipsia, polyphagia, polyuria and hyperglycemia and glycosuria.
2. Psychogenic polydipsia–No polydypsia at night.
3. Nephrogenic DI.
4. Others: CRF, hypercalcemia.

Neurogenic DI is due to deficiency of Anti Diuretic Hormone (ADH) or Arginine Vasopressin. The syndromes associated with DI are Wolfram syndrome with DIDMOAD—Diabetes Insipidus, Diabetes Mellitus, Optic Atrophy and Deafness and septo optic dysplasia. Urine output will be as high as 4-10 L/day with a Sp. gravity of 1005 increasing to 1010 and osmolality upto 300 mOsm/kg during dehydration. Urine osmolality will be ranging between 50-200 mOsm/kg. Plasma ADH will be low, < 0.5 pg/ml. Sweating will not be seen leading to dry skin. DI may occur in HIE, Group B Streptococcal meningitis, intravascular coagulopathy and intraventricular hemorrhage. AVP administration in the form of nasal spray or orally will lead to concentrated urine with osmolality higher than usual or that noted after dehydration.

In psychogenic polydipsia, psychological problems or stress factors may be identifiable and polydipsia and polyuria may not be present in the night during sleep. ADH level will be normal.

In Nephrogenic DI, ADH level is normal but there is end organ defect.

Treatment of DI is Desmopression (DDAVP), AVP analog, as spray or nasal solution (5-15 mcg/day as single or 2 divided doses). DDAVP also releases factor VIII, VW factor and hence higher doses may be useful in Hemophilia A and VW disease to control minor bleeds like epistaxis/mucosal bleeds.

Syndrome of Inappropriate ADH (SIADH) Secretion

It is a common clinical entity secondary to CNS infection, tumors, demyelination, chest infection etc. S. Na will be as low as 110-120 mEq/L with irritability, vomiting or convulsion secondary to dilutional hyponatremia. Hypochloremia and hypouricemia also may be associated. Urine osmolality will remain high in spite of plasma hypoosmolality. The treatment includes fluid restriction, frusemide and 1.5% or 3% NaCl in selected cases, who develop CNS manifestations. Demeclocycline (Ledermycin) is found useful as it interfere with the action of AVP.

Hyponatremia may be hypervolemic (Nephrotic syndrome), Euvolemic (SIADH) or hypovolemic (Diarrhea). Sodium Supplement should be decided depending on this clinical categorisation.

SECTION 13.3

A 6-MONTH-OLD BABY WITH CONSTIPATION AND DEVELOPMENTAL DELAY

A 6-month-old baby was brought with developmental delay. Social smile was inconsistent and there was increased sleepiness. No head control, Baby had hoarse voice and chronic constipation since birth with feeding difficulty. History of choking spells +, History of prolonged neonatal jaundice +.

On examination: Pallor + with dry skin and coarse facies. Weight 6.5 kg. Length 61 cm and OFC 42 cm, as against an expected of 7.8 kg, 68 cm and OFC 43-44 cm, X-ray–knee showed hypoplastic epiphyseal centers at lower end of femur and upper end of tibia and X-ray wrist showed no carpals. Birth weight was 3 kg. Abdomen— distended with umbilical hernia. AF and PF wide open.

DIAGNOSIS AND DISCUSSION

Congenital Hypothyroidism

Normal weight at birth, prolongation of neonatal jaundice due to delayed maturation of glucuronyl transferase enzyme, developmental delay, short stature, coarse facies as in MPS, hoarse voice, feeding difficulty with choking, pallor, dry skin, increased sleepiness and wide open AF& PF and delayed bone age are typical of hypothyroidism. In older babies, beaking of T12, L1 & L2 vertebra may occur as in MPS. In hypothyroidism, Chronological Age > Height Age > Bone age will be the pattern. Mental age will be retarded. S. Cholesterol may be high above 2 years of age and ECG may have shown evidence of low voltage complex and pericardial effusion may occur. TSH will be elevated with low T4. T3 level has less

significance. Low T3 level is seen in sick euthyroid state and high T3 level in T3 toxicosis. Good response occurs with respect to physical and mental growth with thyroid hormone replacement, if given early. In neonatal screening, TSH alone or TSH and T4 are preferably done 4-7 days after birth as it may take some time for TSH to rise. In babies who have high TSH in umbilical cord blood screening, repeat tests should be done for confirmation. Transient hypothyroidism may occur when mother has hypothyroidism due to transplacental transfer of antithyroid antibodies like anti Thyroperoxidase (TPO) antibodies. USS thyroid or radioactive iodine uptake studies may be done to confirm agenesis/ectopic thyroid.

Treatment is usually life long except in doubtful cases when treatment is started empirically. In such cases it may be stopped for a month at 2 years of age, covering the phase of rapid brain growth, followed by estimation of TSH, T4 and S. Cholesterol. The dose is 8-10 mcg/kg/ day as morning dose initially and later it may be stepped down to 4-6 mcg/ kg/day. The dose should be adequate to relieve constipation and to ensure linear growth and developmental milestones. TSH can be monitored in between to adjust the dose.

In **goitrous hypothyroidism**, there may be congenital enzyme defect or excess TSH/ Thyrotropin receptor stimulating antibody (TRS-Ab) level. The term, cretinism is preferably avoided in congenital hypothyroidism. **Myxedema/Acquired hypothyroidism** is usually due to surgical, autoimmune or infiltrative/destructive lesions of the gland. Excess intake of goitrogens

Fig. 46 (Plate 11)

like cabbage and iodide containing cough syrups may cause hypothyroidism. During surgery of thyroglossal cyst, ectopic thyroid may be removed. The clinical features are growth retardation, cold intolerance, loss of lateral eyebrows, myxedema, puffy face, pallor, excessive sleepiness and delayed bone age. Pretibial myxedema is rare in children. Academic performance may be maintained till later stages. USS and FNAC may show evidence of thyroiditis. In thyroiditis, presence of AntiTPO antibody will warrant life long supplementation. In autoimmune/Hashimoto's thyroiditis, initially there may be hyperfunction of thyroid followed by hypofunction. So, frequent monitoring is warranted.

Diffuse goiter and colloid goiter may mark subclinical iodine deficiency or increased demand as in puberty goiter. **Multinodular goitre (MNG)** requires surgery. **Cold hypofunctioning nodule** with or without draining lymph nodes may mark malignancy.

Endemic iodine deficiency can manifest in various ways.

1. **Mild**–goiter in adolescent girls/during pregnancy.
2. **Severe maternal deficiency→intrauterine deficiency→ neurological or myxedematous syndrome.**

Neurological type: MR, goiter, deaf mutism and pyramidal signs. TFT may be normal in this type.

Myxedematous type: MR, myxedema, deaf mutism with no goiter. T4 is low with high TSH in this condition. These children are thought to have Thyroid growth blocking immunglobulin (TGBI).

Apart from iodine deficiency, selenium deficiency also may cause goiter. Iodine deficiency is rampant in hilly areas of India and it is also seen in people of other areas including coastal areas, who consume fish. The reason is due to soil erosion leading to iodine depletion. And the fact that only deep breeding fish concentrate iodine. The source of iodine is from food and drinking water. Universal Iodization of Salt (UIS) is recommended to prevent deficiency. Iodine fortified salt should contain potassium iodate 15 ppm (15 mcg/g) at the beneficiary level and to ensure this around 30 ppm should be added at manufacturer level. Double fortified salt is iodine and iron fortified (ferrous sulphate) without affecting the white color of the salt. Urine iodine excretion can be tested with dipstick and is a good indicator of iodine deficiency. S. iodine is 50-150 mcg/dL and urine iodine is 100 mcg/dL (Refer Chapter 16.13).

Hyperthyroidism is usually due to Grave's disease, increased TSH, Mc Cune Albright syndrome, subacute thyroiditis and hyperfuctioning tumors. **Grave's disease** is due to Thyrotropin receptor stimulating antibodies (TRSAb). TR inhibiting Ab (TRIAb) also may occur in some cases. The ratio between TRS Ab and TRI Ab decides the clinical picture. Transplacental antibodies may cause hyperthyroidism in newborn. C/F of hyperfunction includes hyperthermia, tremors, sweating, weight loss, diarrhoea, emotional liability, poor attention span, tachycardia, proptosis and lid lag. Ophthalmopathy occurs in 2/3 cases and is less severe in children. There will be goiter, splenomegaly and lypmphadenopathy. Associated conditions include Addison's disease, Diabetes Mellitus, myasthenia gravis, pernicious anemia, vitiligo, SLE and rheumatoid arthritis. Total T3, T4 as well as free T3 and T4 will be elevated and TSH will be reduced. **Thyroid crisis or Thyroid storm** is acute thyrotoxicosis, which may rapidly progress to coma and death. Treatment includes Lugol's iodine 1 drop Q8H, Propyl Thirouracil (PTU) 5-10 mg/kg/day and propranolol 2 mg/kg/day. PTU is said to be safe in pregnancy. Administration of radio iodine, surgical resection and neomercazole are useful in refractory cases. USS, thyroid scintigraphy and FNAC are useful tools in the diagnosis of thyroid disorders.

PTU is 10 times less potent than methimazole. PTU is highly protein bound and has to be given 3 times/day compared to once daily methimazole. PTU has lesser ability to cross placenta and into breast milk. PTU inhibits extra thyroidal conversion of T4 to T3 and is advantageous in neonatal thyrotoxicosis.

SECTION 13.4

A 3-MONTH-OLD FEMALE BABY WITH FTT AND AMBIGUOUS GENITALIA

A 3-month-old female baby was admitted with failure to thrive, vomiting and dehydration. BW 2.6 kg. Baby had diarrhea and reduced urine output.

On examination: CFT > 3 seconds, BP 60 systolic, Wt 2 kg. Ambiguous genitalia with enlarged clitoris. AFT depressed, skin pinch =3 seconds, loose skin folds +, no hepato-splenomegaly. Hb 10 g/dL, TC 6000/cu mm, P58, L42, platelet count 2 lakh, B. urea 30 mg/dL , S. Na 118 mEq/L, S. K 6 mEq/L, RBS 60 mg/dlL.

DIAGNOSIS AND DISCUSSION

1. Congenital Adrenal Hyperplasia (CAH)— salt losing type

2. FTT with ADD and severe dehydration

3. Congenital Adrenal Hypoplasia

4. Pseudo hypoaldosteronism.

FTT, Ambiguous genitalia (female pseudo-hermaphrodite with virilization), circulatory collapse, hyponatremia and hyperkalemia point to the diagnosis of CAH. 95% of CAH comprise the salt losing type with 21 Hydro-xylase deficiency. Confirmation is by markedly raised 17 Hydroxy progesterone and urinary 17 Ketosteroids. The different types of CAH are given in Table 13.1.

Due to the enzyme deficiency, there is defective synthesis of cortisone and aldoster-one and excess synthesis of testosterone. Excess testosterone leads to virilization of female infants and excessive genital pigmen-tation in male infant. Other conditions that cause hyponatremia and hyperkalemia such as renal disorders and conditions that cause ambiguous genitalia like exposure to maternal hormones, intersex and malformation of urogenital sinus should be considered in the DD. Early diagnosis of CAH is life saving. 17 OH Progesterone may be mildly elevated in conditions associated with stress, but in CAH, the levels are abnormally very high.

Treatment of CAH: Oral hydrocortisone 10-20 mg/M^2/day Q8H.

Oral Flurocortisone (Florinef) 0.1-0.3 mg /day, start with higher doses.

Access to extra salt should be ensured. Clitoridectomy and reconstructive surgery is usually done later before school entry. Premature pubarche is noticed in most cases. Normal puberty may be delayed in girls due to excess androgen. In some cases with advanced bone age, early puberty may also occur.

In case of shock/dehydration 20-30 ml/kg IV DNS and 5-10 mg/kg Hydrocortisone should be given. Adequate dose of hydrocortisone and Florinef

Fig. No. 47 (Plate 11)

should normalize S.Na & K and suppress 17 OHP to near normal levels.

Prenatal diagnosis is possible by estimating 17 OH levels in amniotic fluid. In mother with one affected baby, dexamethasone should be started at 5 weeks of age and continued if gender of baby is female to prevent virilization. It can be stopped if fetus is male.

Pseudohypoaldosteronism is due to end organ unresponsiveness with high aldosterone and high renin. **Adrenocortical deficiency** can also occur in **congenital adrenal hypoplasia** with hypoglycemia, hyponatremia and hyperkalemia. Due to increased ACTH, there will be hyperpigmentation. In **familial glucocorticoid deficiency**, there will be hyperpigmentation and hypoglycemia without salt loss. This may mimic ketotic hypoglycemia as ketosis is seen in both conditions.

Secondary adrenocortical deficiency occur with adrenal destruction as in hemorrhage, tumors, tuberculosis etc. **Addisons disease** is acquired adrenal deficiency with hypoglycemia, hyponatremia, hyperkalemia and pigmentation. There may be microcardia due to persistent dehydration. **Adrenal leukodystrophy (ALD)** present with pigmentation, spasticity and hyperkalemia and increased VLFA (very long chain fatty acids) in urine.

Adrenal hyperfunction occur in Cushings disease (Pituitary cause) and Cushing syndrome (Adrenal cause). Serum cortisol level and urinary 17 OH corticosteroid will be elevated. **Dexamethasone suppression test** will normally lead to S.Cortisol suppression to level < 5 mg/dL at 8 AM next day after administration of Dexamethasone 0.3 mg/M^2 at 11 pm in the previous night.

Hyperaldosteronism may be primary due to adrenal defect or secondary to renin angiotensin system. In primary defect, hypertension, hypo-

kalemia and low renin are seen. In **secondary hyperaldosteronism** as in nephrotic syndrome, CCF, cirrhosis liver and renal tumors, there is high plasma renin. Treatment includes surgical resection of tumor if any, spironolactone and dexamethasone in selected cases. Virilizing and feminizing tumors also can occur among adrenal tumors.

In the male, **Sertoli cell produces Mullerian inhibitory substance/factor (MIH) and Leydig cells produce testosterone.**

Phenotypic sex, genital sex, gonadal sex and genetic sex should match in a normal individual. If gonads are palpated in the external genitalia, it is testes, unless otherwise proved. In phallus, there is only one median ridge whereas in enlarged clitoris, there are two ridges. In around $^1/_3$ cases with ambiguous genitalia, cause may be obscure. In **testicular feminization syndrome**, female gender is assigned at birth. Testes may be detected during repair of inguinal hernia. At puberty, breast development occurs, but pubic hair is absent and there is amenorrhoea. Testes are removed and are usually reared as females.

Gender assignment at birth is a social emergency. In general, those with 46 XX, should be reared as female. Feminizing genitoplasty may be done in them. Those with 46 XY and complete androgen insensitivity (CAIS) syndrome or those with extreme microphallus, that does not increase to 2.5 cm. even with testosterone injection, 25 mg IM every three weeks, may also best reared as females. In PAIS, it is often easier to assign male gender. There is a view that the patient's choice along with the family choice is also important before doing any corrective surgery. Those with gonadal dysgenesis are usually infertile. Those with CAH are fertile. In true hermaphroditism, maternity can occur, but paternity is very rare. Gonadectomy may be done to prevent malignancy in gonadal dygenesis.

The conditions with ambiguous genitalia are given in Table 13.2.

SECTION 13.5

A CHILD WITH OBESITY AND HYPERTENSION

A 10-year-old girl child was admitted with rapidly progressive obesity.

On examination: Mooning of face +, double chin +, buffalo hump +, purplish striae over abdomen and buttocks +, hypertrichosis+, pubarche+, ance+, Waist/Hip ratio 1:1, Wt 60 kg, Ht 112 cm, BP 130 /90 mm of Hg. Blood: Hb 15 g/dL, TC 5600, P 66, L 24, E 0. FBS 126 mg/dL, 1½ hr PPBS-150 mg/dL.

DIAGNOSIS AND DISCUSSION

Cushing Syndrome

Anthropometry: Wt for Age 60/30 X 100 = 200%, Ht for Age 112/138 X 100 = 81.15%–3 degree stunting.

BMI 48 (morbid obesity).

Stunting, obesity, hypertension, hyperglycemia and the other features suggest Cushing syndrome. Cushing syndrome is due to adrenal hyperactivity and increased cortisone. Pituitary hyperactivity with increased ACTH leads to Cushing disease. ACTH being a pigmentary hormone like MSH, there will be excess pigmentation in Cushing disease. Cushingoid syndrome is due to exogenous/iatrogenic steroids. Clitoromegaly may occur in girls due to associated excess androgen. Menarche also may be delayed due to excess androgen. Ultrasound/CT imaging may show adrenal tumor or hyperplasia in Cushing syndrome and MRI brain may show pituitary tumors in Cushing disease.

Diagnosis can be confirmed by elevated urinary 17 Hydroxy corticosteroids (> 5mg /M² / 24 hrs) and elevated serum cortisol (>5 mg/dL) around 8 AM. Peak level may be noticed at 5 AM. Dexamethasone suppression test is useful to differentiate between ACTH dependent Cushing disease and ACTH non-dependent Cushing syndrome. After a single dose of dexamethasone given at 11 PM in a dose of 0.3 mg/kg and cortisol is done at 8 AM. There will be ACTH and cortisol suppression in Cushing disease, but not in Cushing syndrome.

Treatment includes supportive care and adrenalectomy in Cushing syndrome/pituitary microsurgery or radiation in Cushing disease. ACTH can also be suppressed with cyproheptadine.

In **Nelson syndrome**, which follows adrenalectomy, there will be aggravation of ACTH dependent pigmentation and enlargement of sella tursica due to loss of feedback inhibition of ACTH by cortisone.

Waist Hip ratio—Normal Male <0.95, Female <0.8.

Abdominal obesity—Adult Male > 102 cm (40 inch) and Female > 88 cm (35 inch).

Diet and exercise form the basic pillars of treatment in obesity. The family on the whole should adopt this 'therapeutic lifestyle change (TLC)', rather than forcing the child alone to follow this.

Diuretics, ACE inhibitors and ARB (Losartan) are useful in controlling hypertension.

CHAPTER 13

ENDOCRINOLOGY

SECTION 13.6

A CHILD WITH HEADACHE, SWEATING AND PAROXYSMAL HYPERTENSION

A 4-year-old child was admitted with headache, palpitation, pallor, sweating and paroxysmal hypertension.

On examination: He had cardiomegaly, Grade III PEM and 2nd degree stunting.

DIAGNOSIS AND DISCUSSION

Pheochromocytoma

Differential Diagnosis: Renal Hypertension

Pheochromocytoma is due to catecholamine producing tumor arising from chromaffin cells of adrenal medulla or abdominal sympathetic chain. It may also be an autosomal dominant condition or part of multiple endocrine neoplasia (MEN) syndrome. In pheochromocytoma, there will be headache, sweating hypertension, papilledema, polyuria and polydipsia. Hypertensive encephalopathy, retinal hemorrhage and cranial bleed may occur. DD of pheochromocytoma includes renal hypertension, CAH with hypertension, neuroblastoma, ganglion neuroma, familial dysautonomia etc.

Urinary Vanillyl Mandellic Acid (VMA) and serum catecholamines will be elevated in pheochromocytoma. Vanilla containing foods and fruits should be avoided for 3 days during testing. USS/CT imaging of abdomen may reveal the mass lesion. MIBG Scan using I 131 metaiodobenzyl-guanidine will detect chromaffin cells anywhere in the body.

Treatment includes control of hypertension and surgical resection. Alpha and beta adrenergic blockade is necessary prior to surgery.

SECTION 13.7

A 5-YEAR-OLD GIRL WITH PRECOCIOUS PUBERTY

A 5-year-old girl was brought with precocious puberty.

On examination: There is thelarche, pubarche and cyclical menstruation for last 2 months, Wt 30 kg, Ht 120 cm.

DIAGNOSIS AND DISCUSSION

Precocious Puberty–Probably Idiopathic (Table 13.3)

(Central type: GnRH Dependent)

Menarche before 10 years of age is considered precocious and secondary sexual characteristics before the age of 8 years in girls and 9 years in boys is considered precocious. Delayed puberty is no sexual characteristic by 13-14 years and menarche by 16 years of age.

True precocious puberty is central in origin—**Central precocious puberty (CPP)** due to premature activation of hypothalamic – pituitary-gonadal (HPG) axis, i.e.; GnRH dependent. CPP is always isosexual and follow the sequence of normal puberty. **Peripheral precocious puberty (PPP)** is usually incomplete and GnRH independent. It is also called **pseudo precocious puberty**. It is due to gonadal/extragonadal cause or due to endogenous or exogenous causes. It may be isosexual or heterosexual leading to clitoromegaly in girls or gynecomastia in boys.

Precocious puberty is more common in girls and almost 50% (upto 90% in girls and 30% in boys) may be due to **GnRH dependent central precocity**. Organic lesions in the brain are usually more common in boys. True precocity may be superimposed on pseudoprecocity, when bone age equals that of puberty, irrespective of the chronological age, for e.g., in CAH, increased androgens lead to advanced bone growth and early maturation of HPG axis and early puberty. The earliest sign of puberty in girls is breast development and testicular enlargement in boys (>2 cm/3 ml volume). Testicular size is measured by comparing with different sizes beads in the Orchidometer.

Hypothalamic hamartomas cause CPP and gelastic seizures and onset of puberty is usually > 3 years of age. In **hypothyroidism**, precocious puberty may occur. This is due to increased TSH, which stimulates GnRH receptors. The alpha subunit of TSH and GnRH is the same. Some may also have increased **prolactin** and galactorrhoea. Pseudo-hypertrophy of muscles also may occur in some with hypothyroidism. This is known as **Kochre Debre Semilange syndrome**. Height and skeletal maturation are not advanced in hypo-thyroidism. Thyroxine replacement will lead to regression of precocious puberty.

Precocious puberty may occur in syndromes like Russel Silver. The features are IUGR, asymmetric face or limbs, triangular facies, frontal bossing, variable MR, hypoglycemia, renal anomalies and hypospadias.

Diagnostic Work-up of Precocious Puberty

The points to be considered are the age of onset, the progression as in normal puberty or not, CNS/abdominal or gonadal problems, family history, syndromic appearance like Russel Silver, pigmentation like Mc Cune Albright, neurofibroma, growth and development, intelligence, vision, SMR staging of puberty, features of hypothyroidism and evidence of polyglandular endocrinopathy. Testicular size in boys and palpation of breast in girls for galactorrhea are important. Emotional and mental status should also be evaluated.

Investigations

Bone age and skeletal survey for fibrous dysplasia (Mc Cune Albright) and size of sella turcica and destruction and MRI brain for neurogenic cause. It should not be passed on as physiological or constitutional when the following clues are present.

Investigations are mandatory when

1. Physical growth is accelerated.
2. Bone age is advanced.
3. More than one sign of puberty is evident (Isolated thelarche may be left alone under strict follow-up).
4. New signs of puberty appearing during period of observation.
5. Other features suggestive of ICSOL, abdominal or mediastinal mass lesion are present along with precocity.

In CPP, Leutinising hormone (LH) level will be > 10 IU/L. FSH response is not diagnostic. FSH may be more than LH in isolated thelarche. GH and IGF I levels will also be more during pubertal growth spurt.

In girls, size of uterus, thickness of endometrium and follicles, cysts and tumors in ovaries should be looked for. Oestrogen effect on vaginal mucosa should be looked for in girls. Glistening red mucosa is non estrogenised and pale dull mucosa with secretions is estrogenised.

X-ray chest and USS abdomen are beneficial to look for mass lesions. USS/biopsy of testis may be warranted in boys.

Early morning levels of S. oestradiol < 10 pg/ml and S. testosterone < 25 ng/ml will rule out central precocity. TFT and prolactin are also indicated in suspected CPP. Child should be strictly followed up in view of very slow growing tumors. Reevaluation may be done in 3-6 months S. progesterone levels are usually not indicated. In adrenal lesions, 17 OH progesterone, DHEA/DHEAS will be elevated. In adrenal tumors, dehydroepiandrosterone sulphate (DHEAS) is greatly elevated. S androgen level will be elevated in girls with virilization. HCG and alpha fetoprotein (AFP) will be elevated in HCG secreting tumors. Those with true precocious puberty achieve height velocity early, but ultimate height will be less as the epiphysis fuse early.

Management

Underlying causes like tumors/cysts should be addressed utilizing surgery, radiation and chemotherapy or combination therapy as indicated. Ovarian cysts more than 3 cm diameter or with solid component need excision, while small cysts may be kept under observation. Laparoscopic approach is preferable than conventional surgery.

In CPP, long acting GnRH analogues can stop progression and improve height prospects. GnRH analogue with certain amino acid substitution are several fold more potent than the natural GnRH decapeptide. These block the episodic/pulsatile release of GnRH and down regulate GnRH receptors and GnRH production. **GnRH analogues** are available as short acting and depot injections and nasal spray. Buserilin, Goserilin and Tryptorelin are available in India. Adequate doses will suppress GnRH pulses in 3 months period. Height prospect will improve by about 6 cm and precocity will regress with this. GnRH testing is done at 6-12 months and bone age every 6 months. The dose of Tryptorelin is around 100 mcg/kg/month to a maximum of 3.75 mg and Luperolide is around 10 mg/ month. These are not indicated in PPP.

Other drugs used are medroxy progesterone, testolactone, ketoconazole, cyproterone and spiranolactone. Ketoconazole inhibit androgen and medroxy progesterone inhibits GnRH leading to suppression of breast and testes growth and cessation of menstruation. It has no effect on height or bone growth. It may lead to virilization and Cushingoid features. Dose is 10 mg BD orally or 100 mg/M^2 IM every 2-3 weeks. Testolactone inhibits conversion of testosterone to oestrogen. Dose is 20 mg/kg/day initially followed by 40 mg/

kg/week. It results in regression of ovarian size and menstruation in Mc Cune-Albright syndrome. Spiranolactone and testolactone are together useful in familial GnRH independent precocity. Cyproterone acetate is an antiandrogenic drug, dose is 100 mg/M^2/day PO Q8H. It suppresses signs of precocity.

Sexual abuse and chance for pregnancy and early masturbation and psychosocial problems go hand in hand with precocious puberty. Mental age and emotional age correspond to chronological age only and not to the advanced bone age and sexual maturity. Hence the child and family need extensive emotional support and protection.

SECTION 13.8 A CHILD WITH DIABETIC KETOACIDOSIS

A 10-year-old girl child was admitted with acute onset of vomiting tachypnea, abdominal pain and altered sensorium. She had polyuria and polydypsia for the last 1-2 months.

On examination: Growth–weight 25 kg, height 130 cm. RR 34/mt, pulse 120 /mt, Temp 100° F. RBS 420 mg/dl, urine Alb+, Sugar 2%, Deposit—PC 15-20 /HPF, Acetone ++.

DIAGNOSIS AND DISCUSSION

Diabetes Mellitus with Ketoacidosis and Probably Urinary Tract Infection

25% of DM present initially with ketoacidosis. Others present with infections like pneumonia, infected wounds, UTI, moniliasis etc. or weight loss, growth retardation, hepatomegaly, polydipsia, polyuria and secondary enuresis.

Management

GTT is done by administering 1.75 mg/kg oral glucose (upto 75 g) and taking RBS at 0,1,2,3 hours. Investigations should include S. Lipid profile (SLIP), LFT, RFT, Glycosylated Hb (HbA1C – N < 6%, > 8 % uncontrolled DM), USS Abdomen for pancreatic calculi, blood counts, urine–RE, Urine C&S, X-ray Chest, blood culture and so on.

Treatment should include specific insulin therapy, diet, exercise and psychosocial support. Fluid therapy is most important in ketoacidosis.

Fluid and Electrolyte Therapy (Weight 25 kg)

Deficit Therapy assuming 10% Dehydration (100 ml/kg) = 2500 ml + 24 hours. Maintenance Fluid – (Holiday and Segar Formula) = 1600 ml/24 hours.

Total fluid—2500 + 1600 =3100 ml

Before doing the calculation, 20 ml/kg N saline bolus is initially started 25 x 20 = 500 ml as 1st hour fluid. The rest 2600 ml is given in next 13 hours. From 2nd hour onwards, K Cl 1 ml/100ml IVF is started. Soda bicarb is given only if PH is < 7.2. RBS should be monitored hourly or 2 hourly initially, followed by 4-6 hourly. N Saline can be changed to half N. Saline later if available. When RBS = 250-300 mg/dl, glucose should be given as ¾ N saline initially by adding 125 ml 5% glucose and 375 ml N Saline to be made upto 500 ml followed by ½ N. Saline by adding 250 ml 5% glucose made upto 500 ml. When RBS is remaining high, ½ N.Saline without glucose is preferable after the initial IVF bolus. Fluid therapy aims at reducing the osmolarity and correcting dehydration.

Insulin Therapy

Initial stabilization–0.1Unit/kg/IV bolus (optional), followed by 0.1 U/kg/hour/IV infusion. Step down to 0.05 U/kg/hour once RBS = 250-300 mg/dl followed by 0.2-0.4 U/kg/dose Q6H/SC once RBS =140 mg/dl. Insulin drip is prepared by adding 10 U in 100 ml N. Saline.

Maintenance Insulin Therapy–1-1.5 U/kg/day SC Q12H, 2/3 in the morning and $1/3$ evening before meals (70:30 Lente: Plain) Human mixtard/ Huminsulin. 50:50 insulin is also available.

Glargine is long acting once a day insulin. Actrapid is a highly purified pork or human neutral insulin. Human insulin is preferable as bovine and porcine may evoke insulin antibodies. In those with insulin antibodies, > 2U/kg/day insulin may be required. Prebreakfast, prelunch and presupper blood and urine sugar should be checked initially to decide on the insulin dose. Ketonuria may persist for 48-72 hours due to dissociation of Beta Hydroxy Butric acid to aceto acetic acid.

Proper control of DM will result in Hb A1 C < 7% and > 8% indicates poor control. Metformin is useful in insulin resistance. Especially Type II DM.

Antibiotic Therapy

Prompt treatment of infection is as important as insulin and fluid therapy.

Glycemic Index of Food Items

It is the effect of the food item on blood sugar. It is defined as increase on RBS following ingestion as percentage of increase following standard food like glucose. It is 100% for glucose, 72 for rice, 65 for wheat, 90 for potato, 42 for ice cream, 20 for peanut and soyabean, 40 for apple etc. But, it may vary as per the time of consumption like empty or full stomach etc.

Diet

The golden principle for DM is to adopt **'no fasting or no feasting'**. Also avoid concentrated/ refined sugars and sweet items. The preferred Carbohydrate: Fat: Protein ratio is 55:30:15 and Monounsaturated: Polyunsaturated: Saturated fat may be kept around 20:10:5 instead of the previously suggested 10:10:10 ratio. Complex starch and items with low glycemic index are preferred. Other sweetners like saccharin,

sorbitol, xylitol, aspartamine etc. should be taken in moderation. High fibre content upto 20-35 g/ day will help to reduce RBS and LDL cholesterol.

Number of meals and % of calorie intake

(4-6 meals should be planned).

Breakfast	– 20%
Lunch	– 20%
Dinner	– 30%
Mid morning	– 10%
Mid afternoon	– 10%
Evening	– 10%

Mid morning, mid afternoon portions may be merged with major meals. Those with good glycemic control may be allowed a small fruit or chocolate as a reward for exercise. Sprouted legumes and green, yellow, orange and red (**'GYOR'**) **vegetables** should be included in the diet for antioxidants and micronutrients. Among the cereals, whole wheat is preferred to rice due to the complex nature of the starch and presence of 'Acarbose', that leads to slow absorption of starch. It will also ensure intake of less quantity compared to large quantity intake of rice.

Exercise

Regular exercise should become part of therapy. Exercise can be advised once the child is stable.

Education and Psycho-Social Support

Teaching the child and family regarding diet, exercise, insulin administration, symptoms and treatment of hypoglycemia, hyperglycemia and psycho-social support are very important. This is a life-long disease which warrants life-long monitoring and medication.

Complications

Complications like **microangiopathy, nephro-pathy, retinopathy neuropathy** etc can be prevented by proper glycemic control.

1. **Honeymoon phase:** This refers to complete remission or drop in insulin requirement to 50% or less for a certain period. This is followed by overt diabetic state. This is due to residual beta cell function.

2. **Insulin shock:** RBS <60 mg/dl with tremor, drowsiness, seizure, coma, high bounding pulse, sweating. Treatment: Give 5-10 g sugar or 1 glass sweet drink and reduce insulin dosage by 10%.

3. **Somogy phenomenon:** Nocturnal hypoglycemia with sweating, night terrors/headache followed by morning hyperglycemia and ketosis due to release of counter regulatory hormones. Midnight RBS will be low and morning RBS will be high. Treatment is by reducing the evening dose of insulin by 10%.

4. **Dawn phenomenon:** Morning hyperglycemia without nocturnal hypoglycemia. Both midnight and morning RBS will be high and the night dose of insulin should be increased by 10%.

5. **Brittle diabetes:** Poor control with wide fluctuations in blood sugar is the rule in children due to infections, endocrine factors, emotional stress, puberty, Somogy/Dawn phenomenon etc.

6. **Non-ketotic hyperosmolar coma:** It is rare in children. There is severe hyperglycemia > 600 mg/dl, severe dehydration, lactic acidosis, severe hyperosmolarity, reduced thirst, reduced lipolysis and reduced ketogenesis. Insulin requirement is less in this condition compared to DKA.

The terminologies insulin dependent and non-insulin dependent DM are now questioned. Type I is basically due to insulin deficiency and Type II is due to insulin resistance. The different types of DM are given in Table 13.4.

The CHO content of food items, CHO exchanges and CHO allowances for exercise are given in Tables 13.5–13.7.

The different causes of hypoglycemia are given in Table 13.8.

Table 13.1: Types of CAH

Defect	C F	Remarks
21 OHlase Deficiency	FTT, virilization, salt losing	Common type (95%), high 17 OH Progesterone
11 Beta OHlase Deficiency	Virilization, hypertension later	Rare (5%) , High 11 deoxy cortisone (DOC)
3 Beta OH Steroid Dehydrogenase Deficiency	Severe cases→salt losing+virilization Mild→precocious pubarche	Very rare, High 17OH Pregnenolone and 17 OH Progesterone
17 Alpha OHlase Deficiency	Hypertension, hypokalamia, incomplete virilization	High DOC, High 17 OH Progesterone
20-22 Demolase Deficiency	Hypertension, hypokalamia, incomplete virilization	Cholesterol accumulation in adrenals

Table 13.2: Conditions with ambiguous genitalia

Types	Boys (46 XY)	Girls (46 XX)
	1. Testosterone Biosynthetic defects	1. Congenital adrenal hyperplasia (CAH), Adrenal/ Gonadal tumors
	2. Leydig cell hypoplasia/receptor defect	2. Maternal androgens • Iatrogenic • Virilizing tumors
	3. Androgen insensitivity • Complete Androgen Insensitivity syndrome (CAIS)—due to receptor mutation • Partial Androgen Insensitivity Syndrome (PAIS)—due to receptor mutation (Reifenstein syndrome) • 5 Alpha reductase deficiency (Perineo-scrotal hypospadias)	3. Placental aromatous deficiency

Contd.

Contd.

4. **Gonadal dysgenesis**
   - Partial
   - Complete (Swyer syndrome)
   - True hermaphroditism
5. **Congenital anomalies**
   - Girls: Vaginal agenesis, absent uterus
   - Boys: Persistent Mullerian structures/Mullerian inhibitor gene/receptor mutations
6. **Other anomalies and syndromes**
   - VACTERL association
   - Deny's Drash syndrome
   - Smith Lemli-Opitz syndrome
   - Goldenhar syndrome
   - Trisomy 13, 18

Table 13.3: Causes of precocious puberty	
I. Isosexual	
Central	*Peripheral*
Idiopathic	Ovarian cysts/tumors
Familial	Testicular tumors
Neurogenic	
• Congenital anomalies/cysts • Inflammatory condition	Adrenal causes–hyperplasia/tumors
• Tumors	
Secondary to peripheral precocity	HCG producing tumors
Syndromic: Russel Silver	Exogenous hormones—
	Androgens/oestrogens
	Testotoxicosis–Autosomal dominant
II. Heterosexual	
1. Girls—Virulizing adrenal/ovarian conditions	
2. Boys—Feminizing adrenal/testicular conditions	
III. Incomplete/Variant growth	
Premature thelarche/pubarche/menarche	

Table 13.4: Types of diabetes mellitus

Type	Criteria
1. Insulin dependent DM (Type I)	Glycosuria, ketonuria RBS >200 mg/dl FBS > 140 mg/dl
2. Non-insulin Dependent (Type II)	FBS >126 mg/dl, 2 hours PPBS > 200mg/dl (in oral GTT)
3. Secondary DM (e.g. Cystic Fibrosis, Wolfram syndrome, Leprechaunism)	Associated with other genetic disorders
4. Impaired Glucose Tolerance	FBS < 126 mg/dl, 2 hours PPBS >140–120 mg/dl (in oral GTT)
5. Gestational DM	FBS > 105 mg/dl 1 hour >90, 2 hours>165 3 hours > 145 mg/dl Any 2 or more in oral GTT)

Table 13.5: Carbohydrate (CHO) content of food items

Type	Item
>20% CHO	Cereals, pulses, tubers, potatoes, jam, plantain/banana, jack fruit
5-20% CHO	Agathi, cauliflower, beetroot, beans, ladies finger, plum, papaya, lime
> 5% CHO	Cabbage, spinach, snake gourd, brinjal, bitter gourd, cucumber, drumstick, radish, watermelon, tomatoes

Table 13.6: 10 g CHO exchanges

½ slice bread	Medium apple/orange/plantain/½ banana
2 cream cracker	1 cup porridge
2/3 cup orange juice (unsweetened)	2/3 cup cornflakes
1 small potato	1 cup thin soup
1 glass milk	1 glass curd

Table 13.7: CHO allowances for exercise

Exercise	Allowance	Food item
Mild	10-15 g/hr	1 fruit/l starch exchange
Moderate	25 g before exercise and 10-15 g/hr	½ sandwich + 1 glass milk and 1 fruit/l starch exchange
Severe	50 g before exercise and 10-15 g/hr	I sandwich + 1 glass milk and 1 fruit/l starch exchange

Table 13.8: Causes of hypoglycemia

(Hypoglycemia is RBS <50mg/dl (2.7mMol/l) and in NB, it is < 35mg/dl in term and < 25 mg/dl in preterm)

1. Hyper insulinemic state
   - Islet cell tumors
   - Islet cell dysmaturation syndrome (Nesidioblastosis)
   - Beckwith Wiedemann syndrome
2. Hormone deficiency states
   - Panhypopituitarism
   - GH/ACTH deficiency
   - Glucagon deficiency
   - Epinephirine deficiency
   - Primary adrenal insufficiency
3. Substrate limited states
   - Ketotic hypoglycemia
   - MSUD
   - Organic acidemias (propionic and methyl malonic acidemia)
4. Glycogen storage disorders
5. Gluconeogenesis disorders
   - Fatty acid oxidation defects
6. Other enzyme defects
   - Galactosemia
   - Fructose intolerance
7. Drug induced
   - Oral hypoglycemics
   - Insulin
   - Salicylates
   - Propranol
8. Neonatal conditions
   - IGDM
   - Maternal drugs
   - LBW
   - Prematurity
   - Poor feeding.

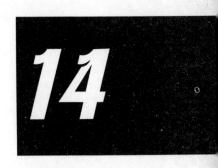

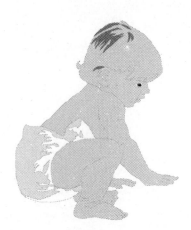

Chromosomal, Genetic and Metabolic Disorders

A CHILD WITH DYSMORPHIC FACIES AND MULTIPLE CONGENITAL ANOMALIES

A 6-month-old baby was brought with dysmorphic facies. He looked like a "Funny Looking Kid" (FLK). The parents were normal, non-consanguinous and were elderly, father 35 and mother 32 years respectively.

On examination: He had growth and developmental retardation. Flat face and occiput, depressed nasal bridge, epicanthic folds, low set ears, upstanted almond shaped eyes, short and broad hands and feet, clinodactyly, transverse Simian crease and a parallel Sidney line, wide space between big toe and others denoting 'sandal or chappel sign' with Kennedy line extending downwards from the space, hypotonia , Brushfield spots on iris and CHD—Endocardial cushion defect.

DIAGNOSIS AND DISCUSSION

Chromosomal Anomaly—Down Syndrome (Trisomy 21): It is the most common chromosomal anomaly.

"Genetic" does not necessarily mean "hereditary". The term implies simply that the genetic material, on a chromosomal or a gene is abnormal or contains one or more mutations which are the cause of the disorder. Once a mutation is present in a patient, particularly if it is constitutional (and thus present in all cells), it can of course be transmitted and thus becomes a hereditary disorder. Fresh mutations can occur any time.

Genetic disorders are generally of four types:

1. *Chromosomal disorders (Numerical/Structural):* Abnormalities of chromosome number are rarely inherited, although affected individuals who reproduce may transmit the extra chromosome to their offspring. Structural abnormalities, such as translocations in which two chromosomes exchange segments (balanced reciprocal translocation), may cause little or no effect in carriers, but predispose to reproductive problems such as miscarriage and infertility. The defect can be transmitted to the offspring.

2. *Single gene/Monogenic ("Mendelian") Inheritance:* It is the result of mutations in single genes, at specific gene "loci". Transmission is observed in monogenic disorders caused by nuclear genes: *autosomal dominant, autosomal recessive* and *X-linked,* which includes X-linked *recessive* (theoretically, only males suffer, given that they are "hemizygous" for the X chromosome) and less frequently, *X-linked dominant* gene mutations (males more seriously affected than females) or rarely Y-linked. A few genes, involved particularly in sex determination and fertility, are localized on the Y chromosome, the transmission of which is only from a father to his XY offspring.

3. *Polygenic or "multifactorial" :* Although this causation is not "as genetic" as are monogenic and chromosomal disorders, the majority of malformations and common

familial disorders have this type of cause. Polygenic implies that the association of several different genes, each one slightly modified, is necessary to produce the disorder. Multifactorial causation means that both genetic and non-genetic (environmental, either pre- or postnatal) factors are associated to produce the pathology.

Some 5-10% of the population will suffer either from a malformation or from a disease in which genetic factors are major determinants.

4. *Mitochondrial disorders:* In recent years a "new" type of inheritance has been proven, that resulting from mutations in the mitochondrial genome. Each cell contains hundreds or thousands of mitochondria, each containing one or several circular chromosomes. These chromosomes can be deleted or suffer other types of mutations which interfere with cellular production of ATP and energy vital for the cell/organ/organism. The symptoms depend on the tissues involved and on the proportion of mitochondria mutated. These involve first the central nervous system and the muscle due to their large energy demands. In many cases the mutation is "de novo" in an affected individual, but hereditary transmission is purely *maternal*, since a fertilized egg's mitochondria originate from the maternal germ cell only.

Chromosomal Anomalies

A chromosome abnormality reflects an abnormality of chromosome number or structure. There are many types of chromosome abnormalities. However, they can be organized into two basic groups:

Numerical Abnormalities

When an individual is missing either a chromosome from a pair (monosomy) or has more than two chromosomes of a pair (trisomy).

Structural Abnormalities

When the chromosome structure is altered. This can take several forms:

- **Deletions:** A portion of the chromosome is missing or deleted.
- **Duplications:** A portion of the chromosome is duplicated, resulting in extra genetic material.
- **Translocations:** When a portion of one chromosome is transferred to another chromosome. There are two main types of translocations. In a reciprocal translocation, segments from two different chromosomes have been exchanged. In a Robertsonian translocation, an entire chromosome has attached to another at the centromere, resulting in only 45 chromosomes.
- **Inversions:** A portion of the chromosome has broken off, turned upside down and reattached, therefore the genetic material is inverted.
- **Rings:** A portion of a chromosome has broken off and formed a circle or ring. This can happen with or without loss of genetic material.

Most chromosome abnormalities occur as an accident in the egg or sperm. Therefore, the abnormality is present in every cell of the body. Some abnormalities, however, can happen after conception, resulting in mosaicism (where some cells have the abnormality and some do not). Chromosome abnormalities can be inherited from a parent (such as a translocation) or be "de novo" (new to the individual). This is why chromosome studies are often performed on parents when a child is found to have an abnormality.

Around 50% of abortions, 50% of congenital anomalies, 50% of mental retardation, 50% of deafness, 50% of blindness, 15% of cancer have chromosomal or genetic background.

Some of the chromosomal anomalies like Down syndrome–Trisomy 21 may be clinically evident as in this case, with all typical features of trisomy 21. In other conditions, a diagnosis of **'Dysmorphic syndrome'** may be made. Chromosomal anomaly is the most likely diagnosis, if the following criteria are satisfied namely: 2 Major anomalies + 1 Minor anomaly or 1 Major anomaly + 2 Minor anomalies or 3 or more Minor anomalies. Upto 3 minor anomalies may be seen in general population. Minor anomalies are markers of major anomalies (1 minor = 3% chance for a major and 2-3 minor = 11% chance and >3 minor = 90% chance for a major anomaly). **Major anomaly** refers to one which affect life span of the individual like CHD, organ function like cleft lip/palate or social function like mental retardation. **Minor anomaly** is one with cosmetic effect only like epicantheic fold, low set ear etc (Table 14.1).

Haploidy refers to 23 chromosomes as in ova or sperm. **Euploidy** refers to exact multiple of 23, i.e., 46 chromosomes as normal human cells and zygote, **Polyploidy** refers to three, four or more exact multiples of 23, i.e., 69, 92 etc. as in leukemic cells and **Aneuploidy** refers to situations with other than exact multiples of 23 like 47, as in Down syndrome. Autosomal trisomies are viable, but monosomies are lethal. The 3 major trisomies are: 21 (Down), 18 (Edward) and 13 (Patau) syndromes. The risk of Down syndrome increases with maternal age (Table 14.2).

Refer Tables 14.3, 14.4 and 14.5 for the various autosomal and sex chromosome defects and deletion syndromes.

There are 3 Types of Down's Syndrome:

1. Non disjunction/Regular Trisomy (90% of cases).
2. Translocation (9%).
3. Mosaicism (1%).

Irrespective of the age of the mother, regular Trisomy 21 is the most common due to anaphase lag. Table 14.2 shows age-related risk. In translocations, G to D translocation has 50% recurrence and G to G translocation has 100% recurrence chance. Maternal defects are more prone for recurrence than paternal.

Care of Down's syndrome involves a multi-disciplinary team approach including special education, physical therapy, cardiac management and support to the family. A child with Down's syndrome is acceptable to many parents as they are less mentally retarded compared to other syndromes and are educable/trainable and sociable. They usually enjoy music and can be reared easily as a **'special child'** with due to attention to their special needs.

The incidence of congenital anomalies is 2-3% and that of genetic disorders is 0.4%. The word **'dysmorphic/congenital'** refers to a defect that is present at birth. It may be due to chromosomal, genetic, sporadic, polygenic/multifactorial or teratogenic effect Table 14.6 summarizes the DD of birth defects. All Congenital need not be genetic and some genetic disorders may manifest very late as in Huntington's chorea.

(**Reference:** *Emery's Elements of Medical Genetics*)

Birth defects present at birth are congenital defects and may be genetic/non-genetic or hereditary/non-hereditary. Genetic disorders may also present at birth or later.

Approach to a child with major chromosomal anomalies includes the following: confirmation by karyotyping, addressing associated problems like CHD, amenorrhoea etc., special education, genetic counselling and prenatal diagnosis in subsequent pregnancies.

Prenatal diagnosis is done in two stages and action is undertaken based on both screens (Table 14.7):

Stage I: First Trimester Screen (12 weeks)— Anomaly scan + Maternal serum PAPPA (Pregnancy Associated Plasma Protein A). PAPPA is low in trisomies and fetal death. Anomaly scan is called **Genetic sonogram** (Table 14.8).

Stage II: Second Trimester Screen (16-18 weeks)—Anomaly scan + Maternal serum **Quad Screen/Triple Test**–HCG, AFP and estriol: AFP and oestriol are low in all trisomies, HCG is high in Trisomy 21, but low in 13 and 18. Very high HCG is seen in molar pregnancy and multiple pregnancy, but low in fetal death and normal in NTD. AFP is very high is NTD, multiple pregnancy and imminent fetal death. High amniotic fluid AFP and acetyl cholinesterase are diagnostic of NTD. Oestriol is normal in multiple pregnancy and neural tube defects (NTD), but low in fetal death. **Dimeric Inhibin A (DIA)** is the 4th test in QUAD and is high in trisomy 21, but low in 13 and normal in 18 and NTD.

The lab values of these tests are expressed as MoM (multiple of median). MoM allows comparison between different labs. Each lab should standardize own data on 200 samples to establish lab median. MoM is obtained by dividing actual value by lab median. MoM of HCG will be >2 in trisomy 21. Maternal weight has inverse correlation with these markers. In multiple pregnancy, correction factor should be applied while interpreting HCG and AFP. PAPP—A is a zinc containing protein and low level is a marker of trisomy and early pregnancy failure and also Cornelia de Lange syndrome.

The current recommendation is to do first trimester USS and PAPPA and record it as initial positive result (IPR) and wait for 2nd trimester USS and QUAD screen. This is in view of false positive tests and if the 2nd test is also positive, confirmation by amniocentesis/fetal karyotyping is advised before declaring final positive result (FPR).

Human Placental Lactogen (HPL)

HPL, also called **human chorionic somatomammotropin,** is a **polypeptide placental** hormone. Its structure and function is similar to that of human **growth hormone**. It modifies the metabolic state of the mother during pregnancy to facilitate the energy supply of the fetus. HPL is an anti-insulin. In bioassay, HPL mimics the action of prolactin, yet it is unclear if HPL has any role in human lactation. HPL affects the metabolic system of the mother. HPL increases production of insulin and IGF-1 and increases insulin resistance and carbohydrate intolerance. Chronic hypoglycemia leads to a rise in HPL. HPL induces lipolysis with the release of free fatty acids, increase in insulin secretion and insulin resistance. With release of HPL, free fatty acids become available for the mother as fuel, so that relatively more glucose can be utilized by the fetus. Also, ketones formed from free fatty acids can cross the placenta and be used by the fetus. These events support energy supply to the fetus in states of starvation.

The ultrasound markers of Trisomy 21 are given in Table 14.8 and the associated medical conditions are given in Table 14.9.

SECTION 14.2

A GIRL WITH SHORT STATURE AND PRIMARY AMENORRHEA

A 16-year-old girl was brought with primary amenorrhea and short stature.

On examination: She had webbing of neck, cubitus valgus leading to increased carrying angle at elbow, wide spaced nipples (inter nipple distance >1/3 of chest circumference). Mentally, she was of average intelligence. She had unexplained acral edema in the newborn period.

DIAGNOSIS AND DISCUSSION

Turner syndrome—45 XO

Barr body was positive in only <10% cells of in buccal smear. This is used as a screening test. Normally >20% will have Barr body, which represents the inactivated 2nd X chromosome. USS showed that ovaries were hypoplastic with infantile uterus. FSH and LH were high with low oestradiol levels. The other features to be looked for are bicuspid aortic valve, coarctation of aorta, hypertension and hypoplastic kidneys. After the age of 13-14 years, cyclical hormones including oestrogen and progesterone (Evalone) may be given to induce withdrawal bleeding. Due to ovarian failure, ovulation and fertilization are remote in Turner's syndrome. Ovum donation can be accepted for becoming pregnant.

Noonan's syndrome is Turner phenotype with normal genotype. It can occur in boys and girls. It may be sporadic/familial (Autosomal Dominant) especially in males, probably with defective gene on chromosome 12q. The cardiac defects are PS and ASD. Hypogonadism and MR may also occur.

Fig. No. 48 (Plate 11)

SECTION 14.3 A BOY WITH MR AND MINOR MALFORMATIONS

A 12-year-old boy was brought with dyslexia and MR.

On examination: He had long face, prominent jaw, large ears, macro-orchidism with 6 cm diameter of testes.

DIAGNOSIS AND DISCUSSION

Fragile X Syndrome (FRAX)

This is a very common inherited cause of MR.

Macro-orchidism may be evident at puberty only. FRAX occur in both boys and girls. It is X-linked condition. Mother may be permutation carrier of CGG trinucleotide repeats upto 50-600 base pairs. In the patients, it is magnified to 2800 base pair repeats.

SECTION 14.4 A CHILD WITH OBESITY, MR AND CHROMOSOMAL ANOMALY

An 8-year-old girl is brought with extreme obesity and MR. Karyotype yielded microdeletion of chromosome 15.

DIAGNOSIS AND DISCUSSION

Prader-Willi Syndrome (PWS)

PWS is an example of a chromosomal anomaly with MR and obesity. There may be associated sleep apnea leading to **Pickwickian syndrome**. The differential diagnosis includes Cushing's syndrome, polycystic ovarian syndrome (PCOS) and Beckwith Wiedemann Syndrome (BWS).

PWS show increased appetite. PWS may be associated with various chromosomal anomalies involving chromosome 15 resulting in only maternal representation due to the following:

1. **Microdeletion** of paternally derived chromosome 15.
2. **Imprinting** of paternally derived chromosome 15 leading to inactivation.
3. **Uniparental Disomy (UPD)** resulting in both copies being inherited from mother (maternal disomy).

The opposite syndrome of PWS is **Angelman (Happy Puppet) syndrome,** with microdeletion/ imprinting of maternally derived chromosome 15/ UPD of both copies inherited from the father (paternal disomy).

Defferential Diagnosis:

1. **Beckwith Wiedemann Syndrome (BWS) is** a fetal overgrowth syndrome due to similar inheritance pattern. In BWS, there is microdeletion/ imprinting/paternal UPD with maternal deficiency of chromosome 11 p15. Fetal overgrowth is due to increased IGF 2 regulated by this area of the chromosome.

2. **Sotos Syndrome:** Prenatal overgrowth with large head, mutation in NSDI gene.

3. **Weaver Syndrome similar to Sotos Syndrome.**

4. **Simpson Golabi Behmel Syndrome:** Prenatal and postnatal overgrowth with macroglossia, skeletal hand anomalies, supernumerary nipples, mutation in Xp26.

CHAPTER 14

CHROMOSOMAL, GENETIC AND METABOLIC DISORDERS

SECTION 14.5

A NEWBORN WITH INBORN ERROR OF METABOLISM (IEM)

A newborn 3 kg at birth born to consanguinous parents developed the '**pentad of symptoms— poor feeding, vomiting and dehydration, lethargy, convulsion and abnormal tone** on 4th post natal day. The couple had lost their first baby due to similar illness. Investigations revealed acidosis, ketosis and hypoglycemia. Baby had a peculiar urine odor. Ferric chloride test showed navy blue color and 2-4 dinitro phenyl hydrazine (DNPH) test yielded yellow precipitate showing ketoacids.

DIAGNOSIS AND DISCUSSION

Refer Table 14.10 for Different Urine Odor and $FeCl_3$ Test Results.

Maple Syrup Urine Disease (MSUD)

MSUD is a disorder of the branched chain amino acids namely valine, leucine and isoleucine. Deficiency of branched chain alpha ketoacid dehydrogenase results in MSUD. There are 4 subunits for this enzyme and the gene is located on chromosome 1 and 7. Body fluids and urine will have the sweet odor of maple syrup similar to that of 'burnt sugar'.

Treatment is unsatisfactory, peritoneal dialysis may be done in acute crisis followed by MSUD formula (Mead Johnson Lab). It is deficient in branched chain amino acids. Vitamin B_1 (Thiamine) 10-200 mg/day is useful. Thiamine pyrophosphate is a co-enzyme of the enzyme. There are different varieties of MSUD. Thiamine responsive type, Intermittent and mild intermediate types.

Hyperglycinemia is an IEM that manifests in newborn period. Hyperglycinemia in the newborn may be a transient condition in the newborn/ nonketotic/ketotic hyperglycinemia. Ketotic hyperglycinemia is secondary to organic acidemias. Non-ketotic type has poor prognosis.

See: Approach to IEM (Figs 14.1(a,b,c), 14.2 and 14.3).

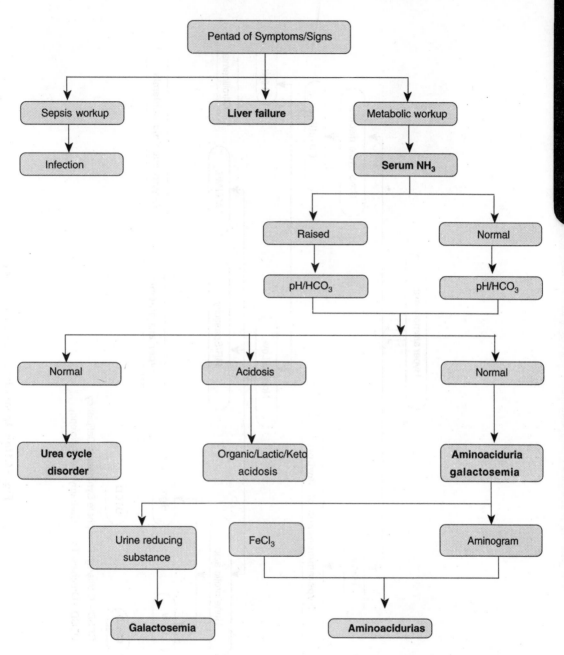

Fig. 14.1(a): Approach to IEM

CHAPTER 14

CHROMOSOMAL, GENETIC AND METABOLIC DISORDERS

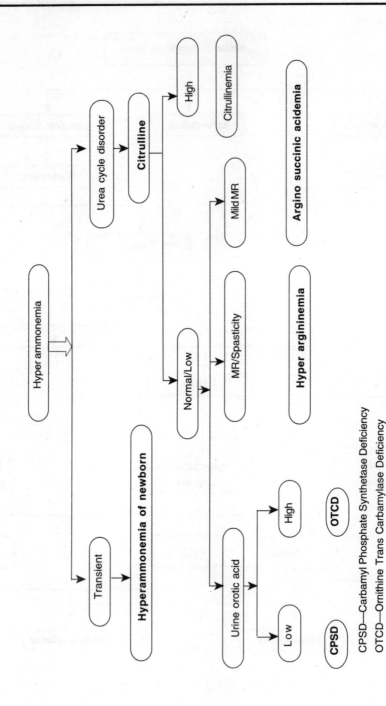

CPSD—Carbamyl Phosphate Synthetase Deficiency

OTCD—Ornithine Trans Carbamylase Deficiency

Fig. 14.1(b): Approach to hyperammonemia

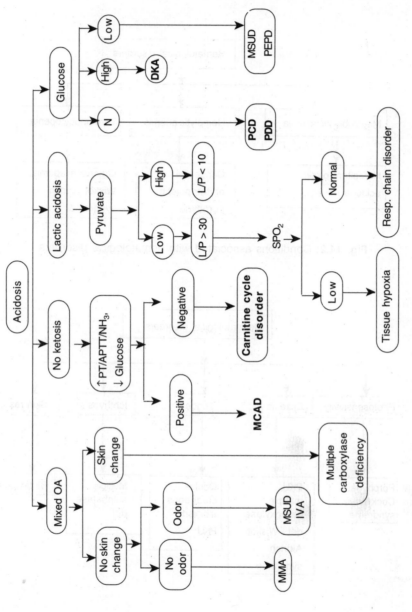

Fig. 14.1(c): Approach to acidosis

MMA: Methyl Malonic Acidemia; MSUD: Maple Syrup Urine Disease; IVA: Isovaleric Acidemia; MCAD: Medium Chain Acyl CoA Dehydrogenase Def.; PCD: Pyruvate Corboxylase Def.; PDD: Pyruvate Dehydrodenase Def.; PEDD: Phospho Enol Pyruvate Def.

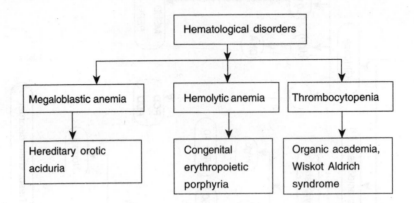

Fig. 14.2: Conditions associated with hematological disorders

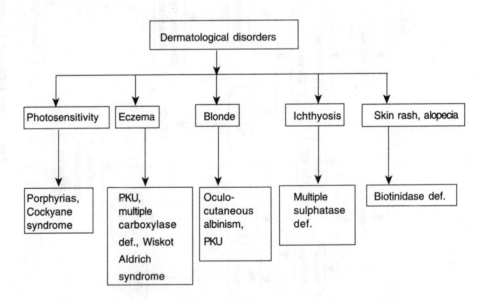

Fig. 14.3: Conditions associated with dermatological disorders

SECTION 14.6

A BLUE EYED BLOND INFANT WITH MR

A 10-month-old baby was brought with development delay and MR. He also had persistent vomiting. Hyperactivity and athetosis were noted. He was the first child of consanguinous parents. He had eczema. He enjoyed rocking and rhythmic movements. He had a mousy order.

Urine ferric chloride test yielded emerald green colour. Guthric test was +ve and serum phenylalanine was increased (> 20 mg/dl).

DIAGNOSIS AND DISCUSSION

Phenylketonuria (PKU)

PKU is hyperphenylalaninemia due to deficiency of alanine hydroxylase or its co-factor, Tetrahydro biopterin (BH4). The defective gene is on 12q. The BH4 deficiency type presents with MR, hyperalaninemia and myoclonic seizures.

Treatment is by low PA diet namely Lofenalac (Mead Johnson Lab), low protein diet and neurotransmitter precursor supplemants like dopa and 5 hydroxy tryptophan. Low PA diet may be relaxed after 5-6 years of age, but should be reintroduced in pregnancy. Affected females can have children with MR if dietary control is poor. So, strict diet is advised in prenatal mothers affected with PKU.

(Refer: Table 14.10 and Figs. 14.1–14.3).

SECTION 14.7 A CHILD WITH CYCLICAL VOMITING

One year old child was brought with history of repeated episodes of vomiting. It was more marked during fever or URI. He was lethargic, anorexic and very drowsy. He also had a brief convulsion prior to admission. He had failure to thrive and was tachypneic. He had not started walking. RBS, LFT and RFT were normal. S. ammonia was increased (200 mg/dl), ABG—No acidosis, S. citrulline—Normal.

DIAGNOSIS AND DISCUSSION

Urea Cycle Disorder Probably OTCD

Hyperammonemia present with refusal of feeds, vomiting, lethargy, coma, convulsion and ataxia. Absence of acidosis clinches the diagnosis of urea cycle disorder as against conditions with organic/lactic/ketoacidosis with both acidosis and hyperammonemia (Refer Algorithm 14.1b and c).

In the absence of raised citrulline and orotic acid, the diagnosis of Ornitine Trans Carbamylase deficiency (OTCD) can be established. In Carbamyl PO_4 Synthetase Deficiency (CPSD), urine orotic acid will be high.

Treatment in acute crisis includes peritoneal dialysis, low protein by mouth, bowel wash, lactulose, IV Fluids and electrolytes. Intralipids (1 g/kg/day) to provide enough calories along with low dose essential amino acids (0.25 g/kg/day) may be tried as partial parenteral nutrition. Sodium benzoate is given in a dose of 250-500 mg/kg/day, usually as a solution or as powder sprinkled on food items. 1 mole of benzoate can remove 1 mole of ammomia as glutamate. When there is no deficiency of arginase and in citrullinemia, arginine may be given in a dose of 300- 400 mg/kg/day. 1 mole of arginine will remove 1 mole of ammonia as citrulline. 1 mole of citrulline can accept 1 mole of ammonia to form arginine. Phenyl butyrate is also beneficial and is given in a dose of 200-500 mg/kg/day. This may displace bilirubin from binding sites in cases with liver failure.

Newborns can have transient hyperammonemia. In case with Reye/Reye like encephalopathy, liver enzymes will be elevated without ketosis. Other causes of cyclical vomiting include migraine and abdominal epilepsy.

SECTION 14.8

A CHILD WITH DYSMORPHIC FEATURES AND HEPATOSPLENOMEGALY

A 2-year-old child born out of consanguinous marriage was brought with developmental delay and abdominal distension. He had hepato-splenomegaly, growth retardation, large head, coarse facies and corneal clouding, no deafness. CVS–Pan Systolic Murmur at apex conducted to axilla, urine, MPS +ve, Skeletal survey—dysostosis multiplex.

DIAGNOSIS AND DISCUSSION

Mucopolysaccharidosis—Hurler Syndrome

Hurler syndrome is called **'gargoyilism'** due to coarse facies similar to hypothyroidism. It is due to deficiency of Alpha 1 Iduronidase deficiency leading to accumulation of mucoploysaccharides like dermatan and heparan sulphates. Gargogyl cells with lysosomal storage are positive in almost all tissues in this condition. The bone findings are characteristic and include dolicocephaly, frontal bossing, prominent metopic sutures, thick skull, J shaped sella turcica, kyphosis, gibbus deformity and lower anterior beaking of L1, L2 vertebrae, shallow hip acetabulam, coxa valga, 'oar' shaped ribs, 'bullet shaped' phalanges with proximal tapering. V shaped radioulnar obliquity etc. Corneal clouding, Mitral and Aortic valve regurgitation and mental retardation are the other features. Deafness is there in X-linked recessive Hunter syndrome. Hurler has AR inheritance. The genetic defect is on chromosome 4. Enzyme deficiency is detec-table in WBC and fibroblasts.There is no specific therapy except BM stem cell transplantation. The different types of MPS and the DD are given in Tables 14.11 and 14.12.

CHAPTER 14

CHROMOSOMAL, GENETIC AND METABOLIC DISORDERS

SECTION 14.9

A 10-YEAR-OLD CHILD WITH MASSIVE SPLENOHEPATOMEGALY

A 10-year-old child born to consanguinous parents was brought with progressive abdominal distension.

On examination: Growth retardation +, average intelligence and huge splenohepatomegaly. No evidence of liver disease, mild leukopenia and thrombocytopenia +.

DIAGNOSIS AND DISCUSSION

Gaucher Disease (Visceral form) with Hypersplenism

This is due to deficiency of glucocerebrosidase enzyme located on chromosome 1. The infantile type presents with early neurological findings.

Juvenile type has late onset of neurological finding and adult type is purely visceral without neurological involvement. The hematological findings are due to hypersplenism or bone marrow infiltration. Gaucher cells will be seen in bone marrow and splenic aspirates. Femur will show 'Erlenmeyer flask deformity'. The neuro findings are ataxia, myoclonus, opisthotonsus, ophthalmoplegia and dementia. Trismus may occur in infantile type.

Adult type may benefit with the placental enzyme ceredase or genetically engineered imiglucerase enzyme (cerezyme).

Conditions with CNS involvement due to genetic defect leading to grey and white matter disease are given in Table 14.13.

SECTION 14.10

A MARFANOID CHILD WITH MR, BLUE EYES AND MALAR FLUSH

A 5-year-old child was brought with tall stature and MR. The child had an affected elder sibling with similar features and blindness. He also had a normal sibling. The child had tall stature, span 6 cm more than height, elongated thumb, arachnodactyly. scoliosis, positive wrist sign and positive Steinberg sign with adducted thumb reaching beyond the palm. The child was unusually fair with blue eyes and malar flush. Eyes showed ectopia lentis, iridodonesis and cataract. He had MR and behavioural disorder. Urine—Homocystine positive.

DIAGNOSIS AND DISCUSSION

Homocystinuria

Similar features without MR are seen in Marfan syndrome. The defective gene for homocystenuria is on chromosome 21.

Type I - Classical type is due to cystathionine synthatase deficiency. High homocystine level predispose to thromboembolic episodes, CVA and increased platelet adhesion. Urine and blood homocystine will be high with low levels of cystine.

Dietary therapy includes restriction of homocystine and high methionine. High dose Vitamin B_6 (160-200 mg/day) and Folic acid (1-5 mg/day) are beneficial. Betaine or trimethyl glycine (6-9 g//day) is also useful as a methyl group donor.

Homocystinuria Type II is associated with megaloblastic anemia and defective formation of methyl cobalamine and may respond to B_{12}, 1-2 mg/day.

Type III is due to Methyl Tetra Hydrofolate reductase deficiency with normal or low methionine levels. Treatment includes vitamin B_6, B_{12}, folic acid, betaine.

Hypermobility syndrome (HMS) is seen in Marfan, Ehlers Danlos syndrome. Table 14.14 summarises the features and diagnosis of HMS.

SECTION 14.11

AN INFANT WITH HEPATIC FAILURE, WHOSE SIBLING DIED OF SIMILAR ILLNESS

A 6-month-old baby was admitted with fulminant hepatic failure and coagulopathy. His sibling died of similar illness in infancy. Developmental delay +, Hepatosplenomegaly+, Cataract +, Viral markers for hepatitis negative. Urine Benedict test for reducing substance +, RBS 20 mg/dl, Urine glucostix –ve.

DIAGNOSIS AND DISCUSSION

Galactosemia

Differential Diagnosis: Tyrosinemia, hereditary fructose intolerance and Alper's disease.

Galactosemia classical type is due to galactose 1 PO_4 uridyl transferase enzyme deficiency with accumulation of galactose 1 PO_4 (GIP) and galactitol. GIP produces MR and hepatotoxicity and galactitol produces cataract. The other features are vomiting, irritability, FTT, aminoaciduria, hepatosplenomegaly, hypoglycemia, convulsion, cirrhosis, ascites etc. Early dietary restriction of all types of milk is rewarding.

Galactosemia due to galactokinase deficiency present with galactosemia, galactosuria and cataract without MR and aminoaciduria. Galactokinase catalyses phosphorylation of galactose.

Type I tyrosinemia is hepato renal tyrosinemia with renal Fanconi syndrome, Vitamin D resistant rickets, self-mutilation and poly-neuropathy. Serum tyrosine and methionine levels are elevated and also alpha feto protein and urinary excretion of Alpha Amino Levulinic acid. Urine ferric chloride test yields transient green color and there is rotten cabbage odor is due to high methonine level. The defective gene is on chromosome 15.

Type II is Oculocutaneous tyrosinemia or Richner Hanhart syndrome with palmar and plantar keratosis, skin lesions and corneal ulcer. The defective gene is located on chromosome 16 and the enzyme is tyrosine amino transferase. High dose Vitamin C is useful with dietary restriction of tyrosine and phenylalanine.

Hereditary fructose intolerance is a rare AR condition with liver damage due to fructose 1, 6.diphosphate.

A 2-YEAR-OLD CHILD WITH HEPATOMEGALY AND EARLY MORNING SEIZURES

SECTION 14.12

A 2-year-old child was brought with occasional seizures in the early morning hours.

On examination: Growth retardation +, development normal, 5 cm palpable liver. FBS 30 mg/dl.

DIAGNOSIS AND DISCUSSION

Glycogen Storage Disease (GSD 0)

GSD 0 or Aglycogenosis is due to glycogen synthetase enzyme deficiency leading to fasting hypoglycemia, hepatomegaly and convulsion. MR may occur secondary to hypoglycemia. Liver biopsy specimen taken in absolute alcohol (not formalin), will give the diagnosis apart from enzyme study. Avoiding fasting, frequent feeding including night feeds with uncooked corn starch are useful. Infants may not have manifestations due to frequent breastfeeding at night.

Types VI and X present with isolated hepatomegaly only. Type X is associated with myalgia. The various GSDs are given in Table 14.15. Also refer Table 13.8 for causes of hypoglycemia.

CHAPTER 14

CHROMOSOMAL, GENETIC AND METABOLIC DISORDERS

SECTION 14.13
A 4-YEAR-OLD CHILD WITH REPEATED HYPOGLYCEMIC SEIZURES IN THE MORNING

A 4-year-old child born to non-consanguinous parents was repeatedly admitted with morning hypoglycemia and seizure. This episode was more common during intercurrent infections and when the child sleeps skipping supper. It also used to occur during midmorning or evening due to skipping of meals, when he was sick. Urine acetone +ve. Plasma insulin < 5 microunits/ml. RBS 20 mg/dl.

DIAGNOSIS AND DISCUSSION

Ketotic Hypoglyclemia (KH)

Differential Diagnosis: Fatty Acid Oxidation Defects

KH is common between 1½ to 8 years and usually regresses thereafter. This is thought to be due to gluoneogenic defect secondary to low alanine level. Alanine is the chief gluconeogenic amino acid. Alanine 250 mg/kg infusion promptly corrects the hypoglycemia. They may present with LBW and neonatal hypoglycemia. Always ketonuria precedes

hypoglycemia and there is no hyperinsulinism. Impaired adrenaline secretion may also be a cause for this. Increase in muscle mass and lowered glucose requirement per unit body mass by 8 years of age leads to regression.

Treatment includes 4 ml/kg 10% Dextrose IV and 5-10 mg/kg IV hydrocortisone. Glucagon, diazoxide, octreotide are also effective in resistant hypoglycemia associated with hyperinsulinism. Other causes of hypoglycemia are given in Table 13.8.

Fatty acid oxidation defects present with **Reye like episodes** and hypoglycemia precipitated by fasting, but there is inappropriately low levels of ketone bodies, e.g., MCAD (Medium Chain Acyl CoA Dehydrogenase deficiency), SCAD (Short Chain), LCAD (Long Chain), VLCAD (Very Long Chain) etc.

Carnitine cycle defects will have associated myopathy and cardiomyopathy. Treatment includes 100 mg/kg/day of L carnitine.

Table 14.1: Major and minor anomalies	
Major anomalies	*Minor anomalies*
Cardiovascular	Preauricular pit or tag
Ventricular septal defect	Epicanthic folds
Atrial septal defect	Lacrimal duct stenosis
Parent ductus arteriosus	Brushfield spots in the iris
Fallot's tetralogy	Lip pits
Central nervous system	Single palmar crease
Anencephaly	Fifth finger clinodactyly
Hydrocephaly	Syndactyly between second and third toes
Microcephaly	Supernumerary nipple
Lumbo-sacral spina bifida	Umbilical hernia
Gastrointestinal	Hydrocele
Cleft lip/palate	Sacral pit or dimple
Diaphragmatic hernia	Choanal atresia
Oesophageal atresia	Tongue tie
Imperforate anus	Polydactyly
Limb	Undescended testis
Transverse amputation	Embryonic cysts
Urogenital	Skin—pigmented anomalies
Bilateral renal agenesis	Lipoma
Polycystic kidneys (infantile)	Imperforate hymen
Bladder exstrophy	Inguinal hernia

Table 14.2: Maternal age related risk for Down syndrome	
Maternal age	*Incidence*
20	1/1500
25	1/1350
30	1/900
35	1/400
36	1/300
37	1/250
38	1/200
39	1/150
40	1/100
45	1/30

Table 14.3: Common chromosomal trisomies		
Type	*Incidence*	*Remarks*
Trisomy 13- Patau	1/20,000	Cleft lip. polydactyly, CNS, cardiac, genital defects
Trisomy 18- Edward	1/8,000	LBW, overlapping fingers, rocker–bottom feet, CNS, cardiac, renal defects
Trisomy 21- Down	1/800	Monologlid facies, hypotonia, CHD, retardation
Trisomy 8- Mosaic	RARE	Long face, prominent forehead, wide upturned nose, micro-retrognathia, MR, osteoarticular anomalies

Table 14.4: Sex chromosome anomalies			
Type	*Remarks*	*Type*	*Remarks*
45 XO-TURNER	Female phenotype, short stature, amenorrhoea Co-arctation of aorta, deafness, Neck webbing	47 XXX - Poly X (Superfemale)	Female with MR
		47 YYY- Poly Y	Tall male, behavioural problems
47 XXY-KLINEFELTER	Tall male, gynecomastia, infertility, female type of hair distribution	Fragile X- FRAX	MR, large ears, macroorchidism at puberty

CHAPTER 14

CHROMOSOMAL, GENETIC AND METABOLIC DISORDERS

Table 14.5: Major deletion syndromes

Type	Remark	Type	Remark
4 p `Wolf-Hirschhorn-`	- Greek helmet face, microcephaly, MR, cleft lip, palate, CHD hypoplastic eye sockets	11p 11.1 `` - Potocki Shaffer	- Microcephaly, exostosis
5p `CRI-DU-CHAT-`	- Cat cry, hypotonia, microcephaly, MR	11p13 ` WAGR	- Wilm's, Aniridia, Gonadoblastoma Retardation
9p ``	- Craniofacial dysmorphology, exophthalmos, MR, cardiac, genital defects	11q 23.3` - Jacobsen	- MR, retrognathia, CHD
		13q 14.1` - Orbeli	- Retinoblastoma
		17 p11.2` - Smith–Meganis	- MR blonde, midfacial hypoplasia
13q ``	- FTT, MR, microcephaly, ptosis, ocular, limb anomalies	17 P13.3` - Miller Dicker	- MR, Lissencephaly
18p`	- MR, ceft lip, palate, ocular defects	22q 11.2` - Di George	- Velocardiofacial, thymic aplasia, hypocalcemia
18q ``	- Frog like position, carp like mouth, MR, ocular defects, ear lobe defects	22q13`	- MR, accelerated growth, joint laxity
21 q ``	- MR, hypertonia, downslant of eyes, skeletal defects, micrognathia	3 p22.3q23` - BPES	- Blephrophimosis/ Ptosis/Epicanthus inversus syndrome
1p.33`	- Severe MR, seizure, facial cleft	5 q 35` - Sotos	- Cerebal gigantism with overgrowth
7q11.23` - William syndrome	- Elfin facies, AS, hypercalcemia	7p13 `` - Greig	- Cephalo polysyndactyly syndrome
8q 24.1` - Langer Giedion	- MR, exostosis	16 p 13.3`- Rubistein Taybi	- Large toe/thumb, microcephaly
		16 p 13.3 ``	- Tuberous sclerosis/ Polycystic kidney
		20p 22` - Alagille syndrome	- Arteriohepatic dysplasia

Table 14.6: Differential diagnosis of birth defects

I. **Malformation**—Arrested or misdirected development of an organ due to inherent abnormality/primary defect—genetic/environmental causes, e.g., NTD,CHD cleft lip/palate etc.

II. **Disruption**—Altered development due to external factors—e.g. Ammonitic band disruption

III. **Deformation**—Distortion due to mechanical force/positional defects e.g. club foot

IV. **Dysplasia**—Abnormal organization of a single type of tissue—e.g. skeletal dysplasia

V. **Sequence**—Consequence of a cascade—e.g. Potter sequence of renal hypoplasia, Pierre Robin sequence

VI. **Syndrome**—Consistent patterns due to a known underlying cause–e.g. Congenital rubella syndrome

VII. **Association**—Non random sporadic occurrence with no known cause – e.g. VATER, VACTRL anomalies (Vertebral, Ano-rectal, Tracheo-esophageal, Renal or Radial, Ano-rectal, Cardiac, Tracheo-esophageal, Renal and Limb anomalies), CHARGE - Coloboma, Heart defect, Atresia Choanae, Retardation of growth and development, Genital and ear effects.

Table 14.7: Prenatal diagnosis: Surrogate markers of pregnancy outcome and Triple/Quadriple test

Condition	AFP	Oestriol	HCG	Inhibin A	PAPP-A
Neural Tube Defect (NTD)	High	Normal	Normal	Normal	Normal
Trisomy 21	Low	Low	High	High	Low
Trisomy 18	Low	Low	Low	Normal	Low
Trisomy 13	Low	Low	Low	Low	Low
Molar preg.	Low	Low	V. High		
Multiple preg.	High	Normal	High		
Fetal death	High	Low	Low		Low

Table 14.8: Sonographic markers of trisomies

Anomaly	Trisomy 21	Trisomy 18	Trisomy 13
Major anomalies	Cardiac defects Duodenal atresia Cystic hygroma	Cardiac Spina bifida Cerebellar agenesis	Cardiac CNS anomalies Facial anomalies
Markers	Nuchal fold thickening	Micrognathia	Cleft lip palate
	Hyperechoic bowel	Omphalocele	Urogenital anomalies
	Echogenic intracardiac focus (EIF)/papillary muscle calcification	Radial aplasia	Echogenic kidneys
	Short limbs—femur, humerus	Cystic hygroma	Omphalocele
	Pyelectasis	Club foot	Polydactyly
	Mild ventriculomegaly	Clenched hand and wrist	Rocker bottom feet
	Clinodactyly	Choroid plexus cyst	Cystic hygroma
	Sandal gap	Brachycephaly-strawberry shaped	Echogenic intra-cardiac focus
	Widened pelvic angle	Short limbs	IUGR
	Pericardial effusion	Single umbilical artery	Pyelectasis
	Right-left heart disproportion		Single umbilical artery
	Macroglossia		
	Brachycephaly		
	Flat facial profile		

Table 14.9: Medical conditions associated with Trisomy 21	
Condition	Incidence %
MR	95
Growth retardation	95
Early Alzheimer's	60
Hearing loss	40
CHD	40
Eye problems	60
Epilepsy	5
GIT malformations	5
Hypothyroidism	5
Leukemia	1
Atlantoaxial dislocation	<1
Infertility	99% (male) and 30% anovulation (female)

Table 14.10: Urine odor and ferric chloride test in IEM		
S. No.	Condition	Urine odor	Colour change in urine test
1. Phenyl ketonuria	Mousy	Emerald green
2. Tyrosinemia	Rotten cabbage	Transient green
3. MSUD	Maple syrup	Navy blue
4. Histidinemia	-	Blue green
5. Glutaric/Isovaleric acidemia	Sweaty feet	-
6. Multiple Carboxylase Def.	Tom cat urine	-
7. Propionic/Methyl melonic acidemia	-	Purple
8. Ketosis	Fruity	Brown red

Table 14.11: Types of mucopolysaccharidosis		
Type		Remarks
I-H	Hurler	– Classical type, Dermatan and Heparan sulphaturia
I-S	Scheie	– No MR, Dermatan SO_4turia, late presentation
I-H/I-S	Hurler-Scheie	– Scheie type with early presentation
II	Hunter	– XLR, MR variable, Hearing defect, no corneal clouding
III	Sanfilippo	– Heparan SO_4turia, No MR, skeletal dysplasia
IV	Moroquio	– Keratin SO_4turia, No MR, skeletal dysplasia, spinal involvement
V		– Keratin and Heparan SO_4turia, MR, vertebra and cornea spared
VI	Maroteaux Lamy	– Dermatan SO_4turia, MR, vertebra and cornea spared
VII	Beta Glucuronidase deficiency	– Hurler type, Chondroitin SO_4turia

Table 14.12: Differential diagnosis of MPS	
Conditions	*Remark*
1. GM1 Gangliosidosis	- 50% Cherry Red spot in fundus
2. Mannosidosis	- Mannosuria (Oligosaccharide)
3. Fucosidosis	- Fucosuria (Oligosaccharide)
4. Multiple Sulphatase deficiency	- Icthyosis
5. Spondylo Epiphyseal Dysplasia	- No Biochemical Changes
6. Kneist syndrome	- AD inheritance, Keratin SO_4aturia
7. Mucolipidosis	- Sialiac aciduria

Table 14.13: Clinical approach to conditions with CNS involvement

I. Grey Matter Disease

A. With Dysmorphism
GM 1, MPS

B. With Visceromegaly
Gaucher, Nieman Pick, Sandhoffs

C. With Megalencephaly
Tay Sachs, Sialidosis

D. With Seizures
GM 1

E. With Cherry Spot
Tay Sachs, GM 1, Sialidosis

F. With Corneal Clouding
MPS, Mannosidosis Mucolipidosis

A. Without Dismorphism
Gaucher, Nieman Pick

B. Without Visceromegaly
Tay Sachs, Menkes Kinky hair

C. Without Megalencephaly
Menkes Kinky hair

D. Without Seizures
MPS, Fucosidosis, Mannosidosis

E. Without Cherry Spot
Gaucher

F. Without Corneal Clouding
Fucosidosis

II. White Matter Disease

A. CNS Only
Canavans, ALD, Pelizaeus Merzbacher Disease

B. With Macrocephaly
Canavans, Alexander

C. With Visual Loss
Canavan

D. With Adrenal Involvement
ADL

E. With Myopathy and Acidosis
Mitochondrial disorders

A.

B. Without Macrocephaly
Alexander

C. Without Visual Loss
Alexander

D. Without Adrenal Involvement
Pelizaeous Merzbacher disease

E. Without Myopathy
Liver failure-Alpers
No Liver failure-Leights

CNS + PNS
1. MLD
2. Krabbes
3. Cockyane syndrome

Features
1. Hypotonia initially
2. Opisthotonus
3. Photosensitivity

Table 14.14: Features of joint hyper extensibility and hypermobility syndromes (HMS)

1. Can you put your hands flat on the floor with your knees straight?
2. Can you bend your elbow backwards? (1 point for each elbow)
3. Can you bend your knee backwards? (1 point for each knee)
4. Can you bend your thumb back on to the front of your forearm? (for each thumb = 2 points total)
5. Can you bend your little finger upto 90 degree (right angle) to the hand (1 point for each finger = 2 points total)

MAXIMUM SCORE IS OUT OF 9, HMS–5 or more

THE DIAGNOSTIC CRITERIA FOR HYPERMOBILITY SYNDROME

Major diagnostic criteria includes:
- Generalised joint hypermobility (floppy/double joints) 5/9 joints.
- Pain or arthralgia for longer than 3 months in 4 or more joints.
  Minor criteria includes:
- Dislocation/subluxation in more than 1 joint or in 1 joint.
- Arthralgia more than 3 months in 1 to 3 joints or back pain.
- Soft tissue rheumatism, > 3 lesions like epicondylitis, tenosynovitis, bursitis.
- Marfanoid habitus/Marfan syndrome, Span: Height ratio will be >1.03 and US: LS ratio will be <0.89. Arachnodactyly, Positive Steinberg/wrist sign.
- Abnormal skin, striae, thin skin, hyperextensibility.
- Eye signs like drooping eyelids, myopia/anti-mongoloid slant.
- Varicose veins, hernia, rectal/uterine prolapse.
- Diagnosis by two major criteria or one major and two minor or four minor criteria.

Table 14.15: Types of glycogen storage disease		
Type	*Name*	*Remarks*
GSD 0	– Aglycogenosis	– Hypoglycemia, hepatomegaly
GSD I	– Glycogenosis	– Doll face, hypoglycemia, hepatomegaly renal involvement, lactic acidosis
GSD I a	– Von Gierke	- Do -
GSD II	– Generalized Pompe	– Cardiomyopathy, hypotonia
GSD III	– Debrancher Glycogenosis/ Forbes disease	– Liver and heart muscle involvement
GSD IV	– Brancher Glycogenosis/ Anderson	– Cirrhosis and liver failure
GSD V	– Mc Ardle	– Muscle phophorylase deficiency, myoglobinuria, muscle cramps
GSD VI	—	– Isolated hepatomegaly
GSD VII	– Tarui	– Phosphofructokinase deficiency (Similar to type V)
GSD VIII	—	– Liver and brain involvement
GSD IX	—	– Liver phosphorylase kinase deficiency (Similar to type VI)
GSD X	—	– Liver involvement, myalgia
GSD XI	– Complex	– Liver and kidney involvement, rickets, galactosuria, hyperlipidemia.

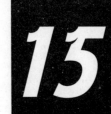

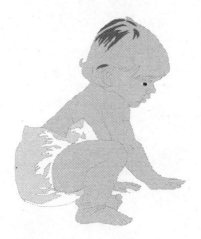

Pediatric Intensive Care

15

Pediatric
Intensive Care

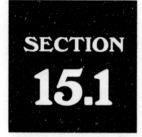

APPROACH TO A SICK CHILD

- Treatment will have to be given earlier than completing history and examination in a critically ill child.
- Stratification of patient by paying special attention to **A**ppearance, **B**reathing and **C**irculation (ABC).
- Check for general danger signs. (Red Flag Sings).

Child with Danger Signs Needs Urgent Attention

I. ASK FOR

- Altered sensorium
- Persistent vomiting
- Feeding difficulty especially inability to drink
- Stridor/cyanosis
- Bleeding tendency
- Seizures
- Looks pale, circulatory collapse
- Decreased urine output.

II. LOOK FOR

Temperature	High	– Consider infectious causes
	Low	– Consider conditions causing shock
Pulse rate	High	– Shock, myocarditis, SVT

	Low	– Raised ICT, odollum poisoning
BP	High	– Hypertensive encephalopathy (AGN)
	Low	– Shock
Respiratory rate	Increased	– Pneumonia, acidosis, CCF

III. FEEL FOR

Vital signs–Normal

Age	Resp rate	HR	Syst BP
Newborn	30-60	90-180	50-70
6 Months	24-40	85-170	65-106
1 Year	20-40	80-140	72-140
3 Years	20-30	80-130	78-114
6 Years	18-25	70-110	80-116
8 Years	18-25	70-110	84-122
10 Years	16-20	65-110	90-130
12 Years	14-20	60-110	94-136

- **Take core temperature**—Axillary + 1°F except in newborn.

CHAPTER 15

PEDIATRIC INTENSIVE CARE

- **Alertness AVPU score**

  A: Awake—Alert

  V: Response to **v**oice—Verbal Response

  P: Response to **p**ain—Pain Response

  U: Unresponsiveness—Unconscious

- **Glasgow coma scale (GCS)—EVM**

Eye opening	Score
Spontaneous	4
To speech	3
To pain	2
None	1

Best verbal response	Score
Oriented	5
Confused	4
Inappropriate words	3
Incomprehensible sounds	2
None	

Best motor response	Score
Obeys	6
Localizes	5
Withdrawal	4
Abn flexion	3
Extensor response	2
None	1

For best infants and toddlers	Score
Appropriate words, smiles fixes and follows	5
Consolable cry	4
Persistently irritable	3
Restless, agitated	2
None	1

GCS <7-Ventilator Support

Clinical Staging of Encephalopathy

1	2	3	4	5
Lethargic	Combative	Comatose	Comatose	Comatose
Follows commands	Inconsistent following of commands	Occasional response to commands	Response only to pain	No response to pain
Pupils reacting	Pupils sluggish	Eyes may deviate	Weak pupillary response	No pupillary response
Normal breathing	May hyperventilate	Irregular breathing	Very irregular breathing	Requires mechanical ventilation
Normal muscle tone	Reflexes inconsistent	Decorticate posture	Decerebrate posture Absent tendon reflexes	

Quick ABC Assessment

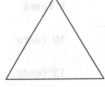

Appearance
Alert, normal tone
Normal posture,
Normal colour

Breathing
Respiratory rate, work
of breathing,
Breath sounds

Circulation
HR, Perfusion (CFT),
Liver span, BP

SECTION 15.2

APPROACH TO A CHILD WITH SHOCK

Shock results from inadequate blood flow and oxygen delivery to meet tissue metabolic demands. Shock progresses over a continuum of severity, from a compensated to a decompensated state.

Signs of Compensated Shock Include

- Tachycardia.
- Cool extremities.
- Prolonged capillary refill (despite warm ambient temperature).
- Weak peripheral pulses compared with central pulses.

Normal Blood Pressure

Signs of decompensated shock include the signs listed above plus hypotension. In the absence of blood pressure measurement, decompensated shock is indicated by the nondetectable distal pulses with weak central pulses in an infant or child with other signs and symptoms consistent with inadequate tissue oxygen delivery.

Hypotension is a systolic blood pressure less than the 5th percentile of normal for age, namely:

<60 mm Hg	– term neonates (0-28 days)
<70 mm Hg	– infants (1 to 12 months)
<70 mm Hg + (2 x age in years)	– children 1 to 10 years
<90 mm Hg	– children ≥ 10 years of age

Clues for Diagnosis of Shock

• Vomiting/diarrhea	:	Fluid loss (Hypovolumic)
• Fever/Rash	:	Dengue/Septicemia
• Urticaria, angioneurotic edema and history of allergen exposure	:	Anaphylaxis
• Cyanosis, unresponsive to Oxygen and signs of CCF	:	Congenital heart disease/cardiomyopathy
• Severe tachycardia	:	Arrhythmias
• Polyuria and acidotic breathing	:	Diabetes/CRF/metabolic disorder
• Immediate history of injury/blood loss	:	Polytrauma, Pneumothorax
• History of drug ingestion/bites/sting	:	Poisoning/envenomation

Lab Investigations

- Complete blood counts, CRP, PCV, Peripheral smear
- Blood sugar
- Renal function tests and Electrolytes
- Liver function tests (ALT, AST)
- Coagulation test (PT, APTT)
- **Various cultures: Blood, CSF, Urine**
- X-ray chest, ECG, USS, ECHO
- Arterial blood gases
- Toxicology

Types of Shock

S - Septic

H - Hypovolemic

O - Obstructive/Others

C - Cardiogenic

K - Kinetic/Distributive

Management of Shock

1. A B C—Appearance, Breathing, Circulation.

2. **Fluids and vasoactive agents:** Crystalloids like Ringer Lactate or Normal saline 20 ml/kg is given as bolus over 20 minutes. Then the patient is reassessed and further boluses are given. Multiple fluid challenges may be needed, especially in patients with septic shock who may require upto 100 cc/kg or more of fluid. Glucose containing solutions are used only in documented hypoglycemia. Blood and blood products, though more efficient volume expanders, are used only in specific conditions like trauma.

How Much Fluid to be Administered

1. **Cardiogenic shock:** Fluids may initially improve cardiac output and peripheral perfusion; however delayed effects may be deleterious with fluid overload. Increasing heart rate or worsening of general condition even after two fluid boluses, consider cardiogenic shock. In the setting of cardiogenic shock, inotropic agents are generally required to improve the underlying problem (5-10 ml/mg bolus is advisable when cardiogenic shock is evident as in arrhythmia/myocarditis).

2. **Hypovolemic shock:** Fluid should be administered to restore the cardiovascular function and inotropic agents should not be used in lieu of appropriate fluid administration to maintain blood pressure (20 ml/kg bolus 30ml/kg bolus in diarrhea).

3. **Septic shock:** In addition to decreased intravascular volume, resulting from increased insensible losses, decreased intake and increased losses. There is endothelial damage and resultant transudation of fluid into extra vascular compartment. The fluid requirements in these patients may be quite large, up to 80-120 ml/kg in the initial phase.

3. **Correction of metabolic abnormalities**

   Acidosis

   Hypoglycemia, hypocalcemia

4. **Inotropic agents**

   Failure to improve after fluid resuscitation, suggests that inotropic support is needed to improve cardiac output.

   a. **Dopamine**

   Dose calculation:

   6 x body wt = mg of dopamine (to be added to 100 ml fluid). 1ml/hr of this fluid provides 1mcg/kg/minute.Initiate at doses of 5-10 mcg/kg/min and gradually increase to a maximum of 20 mcg/kg/minute.

   b. **Dobutamine**

   This is most useful in myocardial dysfunction as in myocarditis with cardiogenic shock, septic shock with myocardial dysfunction. Dose is 5-20 mcg/kg/minute as a constant infusion.

   c. **Adrenaline/Epinephrine (in cold shock)**

   Dose: 0.05-0.1 mcg/kg/min as a constant infusion (inotropic dose) and 0.2 mcg/kg/min vasopressor effect.

   d. **Nor Adrenaline (in warm shock).**

   Dose: 0.01 to 005 mcg/kg/minute.

   Maximum dose 1.0 mcg/kg/minute.

Preparation of Vasoactive Agents

Medication	Dilution	Delivery rate
Dopamine	6 × wt (kg) equals mgs	1 ml / hr delivers
Dobutamine	to be added to 100 ml	1 µg / kg / mt
Epinephrine	0.6 × wt (kg) equals mgs	1 ml / hr delivers
Norepinephrine	to be added to 100 ml	0.1 µg / kg / mt

5. **Steroids Indicated in:** Meningococcemia, CAH.

6. **Antibiotics:** Appropriate antibiotic therapy is indicated for those patients with suspected septic shock. Always start in 1st hour itself after taking 2 samples of blood culture (Cefotaxim, Amikacin + Vancomycin).

Choice of specific antibiotics depends on the specific context (community acquired/Nosocomial).

Indications for Mechanical Ventilation

- Refractory shock.
- Hypoxemia in spite of 100% oxygen.
- Altered mental status with GCS < 8.

Algorithm for the management of shock

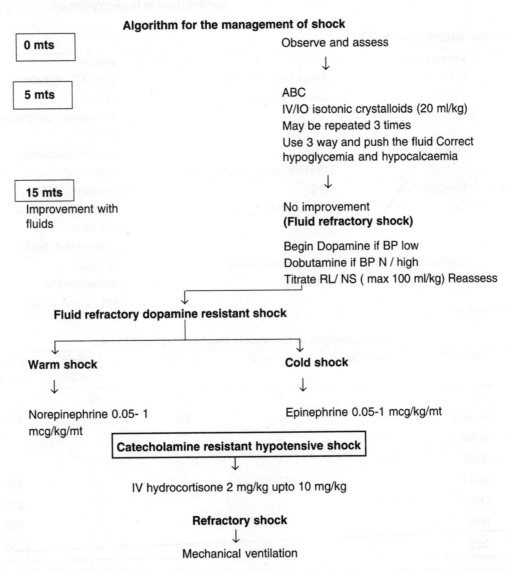

0 mts	Observe and assess ↓
5 mts	ABC IV/IO isotonic crystalloids (20 ml/kg) May be repeated 3 times Use 3 way and push the fluid Correct hypoglycemia and hypocalcaemia ↓
15 mts Improvement with fluids	No improvement **(Fluid refractory shock)** Begin Dopamine if BP low Dobutamine if BP N / high Titrate RL/ NS (max 100 ml/kg) Reassess

Fluid refractory dopamine resistant shock

Warm shock
↓
Norepinephrine 0.05- 1 mcg/kg/mt

Cold shock
↓
Epinephrine 0.05-1 mcg/kg/mt

Catecholamine resistant hypotensive shock
↓
IV hydrocortisone 2 mg/kg upto 10 mg/kg

Refractory shock
↓
Mechanical ventilation

Note: Dobutamine after BP is stabilized.

Always Monitor BP

- Cold shock with normal BP→Give volume replacement and add vasodilators.
- Cold shock with hypotension→Increase volume and add epinephrine.

Role of Crystalloids and Colloids

In refractory cases:

- Hexastarch
- 3.5% in newborns
- 6.5% in older children.

Dose—60 ml/kg/day

Monitor blood glucose levels as hyperglycemia is associated with increased mortality. Small doses of insulin can be given (0.25 U/kg 6th hourly for 4-5 days in hyperglycemia).

Always Anticipate—MODS

Respiratory	ARDS	Oxygen
	Resp muscle paralysis	Early ET intubation
	Central apnea	PEEP
		Permissive hypercapnia
		HFOV
Renal	ARF	Fluid resuscitation,
	Monitor serum electrolytes	Dopamine
Hematological	DIC	Vitamin K, FFP
GIT	Stress ulcer	H_2 blockers or PPIs
	Ileus	NG tube
		Early enteral feeds
Endocrine	Adrenal insufficiency	Steroids
CNS	Seizures	Antiepileptics, antiedema drugs

Composition of Commonly used Intravenous Fluids*

Solution	Na+(meq)	K+(meq)	Cl- (meq)	Lactate (mmols)	Glucose (mmols)
RL	130	4	109	28	-
RL+D5	130	4	109	28	278
½ NS	77	-	77	-	-
3%S	512	-	-	-	-
ISO P	26	20	-	-	278
D5	-	-	-	-	278
D10	-	-	-	-	556
D25	-	-	-	-	1390

* Maintenance fluid is given as per Holliday and Segar Formula (Refer Appendix 6).

SECTION 15.3 APPROACH TO ANAPHYLACTIC SHOCK

Monitoring

- PR/HR
- RR
- BP
- SPO_2
- CFT and urine output
- Sensorium

Early Recognition
Intubation
Aggressive fluid management
Epinephrine

Treatment

1. 100% O_2.
2. Trendelenburg position.
3. Adrenaline—0.01ml/kg of 1 in 1000 solution I/M—I/V which can be repeated every 15 minutes; if given IV the dose is 0.1 ml/kg of 1 in 10000 dilution solution. Repeat at 5-10 minutes intervals x 3 doses. Nebulized adrenaline can be given at a dose of 0.5 ml/kg/dose.

4. Normal saline bolus IV: 20 ml/kg. Upto 2-4 boluses may be given over 1-2 hours.
5. Remove antigen, delay absorption. If penicillin was given IM, tie a tourniquet proximal to the injection site.
6. Steroids: Methyl prednisolone 2 mg/kg stat→1 mg/kg Q 6 hourly.

OR

Hydrocortisone 10 mg/kg IV stat→5 mg/kg Q6 hourly.

7. Anti histamines—Chlorpheneramine 0.35 mg/kg/day in 4 divided doses and ranitidine 1 mg/kg Q 8 hourly.
8. If there is bronchospasm, use Salbutamol nebulization/IV Aminophylline.
9. If still in shock, start IV dopamine infusion through a separate line at 10 micro gm/kg/minute.

SECTION 15.4 APPROACH TO POISONING IN CHILDREN

General Measures

Assess the child and institute resuscitation if indicated. The assessment and intervention should follow the usual order of **ABC** i.e. **A**irway, **B**reathing and **C**irculation.

- Airway is maintained by proper positioning, suction and clearing the airway. 'Head tilt and chin lift or jaw thrust'.
- Breathing is supported by oxygen, bag and mask if indicated.
- Circulation is maintained by IV fluids and vasopressor agents.

Monitor vital signs like respiration, heart rate, blood pressure, temperature and pupillary abnormalities. Refer Table 15.1 for the possible poison depending on the clinical features.

Gastric decontamination: Emesis, gastric lavage, activated charcoal and cathartics are the available options. Charcoal is available in the market as tablets which must be crushed and made into a paste and used. The recommended initial dose is 1 gram/kg prepared as syrup in about 100 ml Sorbitol (1-2 ml/kg of 70% Sorbitol, not more than 150 ml).

Dose of Activated Charcoal

<6 years 15-20 g.

>6 years 30-50 g.

Emesis is contraindicated if the child is unconscious. However gastric lavage may be done.

Toxicology Screens

Qualitative/quantitative toxicology screening tests may be done if facilities are available.

Gastric lavage is contraindicated in corrosives, acids, kerosene ingestion. However, pliable ryles tube/feeding tube may be introduced to prevent stricture if the victim is brought immediately.

'Universal antidote' is powdered charcoal, magnesium and tannic acid (2:1:1).

Common Household Items of Low Toxicity

No treatment required

Bar soap	Lipsticks
Dry cells	Newspaper
Candles	Pencil
Chalk	Shampoo
Clay	Shaving cream and lotions
Crayons	Shoe polish
Dehumidifying packets	Striking surfaces of matches
Detergents	Sweetening agents
Hand lotion	Thermometer
Ink	Toothpaste

Removal Necessary Only if Large Amounts Ingested

After shave lotion	Body conditioners
Colognes	Deodorants
Fabric softeners	Hair dye
Hair tonic	Marker ink
Match stick >20	OCP
Perfumes	Toilet water

Common Poisons (Table 15.1)

Name	Comments	Clinical features	Management
ACIDS	Formic acid (used to process rubber) Oxalic, acetic, carbolic etc.	Intense pain, edema and bleeding in the oral mucosa are characteristic. Child may die of asphyxia due to edema of glottis or larynx. Perforation of stomach may result in peritonitis. Occasionally shock and renal shutdown.	1. Emesis and activated charcoal are contraindicated. 2. Neutralization with alkali like sodium bicarbonate may produce more harm than good. 3. Steroids may prevent future strictures and hence may be used for about two weeks. 4. Surgical opinion as pyloric stenosis is likely sequelae. 5. IV fluids, oxygen, analgesics, antibiotics etc. as is needed.
ALKALI	E.g.: NaOH, KOH, CaOH$_2$	Oral mucosa appears swollen and whitish and the child will be drooling due to difficulty in swallowing.	1. Emesis and activated charcoal are contraindicated. 2. Give milk if child can swallow. 3. Role of steroid is controversial. 4. Stricture of esophagus is likely and hence surgical reference.
BENZYL BEN-ZOATE	Usually used for local application in scabies.	If consumed, it produces CNS stimulation and result in seizures.	1. Gastric lavage. 2. Symptomatic treatment of seizures.
CAMPHOR	Over 50 mg/kg of pure camphor may be fatal.	Odor of camphor in breath, vomiting, headache, irritability and seizures to the extent of status epilepticus.	1. Gastric lavage and activated charcoal. 2. Seizures can be controlled with phenobarbitone.
COPPER SULFATE		Metallic taste in the mouth, vomiting and diarrhea. Massive ingestion may occasionally cause hemolysis and renal/ hepatic dysfunction.	1. Gastric lavage. 2. For massive ingestion, chelation with penicillamine may be tried.
DHATURA	Atropine	Tachycardia, dilated pupils, blurred vision, fever, urinary retention, abnormal behavior.	1. Gastric lavage and activated charcoal. 2. Physostigmine 0.02 mg to 0.06 mg/kg is the specific antidote. However clinical

Contd.

Name	Comments	Clinical features	Management
			effects are short lived, for about an hour or so, and the drug has significant cardiac side effects.
			3. Diazepam may be used to control the CNS manifestations.
			4. Neostigmine may be used but it does not revert CNS symptoms.
			5. Treat fever and seizures symptomatically.
DAPSONE		Produces methemo-globinemia presenting as cyanosis unres-ponsive to oxygen. Pulse oximetry is unreliable for moni-toring in methemoglo-binemia.	1. Gastric lavage and activated charcoal.
			2. Oxygen.
			3. Methylene blue 1-2mg/kg/dose of 1% solution as IV infusion is therapeutic. Response to methylene blue is expected within an hour. When methylene blue is not available, one may resort to partial exchange transfusion.
DIGOXIN (DIGITALIS)	Poisoning can occur due to overdose or acciden-tal ingestion.	Nausea, vomiting, bradycardia, cardiac irregularities ST, T wave changes in ECG etc. Abnormalities of electrolytes may be seen.	1. Gastric lavage and activated charcoal.
			2. Correct electrolyte abnormali-ties if any (particular attention to potassium).
			3. Atropine may be used if heart rate is very low.
			4. Isoprenaline may be indicated for bradycardia, lidocaine or phenytoin for ventricular arrhythmia and for cardiac pacing for AV Block.
			5. Digoxin specific Fab fragment antibodies may be used if available.
			6. Forced diuresis is **not** useful.
ISONIAZID (INH)	Over 40 mg/kg may produce seizures.	Vomiting, Seizure, Metabolic acidosis. In chronic ingestion, optic and peripheral neuritis can occur.	1. Gastric lavage (Activated charcoal may be used).
			2. Oxygen inhalation.
			3. IV fluids with sodium bicar-bonate to tackle acidosis.
			4. Hypotension must be treated with IV fluids and vasopressor as is done in case of shock.

Contd.

Name	Comments	Clinical features	Management
			5. Seizures may be controlled with anticonvulsants like diazepam. *IV pyridoxine in mg equal to mg of INH consumed is the definitive treatment for terminating the seizure.*
			6. Forced diuresis is effective to some extent but must not be used if BP is not stable.
			7. PD and HD are effective.
			8. Hepatic and renal functions must be monitored.
IRON	Dangerous toxicity is possible when **more than 50 mg/kg** of elemental iron is consumed (Fe SO$_4$ is 20% elemental Fe). Estimation of prothrombin time, liver enzymes, blood glucose, electrolytes and bilirubin are to be done.	Up to 6 hrs: Vomiting, diarrhea and hypotension, usually due to hypovolemia. 6-24 hrs: Appears to improve. After 24 hrs: Hepatic dysfunction, Renal failure, Shock, Acidosis. 2-6 weeks: Gastric outlet obstruction.	1. Emesis. Gastric lavage with oro/nasogastric tube is less satisfactory.
			2. Activated charcoal **does not** remove Fe.
			3. Stomach wash with 1 % NaHCO$_3$. One may leave 100 ml 1% solution in stomach after the lavage.
			4. IM or slow IV Deferoxamine must be given to remove Fe from blood in all cases of significant iron poisoning. Repeat the doses must be given if urine is reddish (Vine rose color) till the urine clears.
			5. The dose of Deferoxamine is 50 mg/kg/dose 6-8 hourly (or 10 mg/kg/hr).
			6. In renal failure, chelation therapy may be combined with hemodialysis.
			7. In case of hepatic involvement, standard hepatic support as discussed under hepatic encephalopathy must be instituted.
			8. The child may be discharged if there are no symptoms for 24 hours post ingestion. Liver enzymes should be documented (beyond 1 day) as normal before discharge.

Name	Comments	Clinical features	Management
JATRO-PHA CURCAS	(Kadal-lavanakku, kattavanaku, purging nut, bagberinda)	Vomiting and diarrhea leading on to hypovolemia and electrolyte imbalance.	1. Gastric lavage. 2. IV Fluids.
KERO-SENE	X-ray Chest is best taken **12 hrs** post ingestion.	Cough and dyspnea immediately after ingestion. Respiratory symptoms occurring beyond 24-48 hours is likely to be due to pneumonia due to secondary invaders. Some children may appear drowsy. It is supposed to be due to hypoxia. Since kerosene is highly volatile, it gets aspirated into the lungs to produce hypoxia and pneumonia.	1. No gastric lavage. 2. Activated charcoal has no role. 3. Oxygen inhalation. 4. Salbutamol by nebulization is indicated if wheeze is present. 5. In seriously ill child, steroids and antibiotics may be used empirically although there is insufficient evidence supporting its use. 6. Always rule out another poison if the child is excessively drowsy.
MUSH-ROOMS (Amanita phal-loides)		Mushroom poisoning may fit in with one of the symptom complexes mentioned below: • Cholinergic: (simulates manifestations of Organophosphorus) • Anticholinergic: (simulates manifestations of Dhatura) • Gastrointestinal: (simulates manifestations of jatropha curcas)	1. Gastric lavage followed by activated charcoal. 2. Treatment is depending on the symptom complex identified (refer under relevant sections). 3. Monitor for hepatic and renal functions and for hemolysis.

Contd.

Name	Comments	Clinical features		Management
MULLELI THYLAM	It is a quack remedy consisting of highly hetero-geneous mixture. Even slight overdose produces seizure. Serum electrolytes must be monitored.	Intractable seizures.	1. 2.	Treatment of seizures. Standard measures to reduce intracranial tension (discussed elsewhere).
ODOLLUM (Cerbera odollum)	ECG monitoring must be done. Cardiac pacing must be instituted at the appropriate time.	Vomiting, bradycardia, arrhythmia, BP fall, hyperkalemia.	1. 2. 3.	Gastric lavage. Atropine is given in the dose of **0.05 mg/kg** to keep heart rate near normal. Treat hyperkalemia (Insulin Glucose regimen).
OLEANDER	Monitor ECG (look for brady-cardia, ST depression, AV block etc.) and serum electrolytes.	GIT symptoms, arrhythmia, heart block, BP fall, acidosis, electrolyte abnormalities (especially hyper-kalemia). Nerium odorum can also cause spasms.	1. 2. 3. 4. 5. 6. 7.	Gastric lavage. Activated charcoal may be useful. IV fluids with available alkali (e.g. Ringer Lactate). Treat hyperkalemia if present (e.g. Insulin glucose as described under glomerulonephritis). Treat BP fall by standard methods. Treat arrhythmia. Treat low heart rate (atropine, cardiac pacing).

Contd.

CHAPTER 15

PEDIATRIC INTENSIVE CARE

Name	Comments	Clinical features	Management
OPIATES		Constricted pupils, decreased rate of respiration, hypoxia (leads to cyanosis, seizures and pulmonary edema) vomiting Bowel and bladder retention.	1. Gastric lavage and Activated charcoal. 2. Cathartics may be used as opiates cause intestinal hypomotility. 3. IV fluids containing glucose. 4. Oxygen. 5. Naloxone 0.1 mg/kg/IV. Effect of Naloxone wanes in 30-60 minutes and may have to be repeated or infused in a drip of glucose solution.
ORGANO CHLORIDE (DDT, BHC, LINDANE)	Monitor hepatic/ renal/ CNS functions.	Twitching, para- esthesia, seizures.	1. Gastric lavage and activated charcoal. 2. Oxygen and IV fluids. 3. Treat seizures as per standard protocol. 4. Dialysis and hemoperfusion are **not** effective. 5. Children who recover must be followed up for the rare possibility of aplastic anemia.
ORGANO PHOS- PHORUS (MALA- THION, PARA- THION, TICK 20)	Send blood for estimation of cholin- esterase levels.	Sweating, lacrymation, salivation, wheeze, small pupils, bradycardia, hypotension, incontinence (Muscaranic effects).Twitching, paralysis including respiratory muscles (nicotinic effects). Restlessness, seizures, depression of respiration and circulation (CNS effects).	1. Wash contaminated skin. 2. Gastric lavage. 3. Oxygen and IV fluids. 4. Atropine is given in the dose of 0.05 mg/kg IV repeated every 5-10 minutes till full atropinisation. (dry secretions, dilated pupils, tachycardia etc). 5. Pralidoxime must be given after atropinization has been achiev- ed, ideally within 24 hours at the dose of 25 mg/kg/dose slow IV infusion in normal saline, which may be repeated if needed at 6-8 hourly intervals.

Contd.

Name	Comments	Clinical features	Management
PARA-CETA-MOL	Over 200 mg/kg as a single dose is highly hepatotoxic Adolescent and adult > 7.5g. Ref: Rumack Matthew Normogram for blood levels.	*Clinical course– 4 stages:* *Stage 1:* 0.5–24 hours after ingestion: Anorexia, nausea, vomiting, sweating, abdominal pain, pallor. *Stage 2:* 24-48 hours after ingestion: Hepatic damage– pain in right upper abdominal quadrant; increased liver enzymes, bilirubin and PT (prothrombin time); oliguria. *Stage 3:* 72–96 hours after ingestion: Peak liver function abnormalities; extensive liver damage (necrosis). Liver failure may occur. *Stage 4:* 4 days– 2 weeks: Resolution of hepatic damage.	*Objectives:* 1. Removal of paracetamol from the GIT. 2. Administration of the specific antidote. 3. Prevention of further hepatic damage. 4. Supportive treatment. 1. Gastric lavage. Do **not** give activated charcoal if acetyl-cysteine is administered orally. 2. N acetyl cysteine (as 5% solution via tube or as drink) 140 mg/kg in water/fruit juice followed by 1/2 this dose 4 hourly x 17 times is the standard recommendation. Intravenous preparation is also available in some centers. Initial dose of 150 mg/kg in 5% glucose over 15 minutes followed by 50 mg/kg in 5% glucose as IV infusion over next four hours and then 100 mg/kg in 5% glucose over 16 hours. N acetyl cysteine is best when administered within eight hours of paracetamol poisoning. It may be given orally also.
PHENO-THIA-ZINES	Watch for arrhythmia and hypo-tension.	Extra pyramidal features, oculogyric crisis, small pupils, hypotension, hypothermia. Rarely arrhythmia, respiratory depression, seizures.	1. Gastric lavage. 2. Dystonia may be controlled with diphenhydramine or diazepam. 3. Seizures may be controlled by diazepam; phenytoin etc.
PHENO-BARBI-TONE	Monitor for multi organ failure.	Drowsiness, coma, small and reacting pupils, respiratory	1. Gastric lavage and Activated charcoal. 2. IV fluids and Oxygen.

Contd.

CHAPTER 15

PEDIATRIC INTENSIVE CARE

Name	Comments	Clinical features	Management
		depression, hypotension.	3. Treatment for hypotension (volume expansion, dopamine). 4. Forced alkaline diuresis (as discussed under Salicylates). 5. Peritoneal dialysis and hemodialysis are effective. 6. Ventilation may be required in case of severe respiratory depression.
PHENYTOIN		Nystagmus, ataxia, altered sensorium.	
RAT POISON	Contain zinc/ aluminum phosphide or warfarin like compounds. Monitor renal and hepatic functions and coagulation profiles.	All symptomatic patients are monitored for at least 72 hours, hypotension, respiratory distress etc. Bleeding from various sites like epistaxis, hemetemesis, hematuria or even intracranial bleed is possible if the rodenticide contains warfarin like compounds.	1. Gastric lavage with saline followed by gastric lavage with 1:10000 potassium permanganate solution followed by gastric lavage with 1% $NaHCO_3$. 2. Poisoning by rodenticide with warfarin like compounds is treated by IV Vitamin K, IV Ranitidine and if needed blood or fresh frozen plasma transfusion.
SALI-CYLA-TES (Aspirin)	Over 150 mg/kg of aspirin can be considered to be toxic.	Sweating, flushing, fever, GIT symptoms, tachypnea, seizure, coma, acidosis, hypoglycemia and bleeding manifestations. Prolonged prothrombin time. ABG may show a combined picture of respiratory alkalosis and metabolic acidosis.	1. Gastric lavage and Activated charcoal. 2. Dehydration should be corrected with fluid containing dextrose and bicarbonate and not merely with normal saline. 3. *Forced alkaline diuresis*: It must be attempted after correction of dehydration and stabilizing BP. The aim is to keep urine flow above 5 ml/kg/hr and urinary pH above 7.5 (preferably above 8): Dose of $NaHCO_3$ may be 20-40 meq/L, to be adjusted depending on urine pH.

Contd.

Contd.

Name	Comments	Clinical features	Management
			4. Monitor prothrombin time and give IV Vit.K.
			5. Control seizures as per standard protocol.
			6. Hemodialysis is better than peritoneal dialysis. Alkaline diuresis is better than peritoneal dialysis.
THEO-PHYL-LINE		Vomiting, irritability, seizure, cardiac arrhythmia.	1. Gastric lavage and activated charcoal. 2. IV ranitidine. 3. Correction of hypokalemia. 4. Treat arrhythmia and seizures. 5. Peritoneal dialysis and forced diuresis are **not** very effective.
TRICYCLIC ANTI-DEPRES-SANTS	Even double the thera-peutic dose can be toxic.	Tachycardia, flushing, hyperthermia, urinary retention, hallucinations, delirium etc may occur. Hypotension, tachy or brady arrhythmias, seizures and coma. ECG may show wide QRS, QT prolongation, T-ST abnormalities and various conduction blocks.	1. Gastric lavage and activated charcoal. 2. If conduction defects occur (QRS complex > 0.12 seconds or prolonged QT interval), consult the cardiologist. 3. Cardiac pacing in selected cases. 4. Seizures are managed with phenytoin/phenobarbitone. 5. Hypotension is managed with IV fluids, sodium bicarbonate and other standard methods. 6. Dialysis and hemoperfusion are **not** effective.

SECTION
15.5 APPROACH TO SNAKE BITE

MANAGEMENT

First step in the management is to identify if the bite was by a poisonous snake or not.

If pain, numbness and edema spreading from the site of bite—poisonous snake with 2 close by bite marks.

Evidence of systemic envenomation is:

- CT > 10 minutes
- Bleeding manifestations, Pink serum on clot retraction
- Oliguria/hematuria
- Hypotension
- Ptosis
- Circumoral paresthesia
- Aphonia/dysarthria
- Facial puffiness—forrunner of ARF.

Classification of Envenomation Severity

Grade 0	No envenomation
Grade I	Minimal envenomation
	Local pain and swelling without progression
	No systemic envenomation
Grade II	Moderate envenomation
	Pain, swelling or ecchymosis spreading beyond the site of bite

	Mild systemic or laboratory manifestations
Grade III	Severe envenomation
	Marked local response
	Severe systemic findings
	Significant alteration in laboratory findings.

Investigations

- Blood grouping and cross matching
- Hb; PCV
- CBC—Look for leukocytosis
- Platelet count
- Peripheral smear—Hemolysis
- BT, CT—Serial measurements
- Color of supernatant plasma
- PT, APTT
- Urea, serum electrolytes
- Urine R/E for hematuria/hemoglobinuria
- ECG
- Single breath count.

Monitoring

- Pulse and BP
- Respiration
- Capillary refill
- CT 1/2-1 hourly initially, then 2-4 hourly

- Urine output
- Level of consciousness
- Bulbar muscle weakness.
- Limb circumference for compartment syndrome.

Treatment

Group 0	- Local wound care
	- Injection TT if not immunized
	- Observe for 24 hours
Group I	- Local wound care
	- Injection TT
	- Antibiotics (Injection CP or Ampicillin
	- Observe for 24 hours
Group II and III	- ASV
	- Injection TT
	- Antibiotics (Injection CP or Ampicillin or 3rd generation cephalosporin + Metrogyl)
	- Local anti-edema measures

If the patient comes with a tourniquet, check the pulse beyond and if pulse is present keep the tourniquet till ASV is initiated.

Anti snake venom (ASV): The dose of antivenin is 10 vials polyvalent anti snake venom in most of the cases irrespective of body weight and age. Severe cases with shock and DIC may be given 20 vials. It should be given if there are local reaction, prolonged CT/Hematuria/CNS manifestations etc. The dose may be repeated if needed.

Test dose is a must. Be prepared to tackle anaphylaxis. Intradermal test dose does not correlate with subsequent anaphylaxis. It may be intradermal or IV (one vial in 100 ml NS—few ml slowly).

Skin Test

Done with 0.2 ml of 1:10 solution intra dermally. A small vol of saline on the opposite side as control.

If wheal formation (5-10 mm)—Sensitive.

No wheal formation—Not sensitive.

No Sensitivity

Pretreatment with	Adrenaline (0.01 ml/kg of 1: 1000 soln)
	+
	Methyl prednisolone (2 mg/kg) or Hydrocortisone (5 mg/kg)
	+
	CPM (0.1 mg/kg) or Diphenhydramine (1 mg/kg)

IV Test: ASV can be started by adding one vial in 100 ml NS. After 10 -15 mts of infusion add 9 vials in the same fluid and run over one hour. If coagulation parameters remaining abnormal after 1 hour, administer 10 more vials ASV.

With Sensitivity to ASV

Rapid desensitization with Adrenaline, steroids and antihistamines as with pretreatment.

Then test doses are given with solutions of increasing concentration.

0.1 ml of 1: 100 solution I.D (0.1ml of undiluted ASV made up to 10 ml solution)

0.1 ml of 1: 10 solution I.D. (0.1 ml of undiluted ASV made up to 1 ml solution)

0.1 ml of undiluted solution I.D.

Timing of ASV

Best effects when used with in 4 hours, but can be administered upto 48 hours. It may be effacious even up to 6-7 days, if envenomation persists.

CHAPTER 15

PEDIATRIC INTENSIVE CARE

Response to ASV

- Normalization of BP.
- Bleeding stops in 15-30 mts.
- Upto 6 hours for normalization of coagulation parameters.
- Neurological signs resolve in 30 mts–48 hours.

  In case of inadequate response increase the dose.

Treatment of Complications

I. **Shock**

 a. Central shock

 b. Hypovolemic

 c. Neurogenic

If renal function is normal — I.V. infusion with volume expanders.

20 ml/kg of isotonic solution; maximum of 60 ml/kg - 3 bolus doses. If the shock is not corrected with IVF, then the shock is not hypovolemic.

In central/Cardiogenic shock:

- Raised JVP
- Edema
- Signs of pulmonary edema
- Feeble heart sounds
- Changes in ECG.

  Treat central shock with Dobutamine drip (5-10 microgram/kg/minute). If the shock remains, then the shock can be neurogenic shock. Treat it with Dopamine Drip (10-12 microgram/kg/minute upto 20 microgram/kg/ minutes). If the B.P. is not coming up then treat with Noradrenalin (0.1-0.5 mg/kg—Maxm. 2 mg/kg).

Closely monitor for evidence of fluid overload: Base of lungs–crepitations; Respiratory rate; CVP monitoring.

O_2 inhalation

Foot end elevation

Consider ventilator care.

II. **Renal failure**—Early dialysis is good.

 Anuria

 Hyperkalemia   Consider peritoneal
 Fluid overload   dialysis (PD)
 Uremia

 If coagulation failure—Consider
                     hemodialysis.

III. **Myocardial failure**

 Treat central shock

 Treat CCF

 Avoid fluid overload

 O_2 inhalation

IV. **Shock lung**

 Tachypnea

 Hypoxemia

 Unexplained drowsiness

 Mild acidosis

 O_2 inhalation and put the patient on CPAP— Nasal CPAP or on ventilator.

V. **Bleeding**

- Correction of coagulation failure
- FFP 10 ml/kg
- Correct platelet deficiency
- Whole blood in cases of frank bleeding
- Inj. Ranitidine if G.I. bleeds.

  Closely monitor organ dysfunction. Support vital organ functions.

VI. **Neurotoxins**

Timely administration of Neostigmine along with Atropine will be life saving if neuroparalytic symptoms are seen.

Neostigmine methyl sulphate 100 microgram/ kg/dose

+

Atropine 50 microgram/kg/dose

Can be repeated 4th hourly if needed. Watch for ptosis. If recur more frequent doses may be needed as second line drugs.

VII. **Antibiotics**

Routine antibiotic prophylaxis is not needed. IV Chloramphenicol or IV fluroquinolone can be used as second line drugs.

- *In cobra bite, don't withhold ventilla-tory support even if pupils are dilated.*
- *Any child with suspected snake bite needs observation for at least 24 hours.*
- *The manifestations may be immediate or rarely may be delayed for several days.*

VIII. **Surgical Treatment**

It is important to decompress edema and to clear gangrene/compartment syndrome.

Table 15.1: Clinical feature—Poison	
Probable Poison Involved Depending on Certain Signs	
• Small pupils:	Morphine, organophosphorus (also in chloral hydrate and early stages of barbiturate poisoning)
• Dilated pupils:	Dhatura, sympathomimetics (patient may complain of blurred vision due to dilated pupils). Sometimes in case of antihistamines and very rarely in oleander
• Skin:	increased secretions in Organophosphorus, hot and dry in dhatura
• Loss of vision:	Methyl alcohol
• Pallor:	Sympathomimetics
• Cyanosis:	Dapsone, moth balls etc.
• Delirium with retained consciousness:	Dhatura, atropine, antihistamines
• Ataxia/abnormal movements:	Anticholinergics, antihistamines, phenothiazines, DDT, piperazine etc.
• Bradycardia and conduction blocks:	Digitalis, propranolol, tricyclic antidepressants, phenothiazines, theophyllines etc.

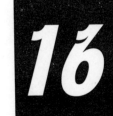

Community
Pediatrics

UNIVERSAL IMMUNIZATION PROGRAMME (UIP)

Community pediatrics is a rapidly emerging relevant subspeciality. Most of the national programmes are community oriented.

UNIVERSAL IMMUNISATION PROGRAMME (UIP)

In addition to the global 'Expanded Programme on Immunisation (EPI), the Universal Immunisation Programme (UIP) was launched in 1985. It is dedicated to the memory of the late Prime Minister, Mrs. Indira Gandhi. It aims at 100% immunisation coverage of all infants against six major killer vaccine preventable diseases (VPDs), namely, tuberculosis, diphtheria, pertussis, tetanus, poliomyelitis and measles. In addition, antenatal mothers are immunised with 2 doses of tetanus toxoid. The primary doses against the VPDs are to be completed before the infant celebrates the first birthday. Cold chain system, vaccine storage and availability of vaccines, syringes and needles are ensured in the programme. The immunisation schedule is given in Appendix 9. The optional vaccines are Hepatitis B, MMR, HIB, Chickenpox, Hepatitis A, Typhoid vaccine, pneumococcal vaccine, meningococcal vaccine etc. HBV is now included in the UIP schedule and is given free of cost in most centres. HIB is called 'meningitis vaccine'. The available meningococcal vaccine does not protect against B serogroup. A cellular pertussis vaccine can be given in those with brain disorder.

A sketch of proper storage of vaccine in a refrigerator is given is Appendix 9.

COMMUNITY PEDIATRICS

CHAPTER 16

There are various feeding programmes. The beneficiaries are underfives, school children and pregnant and lactating mothers. Midday meal programme for the school children is intended to supply one-third of the dail y requirements of calories and half of the daily requirement of proteins. This was started in 1962. In the feeding programmes for the preschool children and antenatal and postnatal mothers a supply of 300 Cal and 10-12 g protein are ensured to the children and 500 Cal and 25 g protein to the mothers. This was started in 1970. These supplementary feedings are given for 300 days in a year. These are undertaken through the Social Welfare and Development Departments, the urban or rural local bodies and voluntary organisations. The examples of such feeding programmes are the ICDS, the urban special nutritional programme (USNP), etc.

SECTION 16.3 INTEGRATED CHILD DEVELOPMENT SERVICES (ICDS) SCHEME

The ICDS scheme was launched in 1975 in some selected blocks. It is expected to cover the whole country by the ninth five-year plan. In the project areas, Anganwadis are set up for 1000 population with community support. The child development project officer (CDPO) is in charge of the programme. Each Anganwadi is run by an Anganwadi worker and a helper. The beneficiaries include all the children 0-6 years old, all antenatal and postnatal mothers and adolescent girls and women in the child bearing age group in the locality. The feeding is mostly targeted to the poor families.

The *package of services include* growth monitoring, medical check up, immunization, referral services, treatment of minor ailments, food supplementation, nonformal education, nutritional supplementation, nutrition and health education (NHE) and home visits.

In supplementary feeding, there is a provision for 'on the spot feeding' and 'take home packets,' for those who cannot attend the feeding sessions, i.e., 0-3 years. ICDS aims at total child development. *Even though, all children 0-6 years are the beneficiaries of ICDS, most of the benefits are availed only by children 3-6 years old who sit in the Anganwadi for nonformal education. Attempts are needed to concentrate on children 0-3 years old, who are more vulnerable and are in need of good supplementation, medical care and growth monitoring.*

The ICDS is now designated as 'Integrated Mother and Child Development Services' (IMCDS) scheme. There is integration between various departments like the Ministry of Human Resources Development, Social Welfare and Health and Family Welfare. Recently emphasis is being given to developmental stimulation, surveillance of developmental milestones and early intervention in children of 0-3 years. Child Development Referral Units (CDRUs) can be set up as referral links for developmental intervention. These centres can be attached to the 'first referral units' (FRUs).

SECTION 16.4

CHILD SURVIVAL AND SAFE MOTHERHOOD (CSSM) PROGRAMME

The various national programmes like Universal Immunisation Programme (UIP), Vitamin A prophylaxis programme, Maternal and Child Health (MCH) programme, Diarrheal Diseases Control Programme, ARI control programme, etc., were integrated and brought under one common programme namely CSSM. It was launched in 1992. The health goals for 2000 AD have been accepted as the goals of the CSSM programme.

The child survival components are essential newborn care including neonatal advanced life support (NALS), UIP, diarrheal diseases control and management, ARI control and management and Vitamin A and anaemia prophylaxis programmes. Treatment of minor ailments, deworming, iron and folic acid tablet distribution are also included in the programme.

The safe motherhood components are antenatal care, immunization, prevention and treatment of anaemia, deliveries by trained persons and institutional deliveries, timing, limiting and spacing of births and management of obstetric emergencies.

The peripheral centers as well as the referral centres need to be strengthened for effective implementation of the CSSM programme.

SECTION 16.5 FIRST REFERRAL UNIT AND NATIONAL RURAL HEALTH MISSION PROGRAMMES

FIRST REFERRAL UNIT (FRU)

The FRU programme was launched in 1995 with the help of UNICEF. District hospitals, major Government hospitals and Community Health Centres (CHCs) are being upgraded as FRUs. The pediatrician, obstetrician, nurse and administrators in these centres are given training in FRU skills. The FRUs are to be equipped with operation theatre, clinical laboratories, blood banking or storage facility and services of anaesthesiologists.

The goal is to establish 1 FRU/1 lakh population. Child development referral units (CDRUs) are also being visualised for early detection and early intervention of development delay. Community participation is ensured in improving the facilities in the FRU and in arranging emergency transport for complicated cases.

NATIONAL RURAL HEALTH MISSION (NRHM)

Recognizing the importance of health in the process of economic and social development and improving the quality of life of our citizens, the Government of India has resolved to launch the National Rural Health Mission (NRHM) to carry out necessary architectural correction in the basic health care delivery system. The Mission adopts a synergistic approach by relating health to determinants of good health, viz., segments of nutrition, sanitation, hygiene and safe drinking water. It also aims at mainstreaming the Indian systems of medicine to facilitate health care. The Plan of Action includes increasing public expenditure on health, reducing regional imbalance in health infrastructure, pooling resources, integration of organizational structures, optimization of health manpower, decentralization and district management of health programmes, community participation and ownership of assets, induction of management and financial personnel into district health system, and operationalizing community health centers into functional hospitals meeting Indian Public Health Standards in each block of the country.

The Goal of the Mission is to improve the availability of and access to quality health care by people, especially for those residing in rural areas, the poor, women and children. The services of the volunteers, on an incentive basis, will be utilized in this venture. They are the accredited social health activists (ASHA). ASHA is to be the 'daughter in law' of each panchayat, who will stay in the area. The services of the Indigenous medicines like Ayurveda, Unani, Siddha and Homeopathy (AYUSH) will be linked with modern medicine.

SECTION 16.6	BREASTFEEDING AND BABY FRIENDLY HOSPITAL INITIATIVE (BFHI)

INITIATION OF BREASTFEEDING

Baby must be put to breast within **half an hour after normal delivery and within four hours after cesarean sections.** Prelacteal feeds like gold rubbed in water, honey, distilled water, glucose etc., should not be given. These items will satisfy the thirst and will reduce the vigor to suck and may lead to diarrhea and helminthic infestation. Soon after birth, the baby is awake, alert and **'biologically ready'** to breastfeed and initiation of breastfeeding is very easy. Later on, the baby goes to prolonged sleep and thereafter initiation may be difficult. Breastfeeding can be initiated even when mother is sedated or on IV fluids. In the first 2-4 days, small **quantity of colostrum (10-40 mL)** that is secreted is all what the baby needs.

Colostrum is rich in protein and immuno-globulins. The mother and baby should be relaxed and comfortably postured during breastfeeding. Initially they may need some help. The baby's head may be resting on the elbow of the mother and she should support the baby with the same hand. She should also support the breast between the index finger and middle finger of the opposite hand during feeding. **'Rooming-in'** is keeping the mother and the baby in the same room, **'bedding-in'** is keeping the mother and baby in the same bed and **'mothering'** is keeping the baby on the abdomen of the mother. These measures ensure **mother infant bonding** the skin-to-skin contact. Skin-to skin contact, eye-to-eye contact and mother-infant bonding leads to successful breastfeeding and emotional adjustment. Sucking should be continued as long as the baby desires to suck. This will satisfy the sucking instinct of the baby and will express the 'hind milk' which is more nutritious. When sucking takes place only for a few minutes, the baby will get only the 'fore milk'. This will satisfy only the thirst of the baby and 'hind milk' has to be fed to satisfy the nutritional demands and to ensure more milk production. It is better to suckle from both the breasts and generally babies finish feeding by twenty minutes.

In case of twin babies, exclusive breastfeeding should be the choice. It is advisable to simultaneously feed them from both the sides or they can be put to breast alternatively one after the other reserving one side for each baby. If weight gain is not satisfactory, they may need extra calories and protein.

Reflexes that Help in Breastfeeding

Three reflexes, namely rooting, sucking and swallowing help the baby in breastfeeding. When the breast nipple is allowed to touch the cheek of the baby, the baby will open the mouth and initiate sucking. This is called rooting reflex. **Sucking and swallowing become coordinated by 34 weeks of gestation.** Sucking by the baby, prolactin **(milk production)** reflex and oxytocin **(milk ejection)** reflex initiate and maintain lactation in the mother. Sucking acts as the afferent stimulus for prolactin and oxytocin reflexes. Oxytocin reflex is also called **'let down reflex'**. Let down reflex will be efficient only when the mother is relaxed and comfortable. Trickling of a few drops of milk from the opposite breast while initiating feeding (let down reflex) gives a positive clue about milk production and ejection. Colostrum is replaced by **'transition milk'** in a few days and later on by **'mature milk'**. It gradually increases till 6 months after delivery and later plateaus off. Average quantity of milk is 500-800 ml/day. Preterm milk secreted by the mother who delivers prematurely is rich in protein to ensure catch up growth. Hind milk is more nutritive than fore-milk.

Common Problems During Breastfeeding

a. **Flat or inverted nipples:** The size of the resting nipple is not important. It is just a guide to show where the baby has to take the breast. The areola and the breast tissue beneath should be capable of being pulled out to form the teat. Occasionally, on attempting to pull out the nipple, it goes deeper into the breast, this is true inverted nipple.

Nipple protractility test should be done during pregnancy if there is any doubt (Fig. 16.1). The nipple usually becomes more protractile (capable of being pulled out) as pregnancy progresses and

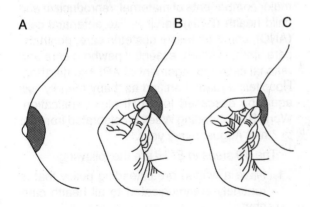

Fig 16.1: Testing a nipple for protractility (A) A short nipple. Is it protractile or not? (B) If you can pull it out like this, then it protracts well (C) If it goes in like this when you try to pull it out, then it is not protractile

mother should be reassured that she will be able to breastfeed.

Normally, the nipple corrects itself as the child suckles. But in a few cases, the problem persists even after that. In such cases, following inverted syringe technique should be tried (Fig. 16.2).

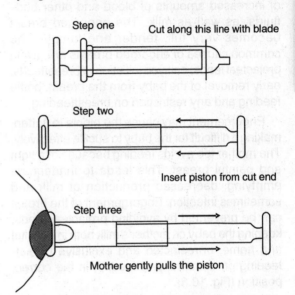

Fig. 16.2: Inverted syringe technique

- Cut the nozzle end of a disposable syringe (10-20 ml).
- Introduce the piston from the ragged cut end side.
- Ask the mother to apply the smooth side of the syringe on the nipple and gently pull out the piston and let her wait for a minute.
- Nipple would then protrude into the syringe. Ask the mother to slowly release the suction and put the baby to breast, at this time it helps the nipple to erect out and baby is able to suckle in the proper position.
- After feeding, the nipple may retract back, but doing it each time before feeding over a period of few days will help to solve the problem.

b. **Fullness and engorgement of the breast:**
Fullness of the breast is a frequent problem. However, milk flow continues and the baby can feed normally. If enough milk is not removed, engorgement of breast may result.

Breast engorgement is due to accumulation of increased amounts of blood and other body fluids, as well as milk. The engorged breast becomes very full, tender and lumpy. The common causes of engorged breasts are giving prelacteal feeds, delayed initiation of breastfeeds, early removal of the baby from the breast, bottle feeding and any restriction on breastfeeding.

Engorgement may cause the nipple to flatten, making it difficult for the baby to suckle effectively. The mother too avoids feeding because of a tight and painful breast. This leads to inadequate emptying, decreased production of milk and sometimes infection. Engorgement of the breast can be prevented by avoiding prelacteal feeds, keeping the baby on mother's milk both in hospital and home, unrestricted and exclusive breast-feeding on demand, and feeding in the correct position (Fig. 16.3).

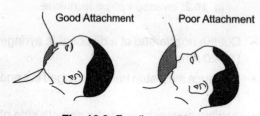

Fig. 16.3: Feeding position

Signs	Signs
• Baby's chin is close to the breast	• Baby sucks only at the nipple
• Baby's tongue is under the lactiferous sinuses and nipple against the palate	• Mouth is not wide open and much of the areola and thus lactiferous sinuses are outside the mouth
• Baby's mouth is wide open and the lower lip turned outwards	• Baby's tongue is also inside the mouth and does not cup over the breast tissue

• More areola is visible above the baby's mouth than below it

• No pain while breast-feeding

• Baby's cheeks are full, not hollow

• Regular, slow, deep sucks

• Chin is away from the breast

• It is painful while breastfeeding

BABY FRIENDLY HOSPITAL INITIATIVE (BFHI)

The BFHI is a global programme organised by UNICEF. It was launched in 1992. It was adopted by India in 1993. Initially, it was started in 12 countries. BFHI certification is done by the National and State BFHI Task Forces. By December 1993, 38 hospitals in India were certified 'baby friendly' and by December 1996, 1040 hospitals were certified. Cochin has been declared the first baby friendly city and Ernakulam in Kerala has been declared as the first baby friendly district. All the hospitals in this area have been accredited as baby friendly. There is a recent suggestion to convert these hospitals into 'mother and child friendly hospitals.

The BFHI plus programme incorporates the major components of maternal, reproductive and child health (RCH) services like antenatal care (ANC), comprehensive obstetric care, postnatal care, immunisation, essential newborn care and rational case management of ARI and diarrhea. Hospitals already certified as 'baby friendly' will again be assessed for BFHI plus certification. World Breastfeeding Week is celebrated from 1st to 7th of August every year.

The *10 steps in BFHI* are the following:

1. Have a written breastfeeding policy that is routinely communicated to all health care staff.

2. Train all health staff in skills necessary to implement this policy.

3. Inform all pregnant women about the benefits and management of breastfeeding.

4. Help the mother initiate breastfeeding within an hour of birth.

5. Show the mothers how to breastfeed and how to maintain lactation, even if they should be separated from their infant.

6. Give the newborn infant no food or drink other than breast milk, unless medically indicated.

7. Practise 'rooming in' and allow mothers and infants to remain together 24 hours a day.

8. Encourage breastfeeding on demand.

9. Give no artificial teats or pacifiers (also called dummies or soothers) to breastfeeding infants.

10. Foster the establishment of breastfeeding support groups and refer mothers to them on discharge from hospital or clinic.

Based on these 10 steps, the hospital policies are formulated and exhibited. The *10 policies of BFHI* are the following:

1. Our hospital has an official policy to protect, promote and support breastfeeding.

2. All maternity and child care health staff in the hospital receive training in the skills to promote breastfeeding.

3. All mothers, both antenatal and postnatal are informed on the benefits of breastfeeding.

4. We assist mothers in the early initiation of breastfeeding, within half an hour of birth for a normal delivery, within 4 hours of birth after a cesarean section.

5. All mothers are shown how to breastfeed and how to maintain lactation, even if they should be temporarily separated from their infants.

6. We give newborns no food or drink other than breast milk. Infant foods and breast milk substitutes are prohibited in this institution.

7. We practise, 'rooming in' by allowing the mothers and babies to remain together 24 hours a day.

8. We encourage all mothers to breastfeed on demand.

9. We strictly prohibit the use of artificial teats, pacifiers, soothers and feeding bottles.

10. We provide follow up support to mothers for exclusive breastfeeding upto 4-6 months after birth and continued breastfeeding upto two years of age. We enlist the cooperation of visiting family members to support breast-feeding mothers. Mothers are also advised on whom to contact for assistance in overcoming any problems in breastfeeding.

The IMS Act is given in Table 16.1.

CHAPTER 16

COMMUNITY PEDIATRICS

SECTION 16.7   PULSE POLIO IMMUNIZATION (PPI)

With a view to eradicate poliomyelitis, India is undertaking PPI along with the other countries of the world. It was started in 1995, and every year in December and January, two doses of OPV are given to all children below 5 years of age, irrespective of their immunization status. In the year 1999-2000, four doses were given at 1 month interval. Initially it was given to only children upto 3 years. A total of 7-13 doses of OPV is given to a child. PPI is undertaken with the help of governmental agencies, non-governmental agencies (NGOs) and local administrations like panchayats and municipalities. In addition to the immunization clinics in the health centres and subcentres, immunization posts are put up in several street corners of the panchayat, municipalities and corporations, bus stations, railway stations and airports for a wide and thorough coverage. So far in India, PPI has been a great success. PPI is carried out on 'National Immunization Days' (NIDs). A country will be declared polio free only when no new cases are reported for three consecutive years. During PPI, a house to house search is also done to ensure coverage.

SECTION 16.8
ACUTE FLACCID PARALYSIS SURVEILLANCE AND POLIO ERADICATION PROGRAMME

Polio eradication is based on four steps. These are: High routine immunization coverage, Pulse polio immunization, Mop-up immunization and Acute Flaccid Paralysis (AFP) surveillance (Fig. 16.4).

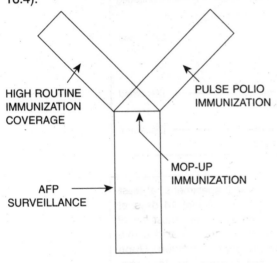

HIGH ROUTINE IMMUNIZATION COVERAGE

PULSE POLIO IMMUNIZATION

MOP-UP IMMUNIZATION

AFP SURVEILLANCE

Fig. 16.4: Strategies for polio eradication

AFP is a flaccid paralysis of an acute onset, less than 4 weeks duration in a child below 15 years of age. The affected limb or limbs are flaccid. Tone is diminished and deep tendon reflexes are diminished or absent. Surveillance is carried out for all cases of AFP and not just for cases of poliomyelitis. AFP in a person over 15 years is unlikely to be poliomyelitis. So surveillance is done in children below 15 years. 'Non-

polio cases' of AFP are Guillain-Barré syndrome (GBS), transverse myelitis (TM) and traumatic neuritis (TN) (Table 16.2).

The role of AFP surveillance is to identify high risk areas and groups, to monitor progress and to certify a country polio free if there are no reports of new cases of polio caused by wild polio virus for three consecutive years, in spite of adequate surveillance. Active surveillance in major centres is by responsible persons called 'Nodal officers'. District immunization officer (DIO) or district RCH officer should make weekly visits to these centres to see if there are new cases of AFP. All AFP cases should be line listed to the DIO with correct addresses, contact telephone numbers and immunization status. The DIO should investigate the case and undertake ring immunization or outbreak response in the locality by giving at least one dose of OPV to children below 5 years among 3000-5000 population in the surrounding urban areas and to children within 5 km radius in rural areas. A minimum of 500 doses are given. It is done within 72 hours to one week of reporting. A second dose of OPV may be given after 1 month. One dose is now considered enough for ring immunization. Two stool samples should be collected from the AFP case for virus study. The clinical and virologic classification schemes are given in Fig. 16.5. Within 10 weeks of onset, all the AFP cases should be reclassified as 'confirmed polio' or discarded as 'nonpolio'.

The keys for AFP surveillance are the following:

CHAPTER 16

COMMUNITY PEDIATRICS

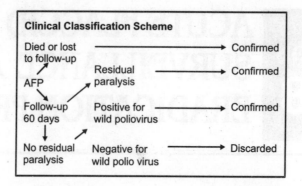

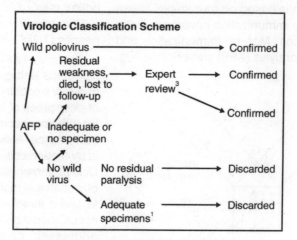

1. Adequate specimens = 2 specimens, at least 24 to 48 hours apart and within 14 days of paralysis onset; each specimen must be of adequate volume (8-10 grams) and arrive in the laboratory in good condition. Good Condition = no desiccation, no leakage, adequate documentation and evidence that the reverse cold chain was maintained.

2. "Compatible" cases represent a surveillance failure and should be scrutinized for clustering in space and time.

3. Cases undergoing expert review and subsequently classified as "discarded" or "compatible" should be line listed.

Fig. 16.5: Clinical and virologic classification of AFP

1. Reporting system should be monitored and revitalised and zero-case reporting must be included weekly. Reports are to be sent on all Mondays from all reporting centres.

2. Immediate response to an AFP report should occur within 48 hours. The DIO is responsible for immediate action.

3. Two stool specimens (8 g or thumb size) should be collected 24-48 hours apart within 14 days of the onset and should reach the concerned National Laboratory for virus isolation within 3 days of being sent.

4. Reported AFP cases should be subjected to a follow-up examination after 760 days to verify the presence of residual paralysis.

5. The stool culture report should be made available within 28 days of receipt of the specimen.

Isolation of wild virus confirms polio. Isolation of vaccine virus is an indirect evidence of the adequacy of the cold chain system and that of nonpolio enteroviruses confirms the adequacy of the cold chain facility during sending of the sample and the credibility of the lab.

High Routine Immunization Coverage

Countries should aim to vaccinate at least 90% of infants against polio by one year of age.

Mopping-Up

Successful NIDs will reduce polio virus transmission to a few final chains of transmission, typically persisting in densely populated areas where inadequate health services lead to both low routine immunization coverage and poor performance during NIDs. Surveillance data are used to identify these final reservoirs of wild virus infection. A case of wild poliovirus in this era is an emergency and is a criterion for mopping-up. This is the key end-stage strategy and includes. 1.5–2 million underfive children in the district and neighbouring districts. A house to house approach is planned after making the houses.

a. **What is "Mopping-up"?** Mopping-up consists of intensive house to house immunization with OPV in areas with persistent polio virus transmission. All children in a specified age group (usually 0–59 months) are immunized during the mopping-up, regardless of their immunization status. Each round is completed in as short a time period as possible.

b. **At what stage is mopping-up done?** Mopping-up immunization is conducted when polio has been reduced from an endemic disease to a disease that occurs only in focal areas. It is usually done in a few neighbouring states/districts when there is a confirmed case of polio.

SECTION 16.9 — NATIONAL NUTRITION POLICY (NNP) AND NUTRITION GOALS

The NNP was adopted in 1993. The policies for intervention are:

1. Fortification of essential foods.
2. Control of micronutrient deficiencies.
3. Improvement of dietary pattern through production and demonstration.
4. Land reforms.
5. Popularization of low cost nutritious food.
6. Public distribution system.
7. Prevention of food adulteration.
8. Health and family welfare.
9. Nutrition surveillance; and
10. Communication and community participation.

The National Plan of Action on Nutrition by the Ministry of Human Resources Development has put up the following nutrition goals for 2000 AD.

1. Reduction in moderate and severe PEM among preschoolers by half of the 1990 levels by 2000 AD.
2. Reduction in undernutrition and stunted growth in children.
3. Reduction of LBW to 10%.
4. Elimination of blindness due to vitamin A deficiency.
5. Reduction in iron deficiency anemia in pregnant mothers to 25%.
6. Universal iodization of salt and to reduce iodine deficiency disorder (IDD) to < 10%.
7. Production of 250 million tonnes of food-grains.
8. Promotion of appropriate diets and healthy lifestyles.
9. Growth promotion and its regular monitoring.
10. Empowerment of all women to breastfeed their children exclusively for 4-6 months and to continue breastfeeding well into the second year.
11. Dissemination of knowledge and supporting services to increase food production to ensure household food security.

The National Nutrition Week is celebrated from 1st to 7th of September every year.

SECTION 16.10 ACUTE RESPIRATORY INFECTION (ARI) CONTROL PROGRAMME

ARI is now identified as the number one killer among children. As pneumonia deaths are more frequent, emphasis is on early diagnosis and treatment of pneumonia.

a. **Prevention of ARI:** Ensure BCG, DPT and measles immunizations and vitamin A prophylaxis to prevent pneumonia. Educate the mothers to avoid exposure to cold and the need for a dust free and smoke free environment. Teach them home remedies for cough and cold and also the 'danger signs' in ARI. Train them to recognise early signs of pneumonia and ensure early antibiotic therapy.

b. **Case Finding and Management:** The various steps in case finding are given in Table 16.3. Children with cough and cold should be evaluated for pneumonia. The respiratory rate should be counted when the child is quiet and after exposing the lower half of the chest. It should be counted by watching and not by palpation. It should be counted for one full minute and should be recounted whenever in doubt. A respiratory rate of 60 per minute or more in an infant less than two months of age, 50 or more in an infant above two months of age and more than 40 or more in a child 1-5 years of age indicates pneumonia. A definite inward motion of the lower chest wall during breathing indicates 'chest indrawing'. Mild chest indrawing is normal in young infants because their chest wall is soft. Severe chest indrawing, deep and easy to see, indicates severe pneumonia. It warrants antibiotic therapy immediately. When there is no fast breathing or chest indrawing, there is no pneumonia.

In children 2 months to 5 years old, fast breathing indicates pneumonia. In such cases, antibiotic therapy is started immediately and the child is reassessed in 2 days for improvement. If there is chest indrawing, it indicates severe pneumonia. The child is initiated on antibiotic therapy and is referred for evaluation and hospitalization.

Irrespective of the age, 'danger signs' like (a) inability to drink, (b) convulsion, (c) drowsiness, (d) noisy breathing or stridor, (e) wheeze, and (f) severe malnutrition indicate very severe disease, which needs immediate referral, hospitalization and antibiotic therapy. In young infants less than two months of age fever and hypothermia are also considered as signs of very severe disease. In them, fast breathing with or without indrawing indicates severe pneumonia.

The home treatment of ARI includes frequent feeding of breast milk and extra fluids. Clearing the nose using saline or a moistened wick and soothing the throat using home remedies like lime, honey, ginger, tulsi or hot water are beneficial.

Keeping the baby warm and control of fever by giving paracetamol are important. Cotrimoxazole is considered the first line of drug. Ampicillin 50 mg/kg/dose × 4 doses/day is considered ideal in hospitalized patients. Penicillins with or without aminoglycosides and chloramphenicol are considered as the second line of drugs. Cloxacillin is added when there is suspicion of staphyl-ococcal infection in the form of skin infections like abscess, boils or carbuncles.

'Danger signs' like breathing becoming faster and difficult, inability to drink, drowsiness, convulsions, stridor or wheeze and fever or hypothermia in a young infant warrant hospitalisation in a critical care facility.

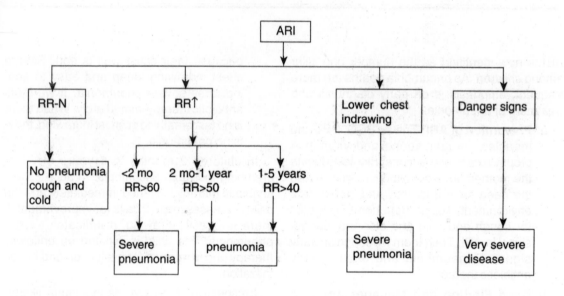

Fig. 16.6: Algorithm for ARI classification

SECTION 16.11

CONTROL OF DIARRHEAL DISEASE (CDD) PROGRAMME

Diarrheal disease is a major cause of morbidity and mortality among underfive children. A child on an average suffers from 2-3 attacks of diarrheal episodes every year. Prevention of diarrhea requires multidimensional interventions like sanitation and safe drinking water. Prevention of death is possible by simple interventions like oral rehydration therapy. Oral rehydration therapy (ORT) includes oral rehydration salt (ORS) solution and home available fluids (HAF). ORT has reduced morbidity and mortality due to diarrheal disease. ORT prevents and treats dehydration.

Diarrhea is passage of liquid or watery stools usually more than three times a day. But, even a single large watery stool can be labelled as diarrhea. Diarrhea may thus be defined as *'increase in frequency, fluidity and bulk of stool when compared to the normal bowel habit of a particular individual.'* Passage of blood and mucus along with stools is termed 'dysentery'. Diarrhea lasting for more than 14 days is called 'persistent diarrhea'.

Acute diarrheal disease (ADD) is usually selflimited and lasts for 3-7 days. Among those with diarrhea, 90% of them do not develop dehydration, 9% develop some dehydration and only 1% develop severe dehydration requiring IV fluid therapy. The child should be assessed for dehydration using the tools, **ask, look and feel** (Table 16.4). The key or star signs of dehydration are general condition, thirst and skin turgor. Appropriate management should be given according to the degree of dehydration and according the plan of therapy (Table 16.5).

In plan A, children with no dehydration are included. Give more fluids to prevent dehydration. Give half glass extra fluid to children below two years of age and one glass extra fluid to older children after each purge. Continue feeding to prevent malnutrition. Watch for signs of dehydration and 'danger signs' *like excessive thirst, irritability, repeated vomiting, high purge rate, oligo anuria, not feeding well, fever, drowsiness, convulsion and collapse.* ORS or HAF like salted kanji water can be given. Among HAF, 'the recommended home fluid' (RHF) varies from place to place. It is the most widely accepted HAF in a locality. It is important to set up ORS depots in every village. The depot holders of contraceptives and chloroquine tablets and the public health nurses, Anganwadi workers and Mahila Swasthya Sangh workers can act as ORS depot holders.

In plan B, there is some dehydration. Give 70-100 ml ORS in 4 hours. More fluids may be given in order to satisfy the thirst of the child. ORS is given minute by minute using a glass and a spoon. If the child vomits, stop for 10 minutes and again restart slowly. Vomiting more than three times in an hour is considered severe vomiting.

The WHO ORS packet contains 20 g glucose, 3.5 g sodium chloride, 2.9 g sodium citrate and 1.5 g potassium chloride (Appendix).

This is dissolved in 1 litre or 5 glasses of water. Every day ORS should be prepared fresh. 2.5 g sodium bicarbonate can also be used instead of sodium citrate. Citrate ORS is not hygroscopic. It is more stable and is claimed to decrease stool output by 8-14%. The WHO-ORS ensures a 2% solution for optimum 'substrate mediated electrolyte absorption'. One litre of ORS supplies:

119 mEq of glucose
90 mEq of Na^+
20 mEq of K^+
80 mEq of Cl^- and
30 mEq of HCO_3^- or
10 mEq of citrate

In Plan C and in ORT failure, 100 ml/kg Ringer lactate or N. saline is given in 2 rations. First ration 30 ml/kg is given in 1 hour in infants and in half an hour in others. Second ration 70 ml/kg is given in 5 hours in infants and 2½ hours in others. During IV fluid therapy, ORS can also be given orally.

As soon as dehydration is corrected, oral feeding should be started. The child requires an extra meal/day for 1-2 weeks after the illness, to regain weight loss and to prevent malnutrition. Prevention of diarrhea should also be taught to the mother. The interventions to reduce diarrheal morbidity and mortality are:

1. Breastfeeding—exclusive breastfeeding for four months and partial breastfeeding for four months and partial breastfeeding till 2 years age.
2. Improved weaning practices.
3. Use plenty of clean water.
4. Hand washing.
5. Use of latrines.
6. Proper disposal of stools of young children.
7. Immunization especially against measles.
8. Vitamin A prophylaxis.

Drugs are unnecessary in ADD except in cholera. In cholera, furazolidone or tetracycline can be given. Tetracycline is avoided in children below 8 years of age. Acute dysentery is treated with Cotrimoxazole or nalidixic acid for 5 days. Erythromycin is useful in Campylobacter (Helicobacter) jejuni infection. Furazolidone or metronidazole are given in giardiasis. Metronidazole is given in amoebiasis. Amoebiasis is rare in young children.

When there is high fever, severe malnutrition, dysentery or persistent diarrhea, the child requires investigations and appropriate drug therapy. These are included in Plan D. In persistent diarrhea, stool is tested for pH and reducing sugars. Stool microscopy and cultures also may be done. Other investigations include Mantoux test, X-ray chest, blood counts and urine test. Presence of more than 1% sugar and an acidic pH less than 5.6 on two occasions indicate lactose intolerance. Perianal excoriation is another clue for the diagnosis of lactose intolerance.

Dietary manipulation is beneficial in persistent diarrhea. Diet A includes a low lactose, low milk diet using curd, cereal—pulse gruel, oil, etc. Diet B includes a lactose, milk free diet using cereal—pulse, oil, soya milk, etc. Diet C indicates a lactose, sucrose and starch free diet using egg protein, chicken based diet, oil glucose, etc. (Refer Chapter 9). Various other types of ORS are given in Appendix 7.

SECTION 16.12 VITAMIN A PROPHYLAXIS PROGRAMME

Vitamin A deficiency is identified as the most common deficiency among children in India. It is the most common cause of preventable blindness in children. Vitamin A prophylaxis programme ensures five megadoses of vitamin A given at 6 months interval to children between 9 months and 3 years. In infants, the dose is 1 lakh units and in older children, the dose is 2 lakh units. Vitamin A concentrate contains 1 lakh unit/ml. The vitamin A prophylaxis programme is now integrated with the immunization programme. The first dose of vitamin A is given during measles vaccination and the second dose is given during DPT first booster injection. The third dose is given at 2 years, the fourth dose is given at 2½ years and the fifth dose is given at 3 years. Care has to be taken not to give vitamin A containing tonics and capsules to these children to prevent hypervitaminosis A. In some states like Tamilnadu, vitamin A is given as pulse doses at 6 months interval in June and December. This will ensure regular supply and will avoid repeated dosing from different sources. In some states, 6 months to 5 years old children are given vitamin A prophylaxis.

CHAPTER 16

COMMUNITY PEDIATRICS

<table>
<tr><td>**SECTION**
16.13</td><td># IODINE DEFICIENCY DISORDERS (IDD) CONTROL PROGRAMMES</td></tr>
</table>

Iodine deficiency disorders (IDD) are more common in mountainous areas. Two-thirds of the iodine requirement is derived from drinking water. Chronic iodine deficiency causes endemic goitre. Intrauterine iodine deficiency may led to mental retardation. IDD control programme utilises iodized common salt for prevention. Iodized salt fortified with potassium iodate (15 mcg/g or 15 ppm) is useful to meet the requirements even in mountainous areas. In commercial iodised salt, upto 30 ppm iodine is added to cover the losses and the requirements. The usage of iodine fortified salt is accepted as a universal policy in most of the states of India. However, there is controversy in some states due to the high price of iodised salt and due to the fact that iodine deficiency is common only in certain parts of India.

Double fortified salt is both iodine and iron fortified.

Urinary iodine excretion can be used to quantify deficiency. Value < 20 mcg/L indicates severe IDD, 20-50 moderate, 50-100, mild and >100 mcg/L indicates normal status. Grading of goiter is as follows:

Grade O—No visible/palpable goiter.

I-palpable thyroid swelling, moving while swallowing.

II-visible and palpable thyroid swelling.

III-large visible from a distance.

SECTION 16.14

THE RIGHTS OF THE CHILDREN

As per the UN Declaration, the rights of the child are concerned with:

1. Right to love and affection.
2. A sense of belonging and security.
3. Increasing independence within the limitations imposed by the society.
4. Promotion of self respect and confidence.
5. Right to play and recreation.
6. Right to take pride in achievements.
7. Generate social and emotional interaction with parents.

These were adopted in the convention on Rights of the Child' by the UN General Assembly on 20th November, 1989. It has been ratified by most of the countries by 1996. It was ratified by the Government of India on 12th November 1992. Ninety-six per cent of the world's children live in states that have a legal obligation to protect the rights of the child.

These are 54 articles in the 'Convention on the Rights of the Child'. These can be grouped into four sets (Table 16.6).

Article 39 of the Constitution of India and the National Policy of Children passed in 1974 ensure constitutional provisions regarding the Rights of the Child.

CHAPTER 16

COMMUNITY PEDIATRICS

SECTION 16.15 THE DISABLED CHILD

A disabled child should get privileges as a 'special child'. Any disability in a child is of serious concern to the parents. They need correct information, social, family and professional support and facilities to give them confidence in looking after their 'special child'. A 5-10% of the child population is estimated to be handicapped.

1. Types of Disabilities

According to the WHO classification, the disabilities are divided into 7 groups:

1. Orthopedic/movement disability
2. Visual disability
3. Speech and hearing disability
4. Mental retardation
5. Fits related disability
6. Feeling related disability and
7. Strange behaviour (mental illness).

The 'UN Declaration of the Rights of the Disabled Persons' states that they are not really handicapped. They are just disabled in certain areas and they became handicapped when society imposes restrictions on them. The UN Rights of the handicapped are given in Table 16.7. Parental awareness, public education and continued support from governmental and non-governmental organizations (NGOs) are needed to enforce these rights.

2. Facilities for the Disabled

Various facilities are needed to develop the child's full potential. These facilities include:

a. Multidisciplinary disability assessment and intervention.
b. Special education.
c. Vocational training and employment, and
d. Social support and welfare schemes.

The Act for the Disabled Persons, 1995 ensures equal opportunities, protection of rights and full participation.

3. Multidisciplinary Disability Assessment and Intervention

One centre should be available at each district, which may be named 'disability intervention referral unit (DIRU). Local adaptations for early diagnosis and interventions are desirable in these centres. The aims of the centre are the following:

a. Early recognition and evaluation of disabilities.

b. To plan and undertake interventional strategies to correct, overcome, bypass or minimise the effects of the disabilities using methods like physiotherapy, occupational therapy, behaviour therapy, stimulation therapy, speech therapy, hearing aids, visual aids, spectacles, surgery etc.

c. To prepare the child for appropriate schooling. The multidisciplinary assessment team should ideally include a pediatrician, neurologist, psychiatrist, clinical psychologist, ophthalmologist, ENT specialist, audiologist, speech therapist, special educator, social worker, etc. When so many experts cannot be made available, a medical specialist, a paramedical and a rehabilitation cum social worker can run the centre with appropriate training. A 'trained peripheral disability worker' can do a lot of help, especially in the underprivileged communities. A questionnaire designed by WHO is found very useful for early diagnosis of disabled persons in the community (Table 16.8).

4. Special Education

The parents should be given advice and access to an appropriate educational centre that will help the child to achieve and express one's maximum potential. As each child's needs and requirements are unique, decision should be based on an assessment by the developmental therapist, psychologist and special educator. The following points are to be considered before giving the advice.

a. The severity and nature of the handicap.

b. The available resources in the local schools.

c. The facility for institutional or special care.

d. The effects of home/institutional care on the child as well as his/her family.

The four major options for teaching are:

1. Home based training programmes or **home based rehabilitation (HBR).**

2. Community based rehabilitation (CBR).

3. Special schools, and

4. Integrated schooling or 'mainstreaming'.

1. **Home Based and Community Based Rehabilitation (HBR and CBR):** In home based training programme, the parents are given training and are empowered to train the child. The disability worker/the multipurpose worker in a community based rehabilitation (CBR) programme or home based rehabilitation (HBR) programme can help the parents in this respect. Home based training programme is best suited for severely handicapped and retarded children.

2. **Special Schools:** They have the advantages of specially trained teachers, special training materials, less number of students, less academic pressure, individualized attention, realistic academic expectations and special training in social and vocational skills. The major disadvantages of special schools is that such schools are only very few in number and situated only in bigger cities.

3. **Mainstreaming:** In integrated schooling or mainstreaming, the handicapped children are sent to normal schools along with the nondisabled children. But they need additional support and additional trained staff. Integration in the usual classes is possible with physically handicapped children who have normal vision, hearing and intelligence. Some may need special seats and special equipment for movement. Blind children may need books written in 'Braille' and tape recorders. Mentally subnormal children can be accommodated in lower classes. Moderate to severely retarded children cannot be sent to normal schools.

Within the normal school, 'special classes' may be arranged for the disabled children with the help of specially trained teachers. They should have access to noncurricular activities like sports, games, craft, art, entertainments, food, etc., along with the normal children.

Integrated schooling has several advantages over segregated special schooling. Integrated schooling is the most feasible method to educate the disabled children scattered throughout the country. It is less costly, easy to maintain and can be run using the same campus, building and staff. The disabled children learn more by competing with normal children and the normal children learn about the needs of the disabled children and develop the attitude to help them.

Residential special schools may be housed close to normal schools with special arrangement to allow intermingling with the normal children during common functions, sports, meet, etc.

5. **Vocational Training and Employment:** Disabled children, especially adolescents need proper vocational training for suitable employment. They should develop self-esteem and confidence to support themselves and their families. The physical and sensory abilities of the child, the aptitude of the child and the interest of the family should be taken into consideration. Printing, textile, paper binding, art, crafts, telephone, telegraph, farming, etc., are suited to most of them. The 'abilities in the disabled' should be fully developed and made use of. Some of the advances in technology may be extremely helpful to them. An 'office or a workshop setting' is preferable for work under supervision. Self-employment, government and private sector employment and sheltered workshops run by the disabled or their parents are specifically suited to them.

6. **Socialization, Community Support and Welfare Schemes:** Disabled children should not be hidden from the society, but they should be exposed to normal social activities. They should be taken out to place of worship, playgrounds, zoo and market places. They should also attend functions like parties and camps. These steps are important for socialization and social acceptance. The people whom they meet can contribute to their development. 'Social acceptance' is very important in total rehabilitation.

There are a lot of welfare programmes for the disabled, at National, State and local levels.

a. Railway and bus fare concessions for the disabled and accompanying persons.

b. Income tax benefits.

c. Reservations for education and employment.

d. Scholarship for education.

e. Preferential allotment of agencies and employment.

f. Allowances for underemployment and unemployment.

g. Parental allowances.

In addition to the above, there are several welfare schemes run by individuals and NGOs as the 'Spastic Society' and the 'Hemophilia Society'.

REPRODUCTIVE AND CHILD HEALTH (RCH) PROGRAMME

This 'Target free approach' programme was started in 1996. It is a 'need based, client oriented, demand driven, high quality' family centred approach. It has a self generated target.

Definition

RCH is defined as a state in which people are empowered to regulate fertility, women are able to go through pregnancy and child birth safely, the outcome of pregnancy is successful in terms of infant and maternal survival and well being, couple can have sexual intercourse free of fear of pregnancy and contracting sexually transmitted diseases.

Components

1. **Child Survival**
   Essential NB care
   Successful breastfeeding and Complementary feeding
   Universal Immunization
   IMNCI–Horizontal integration of all vertical programmes
   Referral Services
   Developmental Surveillance and early stimulation.

2. **Safe Motherhood**
   Antenatal care
   Essential obstetric care

   Emergency obstetric care
   Referral services
   Post natal care.

3. **Adolescent Care and Counselling**
   Family life education
   Teenage care and counselling
   Adolescent nutrition and anemia prophylaxis
   Personal and menstrual hygiene
   Prevention of RTI and STI (Reproductive Tract Infection and Sexually Transmitted Infection).

4. **Family Health**
   Safe abortion
   Infertility treatment
   RTI and STI treatment and prevention
   Timing limiting and spacing births
   Screening and management of cervix and breast cancers.

5. **Community Participation.**

Implementation

The existing health workers, supervisors and medical officers are given training for the implementation of RCH and sub centres are redesignated as RCH centres. The District Immunization Officer is in charge and is designated as RCH officer.

CHAPTER 16

COMMUNITY PEDIATRICS

SECTION 16.17 THE INTEGRATED MANAGEMENT OF NEONATAL AND CHILDHOOD ILLNESS

The Integrated Management of Neonatal and Childhood Illness (IMNCI) is a strategy that ensures horizontal integration of a range of vertical programmes like preventive, promotive and curative services among infants and children. It focuses on proper growth and reduction in morbidity and mortality among newborns and underfives, both in the community and hospital settings.

Initially it was IMCI, later on essential newborn care was also incorporated in it leading to the current IMNCI strategy. IMNCI is undertaken through guidelines and two checklists for sick young infants 0-2 months and sick children 2 months–5 years of age. IMNCI includes programmes like essential newborn care, neonatal sepsis, jaundice, low birth weight (LBW) and early referral, ARI, diarrheal disease and ORT, acute febrile illness, measles, malaria, ear infections, meningitis, immunization, infant feeding including breastfeeding, nutrition surveillance and counselling, micronutrient supplements and rational drug therapy.

The benefits of IMNCI are the following:

1. IMNCI addresses most of the common neonatal and childhood conditions and responds to the demand with respect to morbidity and mortality. The check list also has a column to note non IMNCI conditions like heart disease, seizure etc.

2. IMNCI allows the child to be seen in toto and not just with the disease or condition with which the child presents with. Thus, it reduces missed opportunities for immunization, breastfeeding, nutritional counselling, iron, folic acid and vitamin A supplementation.

3. IMNCI ensures health promotive, preventive and curative services and will prove to be a great investment with a positive impact on disease burden and mortality.

4. IMNCI is very cost effective as it does not involve costly equipments or complex technologies, but is based on clinical clues, general danger signs and systematic checklists. Training of the health workers will be the only investment required along with strengthening the existing facilities.

5. IMNCI will achieve equity in health care, case finding, disease classification, management and referral services.

The Indira Gandhi Open University (IGNOU) course for Postgraduate Diploma in Maternal and Child Health (PGDMCH) includes IMNCI in its syllabus. IGNOU has a Programme Study Centre (PSC) attached to Thiruvananthapuram Medical College. The IGNOU counsellors have undergone special training in IMNCI.

In short, IMNCI is the need of the era as it focuses on newborns and children with a holistic approach. It will help to ensure optimum growth, to reduce missed opportunities and disease burden and deaths. IMNCI is unique as it is suitable for both community and hospital settings. It will integrate the various vertical preventive and curative services. It will ensure equity and quality services at very low costs. It will achieve reorientation and empowerment of health workers and a definite positive outcome.

The IMNCI Check List and Recording Forms are available in:

1. WHO, Integrated Management of Childhood Illness, Information Pack, Child and Adolescent Health and Development Division, Geneva, 1998.

2. O.P. Ghai, Essential Pediatrics, CBS Publishers, N. Delhi.

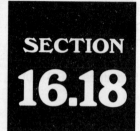

SECTION 16.18 VITAL STATISTICS

The National Vital Statistics Indices are given in Table 16.9.

HEALTH INDICATORS

1. Crude Birth Rate (CBR)

$$\frac{\text{No. of live births}}{\text{Mid year population}} \times 1000$$

2. Crude Death Rate (CDR)

$$\frac{\text{No. of deaths}}{\text{Mid year population}} \times 1000$$

3. Infant Mortality Rate (IMR)

$$\frac{\text{No. of infant deaths}}{\text{No. of live births}} \times 1000$$

4. Maternal Mortality Rate (MMR)

$$\frac{\text{No. of deaths due to peurperial cause}}{\text{No. of live births}} \times 1000$$

5. Age Specific Mortality Rate

$$\frac{\text{No. of deaths in a given age group during a year}}{\text{Mid year population of the same age group}} \times 1000$$

6. Neonatal Mortality Rate (NMR)

$$\frac{\text{No. of infant deaths under 28 days of age}}{\text{No. of live births}} \times 1000$$

7. Postnatal Mortality Rate (PNMR)

$$\frac{\text{No. of deaths after 28 days to the first year of life}}{\text{No. of live births}} \times 1000$$

8. Perinatal Mortality Rate (PMR)

$$\frac{\text{No. of late foetal deaths of 28 or more weeks of gestation and neonatal deaths below the age of 7 days}}{\text{No. of live births and foetal deaths of 28 or more weeks of gestation}} \times 1000$$

9. Underfive (U5) Mortality Rate (U5 MR)—
Probability of dying by 5 years of age.

$$\frac{\text{No. of deaths in 0-5 years age group}}{\text{No. of live births}} \times 1000$$

It is a critical indicator of the well-being of children. The countries are listed and ranked in descending order; Sierra Leone U5MR-283-Rank 1, India U5MR-83-Rank 52, Sri Lanka-U5MR-14-Rank 135, United States U5MR-8-Rank-152, Japan and Sweden U5MR-4-Rank 185, Singapore U5MR 3-Rank-192.

The IMR and the U5MR of Sweden are 4. CDR is 11 and CBR is 12.

In Japan, IMR is 4 and U5MR is 6, CDR is 7 and CBR is 10. In USA< IMR and U5MR are 8, CDR is 9 and CBR is 14.

ESTIMATION OF BENEFICIARIES/AGE-WISE POPULATION

It is important to estimate the age-wise population in order to compute the beneficiaries for the various national programmes.

1. *Pregnant women:*

   It is estimated as follows:

   Birth rate x population + 10%

   ──────────────────────────

   1000

   10% of the calculated number is added to cover still birth. The proportion of pregnant women in a population is estimated 3.2%. It is lowest in Kerala (1.9%).

2. *Live births (postnatal cases)*

   The proportion of live births and postnatal cases is around 3% (Kerala 1.8%).

3. *Infants alive at 1 year*

   This is estimated to be 92% of the live births. It can be calculated as follows: (1-IMR) × Birth rate. It is highest in Kerala (98.3%).

4. *Children below 3 years of age*

   The proportion of children below 3 years is estimated to be 8% (Kerala 5.5%).

5. *Children below 5 years of age*

   It is around 13% in India and 9% in Kerala.

6. *Children 5-9 years of age*

   It is around 7.6% in Kerala.

Table 16.1: Infant Milk Substitutes Act

The Infant Milk Substitutes, Feeding Bottles and Infant Food (Regulation of Production, Supply and Distribution) Act, 1992 is in force since August 1, 1994. It extends to the whole of India. Certain highlights of the Act are as follows:

1. *Advertisments:* No advertisement of infant milk substitutes or feeding bottles.

2. *Incentives:* No incentives of any kind for the purpose of promoting the use or sale of infant milk substitutes or feeding bottles. No free samples to mothers.

3. *Donations:* No donation or subsidised supplies of infant milk substitutes or feeding bottles to any person except to an orphanage.

4. *Healthcare system:* No display of placards or posters for the purpose of promoting the use or sale of infant milk substitutes, feeding bottles or infant foods (weaning foods).

5. Information to health workers should be scientific and factual.

6. *Health worker:* No inducement to health worker for promoting the use of infant milk substitutes, feeding bottles or infant foods.

7. Any direct or indirect expenditure incurred on a health worker by the manufacturer, distributor or retailer of infant milk substitutes, feeding bottles or infant foods should be disclosed (both by the giver as well as the health worker) to the institution or organization to which such health worker is attached.

8. *Labels:* Containers of infant milk substitutes or infant foods should indicate in a clear, easily, readable manner, the words "Important Notice" in capital letters in English and Hindi (use of any local language in addition to these can be made). The labelling must include certain details outlined in the Act.

9. No container or label of infant milk substitutes shall:

   a. Have pictures of an infant or a woman or picture of phrases designed to increase the saleability of the product.

   b. Use of the word "humanized" or "maternalized" or any other similar word.

Table 16.2: Differential diagnosis of acute flaccid paralysis (AFO)

Signs and symptoms	Polio	GBS	Transverse myelitis	Traumatic neuritis
Progression of paralysis	24-28 hours onset to full paralysis	From hours to 10 days	From hours to 4 days	From hours to 4 days
Fever onset	High, always present at at onset of flaccid paralysis	Not common	Rarely present	Commonly present before, during and after flaccid paralysis
Flaccidity	Acute, asymmetrical, proximal ↓	Acute, symmetrical, distal ↓	Acute, lower limbs, symmetrical ↓ in lower limbs	Acute, asymmetric limb ↓ in affected limb
Muscle tone				
DTRs	Decreased or absent	Absent	Absent early followed by hyperreflexia	Decreased or absent
Sensation	Severe myalgia and backache, no sensory changes	Cramps, tingling, hypoanaesthesia of palms and soles	Anaesthesia of lower limbs with sensory level	Pain in gluteal region
Cranial nerve	Only when bulbar and bulbospinal	Often present, affecting VII, IX, X, XI, XII	Absent	Absent
Respiratory insufficiency	Only when bulbar and bulbospinal	In severe cases	Sometimes	Absent
CSF: WBCs protein	High WBCs	<10 WBCs High in 2nd week	Normal Normal or elevated	Normal Normal
Bladder dysfunction	Absent	Transient	Present	Never
Nerve conduction velocity: Third week	Abnormal, anterior horn cell disease (normal initially)	Abnormal, demyelination	Normal or abnormal no diagnostic value	Abnormal in sciatic nerve
EMG - 3 weeks	Abnormal	Normal	Normal	Normal
Sequelae at 3 months and upto a year	Severe, asymmetrical, atrophy, skeletal deformities later	Symmetrical atrophy of distal muscles	Flaccid diplegia, atrophy after years	Moderate atrophy, only in affected lower limb

Table 16.3: Case finding strategies in ARI control programme

Any group	Fast breathing	Chest indrawing	Danger signs	Diagnosis
2 months to 5 years	Present	Present/Absent	Present	Very severe disease
	Present	Present	Absent	Severe pneumonia
	Present	Absent	Absent	Pneumonia
	Absent	Absent	Absent	No pneumonia
0 to 2 months	Present	Present/Absent	Present	Very severe disease
	Present	Present/Absent	Absent	Severe pneumonia
	Absent	Absent	Absent	No pneumonia

* Respiratory rate
- \> 60/minute in 0-2-month-old infants
- \> 50/minute in infants
- \> 40/minute in children

Table 16.4: Clinical signs and classification of dehydration

	A	B	C	D
1. Look: Condition	Well, alert	*Restless irritable*	*Lethargic or unconscious; floppy*	Persistent diarrhea
Eye	Normal	Sunken	Very sunken and dry	> 2 week's duration
Tears	Present	Absent	Absent	
Mouth and tongue	Moist	Dry	Very dry	Severe PEM
Thirst	Drinks normally not thirsty	*Thirsty, drinks eagerly*	*Drinks poorly or unable to drink*	High fever
2. Feel, skin pinch	Goes back	*Goes back slowly*	*Goes back very slowly* (3 or more sec)	Blood and mucus in stool
3. Decide	The patient has no signs of dehydration	If the patient has two or more signs, including at least one* *sign*, there is SOME DEHYDRATION	If the patient has two or more signs, including at least one* *sign*, there is SEVERE DEHYDRA-TION	Child may need hospitalisation and investi-gations
4. Treat	Use treatment plan A	Weigh the patient, if possible, and use treatment Plan B	Weigh the patient and use treatment Plan C Urgently	Use Plan D

* Antibiotics may be indicated in plan D

Table 16.5: Management of ADD

Plan	Hydration	Quantity	Fluid
Plan A	No dehydration	1/2-1 glass/purge	ORS/HAF
Plan B	Some dehydration	70-100 ml/kg in 4 hours	ORS
Plan C	Severe dehydration	100 ml/kg in 3-6 hours (30 ml/kg 1st ratio in 1/2-1 hour 70 ml/kg second ratio	IVF-RL/NS
Plan D	Admit and investigate	in 2½-5 hours)	

HAF-Home Available Fluids, RL—Ringer Lactate, NS—Normal Saline

Table 16.6: The rights of the children

1. The right to survival
   - The right of life.
   - The highest attainable level of health and nutrition.
2. The right to protection
   - Freedom from all forms of exploitation, abuse inhuman or degrading treatment and neglect.
   - Special protection in situations of emergency and army conflicts.
3. The right to development
   - Right to education.
   - Support for early childhood development and care.
4. The right to participation
   - Respect for the views of the child, freedom of expression.

   - Access to information.
   - Freedom of thought, conscience and religion.

Table 16.7: The UN declaration of the rights of the disabled persons

S.No.	Items
1.	To the same fundamental rights as other human beings to enjoy a decent life, as normal as possible.
2.	To the same civil and political rights as their fellow citizens.
3.	To measures enabling them to become as self reliant as possible.
4.	To medical, psychological and functional treatment, rehabilitation and placement services.
5.	To economic and social security to work according to their capabilities in a useful, productive and remunerative occupation.
6.	To their special needs in all stages of social and economic planning.
7.	To live with their family and participate in all social, creative and recreational activities.
8.	To protection against exploitation and discrimination.
9.	To legal heirship.
10.	To enjoy these rights regardless of race, colour, sex, religion, national and social origin.

CHAPTER 16

COMMUNITY PEDIATRICS

S.No.	Items
1.	Does any person has fits?
2.	Does any person has difficulty with learning?
3.	Does any person has difficulty with speech and hearing?
4.	Does any person has difficulty with seeing?
5.	Does any person shows strange behaviour?
6.	Does any person has difficulty with moving?
7.	Does any person has no feeling in hands and feets?
8.	Does any person has any other disability?

Table 16.8: The WHO questionnaire to identify disabled persons

Item		India (2005)	Kerala (2005)	World
IMR/1000 live births		58	14	54
PMR/1000 live births		48	7	
U5 MR/1000 live births		85	32	71
MMR/1000 live births		4.4	0.23	
Low birth weight—LBW%		30	17	16
Crude birth rate—CBR/1000		22	17	
Immunization	Infants%	85	90	
	Antenatal%	80	100	
Antenatal care—ANC%		80	100	
Deliveries% by trained persons		34	100	
Vitamin A deficiency blindness%		–	–	
Total fertility rate		3.2	1.8	
GNP		$450	–	
Life expectancy		63	74	64
Adult literacy%	Male	71	93	85
	Female	44	86	74
	Combined	58	90	
Goitre rate% (6-11 years)		9	–	
Moderate and severe PEM% (under fives)		47	26	
Moderate and severe stunting%		46	27	31

Table 16.9: National MCH indices

Contd.

Contd.

Moderate and severe wasting%	16	12	10
Crude death rate CDR/1000	7	6	9
Age at marriage	19	22	
Annual growth rate	2.1	1.34	
Total fertility rate	3.8	1.7	2.7
Crude birth rate/1000	24	15	22

IMR—Infant mortality rate, PMR—Perinatal Mortality Rate.

U5MR—Under five Mortality Rate, < MMR-Maternal Mortality Rate, U5 Mortality Rank India 52.

Source: The State of the World's Children, UNICEF, 2006, Sample Registration Survey (SRS) 2005.

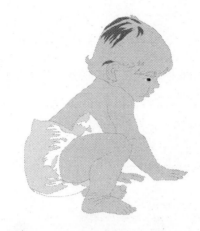

Appendices

Appendices

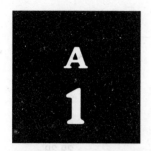

BMI CHARTS

1. Classification of body mass index (BMI) for adults

Classification	BMI (Kg/m²)	Risk of co-morbidities
Underweight	< 18.5	Low (but risk of other clinical problems increased)
Normal range	18.5-24.9	Average
Overweight	≥ 25.0	—
Pre-obese	25.0–29.9	Increased
Obese class I	30.0–34.9	Moderate
Obese class II	35.0–39.9	Severe
Obese class III	≥ 40.0	Very severe

2. International obesity task force (IOTF) cut-off points of BMI for the diagnosis of overweight and obesity in children defined to pass through BMI of 25 and 30 Kg/m² at age 18

Age (years)	BMI 25 kg/m²		BMI 30 kg/m²	
	Males	Females	Males	Females
2	18.41	18.02	20.09	19.81
2.5	18.13	17.76	19.80	19.55
3	17.89	17.56	19.57	19.36
3.5	17.69	17.40	19.39	19.23
4	17.55	17.28	19.29	19.15
4.5	17.47	17.19	19.26	19.12
5	17.42	17.15	19.30	19.17
5.5	17.45	17.20	19.47	19.34
6	17.55	17.34	19.78	19.65
6.5	17.71	17.53	20.23	20.08
7	17.92	17.75	20.63	20.51
7.5	18.16	18.03	21.09	21.01
8	18.44	18.35	21.60	21.57
8.5	18.76	18.69	22.17	22.18
9	19.10	19.07	22.77	22.81
9.5	19.46	19.45	23.39	23.46
10	19.84	19.86	24.00	24.11
10.5	20.20	20.29	24.57	24.77
11	20.55	20.74	25.10	25.42

Contd.

Contd.

11.5	20.89	21.20	25.58	26.05
12	21.22	21.68	26.02	26.67
12.5	21.56	22.14	26.43	27.24
13	21.91	22.58	26.84	27.76
13.5	22.27	22.98	27.25	28.20
14	22.62	23.34	27.63	28.57
14.5	22.96	23.66	27.98	28.87
15	23.29	23.94	28.30	29.11
15.5	23.60	24.17	28.60	29.29
16	23.90	24.37	28.88	29.43
16.5	24.19	24.54	29.14	29.56
17	24.46	24.70	29.41	29.69
17.5	24.73	24.85	29.70	29.84
18	25	25	30	30

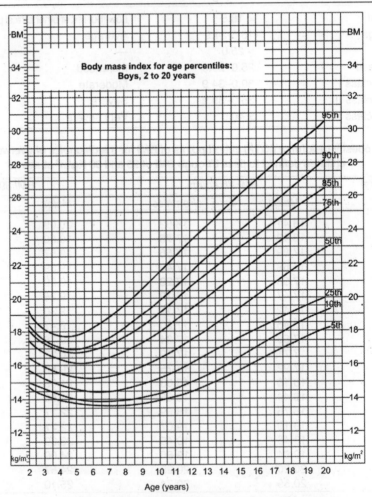

3. Body mass index for age percentiles: Boys, 2-20 years
Source: NCHS and CDC (US), 2000

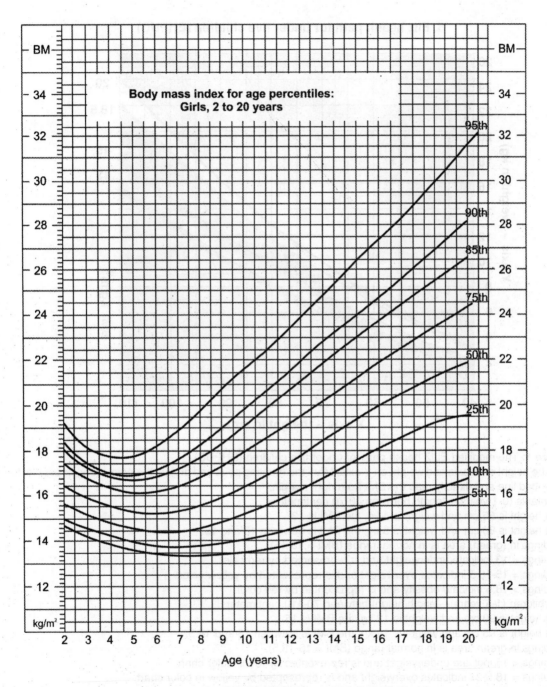

Body mass index for age percentiles: Girls, 2 to 20 years

4. Body mass index for age percentiles: Girls, 2-20 years

Source: NCHS and CDC (US), 2000

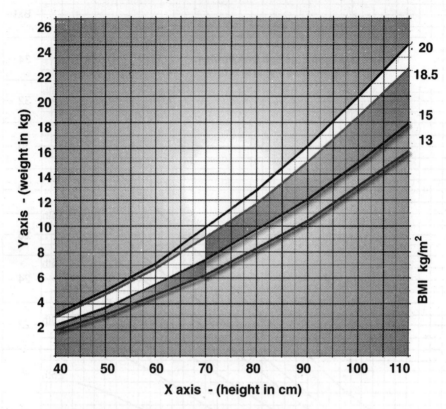

Figure 1: The modified ELIZ health path for under five children (EHPUC).

Plot the height on X axis and weight on Y axis. Mark the meeting point and project the point along or parallel to the dotted line and directly read the BMI from right margin.

For infants (0-1 years)—length between 40-70 centimeters.

If the height is 55 cm and weight is 4 kg, the BMI is 13.

If the height is 60 cm and weight is 5 kg, the BMI is between 13 and 15.

Readings in (green) area is in normal range (BMI = 13-15).

Readings < 13 indicate underweight and is represented by red color.

Readings = 15-18.5 indicates overweight and is represented by yellow color.

Readings > 18.5 indicate obesity and is represented by red color.

For children (1-5 years)—length/height between 70-110 centimeters.

If the height is 90 cm and weight is 12 kg, the BMI is 15.

If the height is 95 cm and weight is 14 kg, the BMI is between 15 and 18.5.

Readings in green area is in normal range (BMI = 15-18.5).

Readings < 15 indicate underweight and is represented by red in color chart.

Readings = 18.5-20 indicates overweight and is represented by yellow in color chart.

Readings > 20 indicate obesity and is represented by red in color chart.

6. Eliz health path for older children (EHPOC)

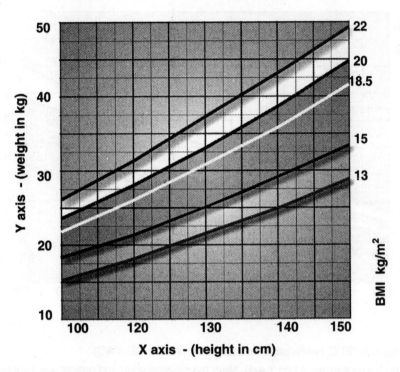

Figure 2: The modified ELIZ health path for older children (EHPOC).

Plot the height on X axis and weight on Y axis. Mark the meeting point and project the point along or parallel to the dotted line and directly read the BMI from right margin.

For children (5-10 years)—height between 110-150 centimeters.

E.g.: If the height is 130 cm and weight is 25 kg, the BMI is 15.

If the height is 140 cm and weight is 35 kg, the BMI is between 15 and 18.5.

Readings in shaded (green) area is in normal range (BMI = 15-20).

Readings < 15 indicate underweight and is represented by red in color chart.

Readings = 20-22 indicates overweight and is represented by yellow in color chart.

Readings > 22 indicate obesity and is represented by red in color chart.

7. Eliz health path for adolescent children (EHPAC)

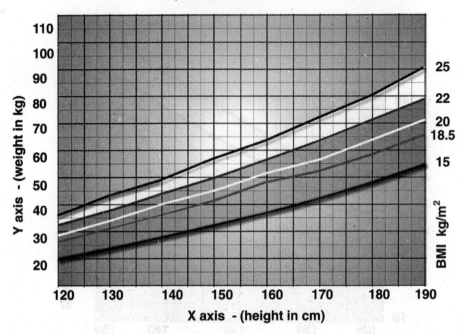

Figure 3: The modified ELIZ health path for adolescent children (EHPAC).

Plot the height on X axis and weight on Y axis. Mark the meeting point and project the point along or parallel to the dotted line and directly read the BMI from right margin.

For children (10-18 years)—height above 120 centimeters.

E.g.: If the height is 130 cm and weight is 25 kg, the BMI is 15.

If the height is 140 cm and weight is 35 kg, the BMI is between 15 and 18.5.

Readings in (green) area is in normal range (BMI = 15-22).

Readings < 15 indicate underweight and is represented by red in color chart.

Readings = 22-25 indicates overweight and is represented by yellow in color chart.

Readings > 25 indicate obesity and is represented by red in color chart.

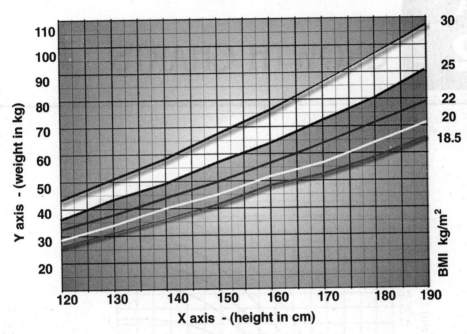

8. Eliz health path for adults (EHPA)

Figure 4: Modified ELIZ health path for adults (EHPA).

Plot the height on X axis and weight on Y axis. Mark the meeting point and project the point along or parallel to the dotted line and directly read the BMI from right margin.

For adults—height above 120 centimeters.

E.g.: If the height is 150 cm and weight is 50 kg, the BMI is 22.

If the height is 155 cm and weight is 55 kg, the BMI is between 22 and 25.

Readings in shaded (green) area is in normal range (BMI = 18.5-25).

Readings < 18.5 indicate underweight and is represented by red in color chart.

Readings = 25-30 indicates overweight and is represented by yellow in color chart.

Readings > 30 indicate obesity and is represented by red in color chart.

Reference: Elizabeth K E. Three-in-one Weight, Height and BMI Charts for children and Adults, Journal of Tropical Pediatrics, Oxford University Press, London, 2003, 49:224-227.

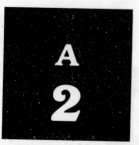

APPENDIX 2

A 2

GROWTH CHARTS

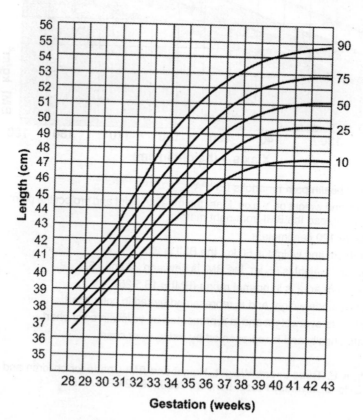

1. Intrauterine growth: Length, 28-43 weeks (both sexes)

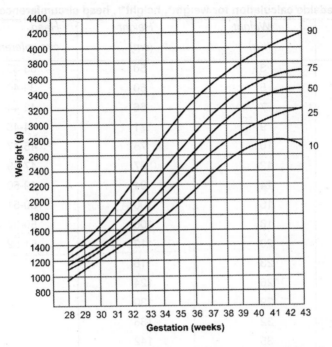

2. Intrauterine growth: Weight, 28-43 weeks (both sexes)

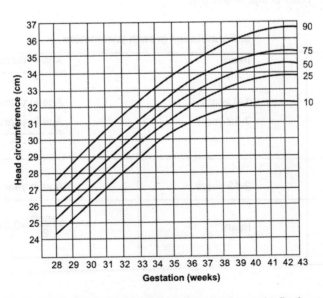

3. Intrauterine growth: Head circumference, 28-43 weeks (both sexes)

4. Bedside calculation for weight*, height**, head circumference

Age (years)	Weight (Kg)	Height (cm)	Head circumference (cm)
Birth	3	50	33-35
3/12	5	60	39-40
6/12	7	66	42-44
9/12	9	71	44-45
1	10	75	45-47
2	12	87	47-49
3	14	94	49-50
4	16	100	50-51
5	18	106	50-52
6	20	112	51-52
7	23	118	
8	26	124	
9	29	130	
10	32	136	
11	35	142	
12	38	150	

* Add 2 kg/year in 1-6 years of age and add 3 kg/year thereafter till puberty.

**Add 6 cm/year after 2 years of age till puberty.

5. Formula for growth parameters

Weight (Kg) (Weech's)	Infant	$\dfrac{\text{Age in months} + 9}{2}$
	1-6 years	Age in years $\times$ 2 + 8
	7-12 years	$\dfrac{\text{Age in years} \times 7 - 5}{2}$
Height (cm) (Weech's)	2-12 years	Age in years $\times$ 6 + 77
Head circumference (Dine's)	Infant	$\dfrac{\text{Length}}{2} + 9.5 \pm 2.5$

6. Growth parameters recommended by WHO
NCHS reference standards: 50th centile, agewise

Male				Female		
Wt	Length	OFC	Age	Wt	Length	OFC
Kg	cm	cm	mo	Kg	cm	cm
3.3	50.5	34.8	0	3.2	49.2	34.3
4.3	54.6	37.2	1	4.0	53.5	36.4
5.2	58.1	40.3	2	4.7	56.8	38.0
6.0	61.1	40.6	3	5.4	59.5	39.5
6.7	63.7	42.0	4	6.0	62.0	41.0
7.3	65.9	43.0	5	6.7	64.1	42.0
7.8	67.8	43.8	6	7.2	65.9	42.4
8.3	69.5	44.5	7	7.7	67.6	43.5
8.8	71.0	45.0	8	8.2	69.1	44.0
9.2	72.3	45.8	9	8.6	70.4	44.3
9.5	73.6	46.0	10	8.9	71.8	45.0
9.9	74.9	46.5	11	9.2	73.1	45.4
10.2	76.1	47.2	12	9.5	74.3	45.6
10.4	77.2	47.5	13	9.8	75.5	45.9
10.7	78.3	47.8	14	10.0	76.7	46.2
10.9	79.4	48.0	15	10.2	77.8	46.5
11.1	80.4	48.2	16	10.4	78.9	46.8
11.3	81.4	48.3	17	10.6	79.9	47.0
11.5	82.4	48.4	18	10.8	80.9	47.1
11.7	83.3	48.6	19	11.0	81.9	47.2
11.8	84.2	48.8	20	11.2	82.9	47.4
12.0	85.1	49.0	21	11.4	83.8	47.5
12.2	86.0	49.1	22	11.5	84.7	47.7
12.4	86.8	49.2	23	11.7	85.6	47.9
12.6	87.6	49.3	24	11.9	86.5	48.1
13.6	92.3	49.9	30	12.9	91.3	48.8
14.6	96.5	50.5	36	13.9	95.6	49.3
15.5	99.0	50.7	42	15.0	98.0	49.5
16.0	103.0	51.0	48	15.9	102.0	50.0
17.7	106.6	51.4	54	16.8	105.1	50.5
18.7	109.9	51.9	60	17.7	108.4	50.8

OFC—Occipitofrontal circumference

7. Growth chart percentiles: Weight (kg), height (cm), head circumference (cm): 97th, 50th and 3rd centiles, agewise upto 18 years

	Boys			Girls		
	Kg	*cm*	*cm*	*Kg*	*cm*	*cm*
Birth	4.2	54.8	37.2	3.9	53.9	35.9
	3.3	50.5	34.8	3.2	49.9	34.3
	2.5	46.2	32.6	2.3	45.8	32.1
3 months	7.6	66.1	43.1	6.9	64.2	41.7
	6.0	61.1	40.6	5.4	59.5	39.5
	4.2	56.1	38.4	4.0	54.9	37.3
6 months	9.7	72.9	46.2	8.9	70.9	44.6
	7.8	67.8	43.8	7.2	65.9	42.4
	6.0	62.8	41.5	5.6	61.0	40.3
9 months	11.1	77.3	48.1	10.4	75.6	46.4
	9.2	72.3	45.8	8.6	70.4	44.3
	7.4	67.4	43.5	6.7	65.3	42.3
1 year	12.2	81.2	49.4	11.5	79.6	47.6
	10.2	76.1	47.0	9.5	74.3	45.6
	8.2	71.0	44.8	7.6	69.0	43.5
1½ years	13.8	88.1	50.6	13.0	85.7	49.1
	11.5	82.4	48.4	10.8	80.9	47.1
	9.3	76.7	46.3	8.6	75.1	45.0
2 years	15.0	94.0	51.4	14.3	92.6	50.1
	12.6	87.6	49.2	11.9	86.5	48.1
	10.1	81.3	47.3	9.6	80.3	46.1
2½ years	16.2	98.7	52.2	15.7	97.7	50.8
	13.7	92.3	49.9	12.9	91.3	48.8
	10.9	85.8	48.0	10.5	84.9	47.0
3 years	17.5	103.2	52.8	17.0	102.3	51.4
	14.7	96.5	50.5	13.9	95.6	49.8
	11.8	89.9	48.6	11.3	88.8	47.6
3½ years	19.3	106.7	53.0	19.1	105.3	52.2
	15.7	99.1	50.8	15.1	97.9	49.8
	12.4	91.5	48.2	12.1	90.6	47.4
4 years	20.5	111.0	53.8	20.4	109.2	52.6
	16.7	102.9	51.2	16.0	101.6	50.2
	13.1	94.9	48.6	12.8	94.0	47.8
4½ years	21.8	114.9	53.9	21.6	113.0	52.9
	17.7	106.6	51.4	16.8	105.1	50.5
	13.9	98.2	48.9	13.4	97.2	48.1

Contd.

Contd.

5 years	23.2	118.6	54.1	22.9	116.7	53.2
	18.7	109.9	51.6	17.7	108.4	50.8
	14.7	101.3	49.1	14.0	100.1	48.4
6 years	26.2	125.2	54.4	25.8	123.9	53.6
	20.7	116.1	51.9	19.5	114.6	51.2
	16.3	107.0	49.4	15.3	105.4	48.8
7 years	29.8	131.3	54.6	29.7	130.9	53.9
	22.9	121.7	52.1	21.8	120.6	51.5
	17.9	112.1	49.6	16.7	110.3	49.3
8 years	34.1	137.0	54.8	35.0	137.7	54.1
	25.3	127.0	52.3	24.8	126.4	51.7
	19.5	116.9	49.8	18.3	115.0	49.3
9 years	39.2	142.8	55.0	41.3	144.5	54.3
	31.4	137.5	52.8	28.5	132.2	51.9
	22.7	126.0	50.3	20.2	120.0	49.5
10 years	45.2	149.0	55.3	48.2	151.2	54.7
	31.4	137.5	52.8	32.5	138.3	52.2
	24.8	130.6	50.4	22.5	125.4	49.7
11 years	51.7	155.9	55.8	55.3	157.8	55.2
	35.3	143.3	53.1	37.0	144.8	52.7
	24.8	130.6	50.4	25.2	131.7	50.2
12 years	58.7	163.8	56.4	62.0	164.4	55.6
	39.8	149.7	53.6	41.5	151.5	53.2
	27.6	135.5	50.8	28.3	138.7	50.8
13 years	65.9	172.0	57.0	68.0	169.7	56.0
	45.0	156.5	54.1	46.1	157.1	53.6
	31.2	140.9	51.2	31.7	144.6	51.2
14 years	73.2	179.2	57.5	73.0	172.9	56.2
	50.8	163.1	54.6	50.3	160.4	54.0
	35.9	147.0	51.7	35.2	147.8	51.8
15 years	80.1	184.2	57.6	76.8	174.5	56.3
	56.7	169.0	54.8	53.7	161.8	54.2
	40.9	153.8	52.2	38.3	149.1	52.1
16 years	86.4	187.1	57.7	79.1	175.0	56.4
	62.1	173.5	55.0	55.9	162.4	54.3
	45.7	160.0	52.3	40.8	149.9	52.2
17 years	91.6	188.6		80.8	175.0	
	66.3	176.2		56.7	163.1	
	49.6	163.9		42.3	151.1	
18 years	95.3	189.2		79.9	174.9	
	68.9	176.8		56.6	163.7	
	52.0	164.4		42.9	152.5	

US NCHS Reference Standards recommended by WHO.

8. 2 to 20 years (Boys) Stature-for-age and weight-for-age percentiles

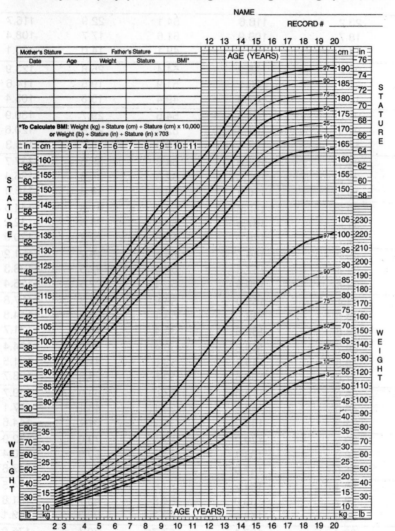

Source: Developed by the National Centre for Health Statistics in Collaboration with the National Centre for Chronic Disease Prevention and Health Promotion (2000).

9. Weight-for-stature percentiles: Boys

NAME _____

RECORD # _____

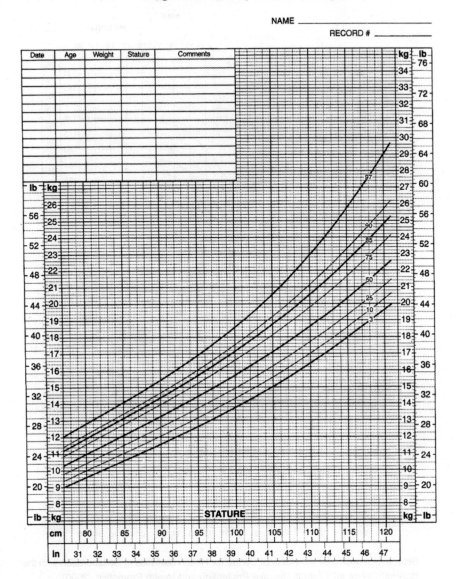

Source: Developed by the National Centre for Health Statistics in Collaboration with the National Centre for Chronic Disease Prevention and Health Promotion (2000).

10. 2 to 20 years (Girls) Stature-for-age and weight-for-age percentiles

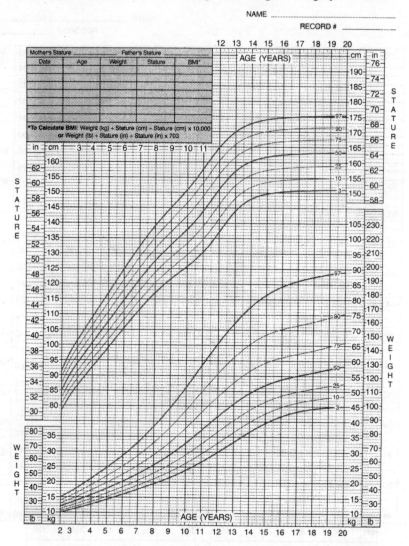

Source: Developed by the National Centre for Health Statistics in Collaboration with the National Centre for Chronic Disease Prevention and Health Promotion (2000).

11. Weight-for-stature percentiles: Girls

NAME _____

RECORD # _____

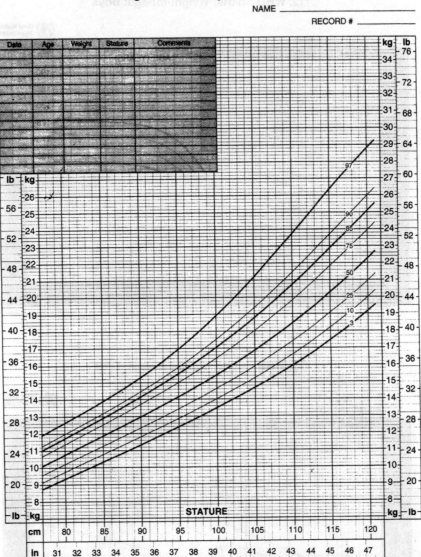

STATURE

Source: Developed by the National Centre for Health Statistics in Collaboration with the National Centre for Chronic Disease Prevention and Health Promotion (2000).

12. WHO Charts: Weight-for-age: Boys

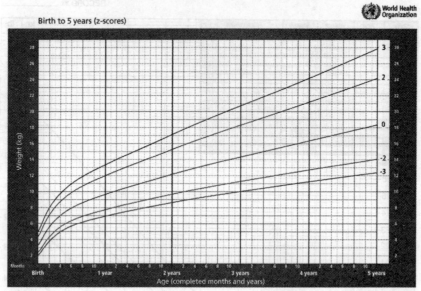

13. WHO Charts: Weight-for-age: Girls

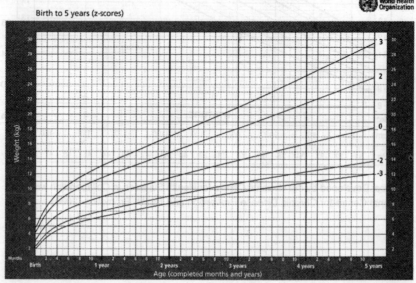

14. WHO Charts: Length/height-for-age: Boys

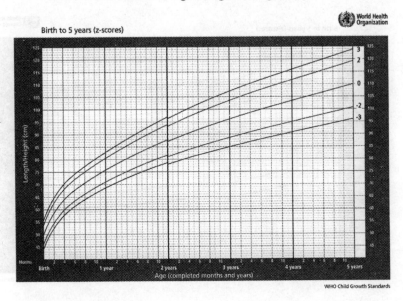

15. WHO Charts: Length/height-for-age: Girls

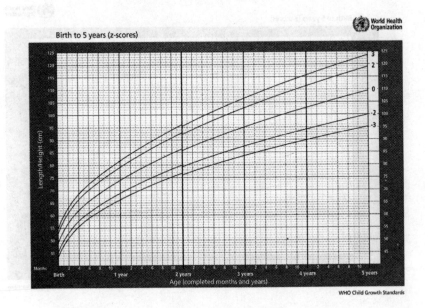

APPENDIX 2

16. WHO Charts: BMI-for-age: Boys

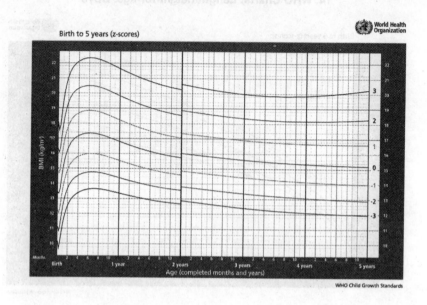

17. WHO Charts: BMI-for-age: Girls

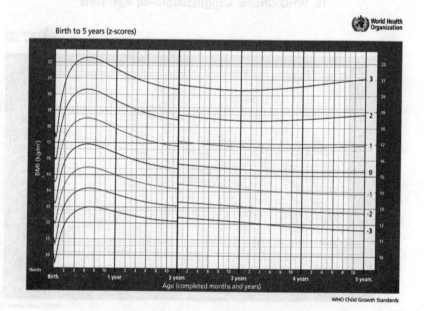

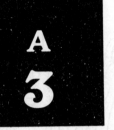

BONE AGE CHARTS

I. Male hand and wrist, birth to 17 years

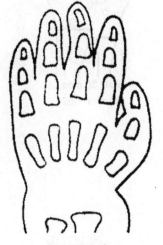

Male newborn

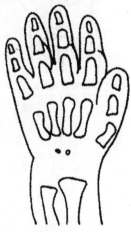

Male 3 mos.
3.01±0.69

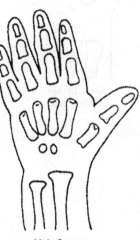

Male 6 mos.
6.09±1.13

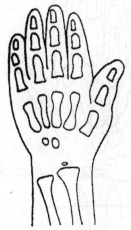

Male 9 mos.
9.56±1.43

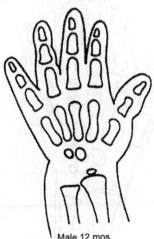

Male 12 mos.
12.74 ± 1.97

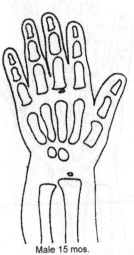

Male 15 mos.

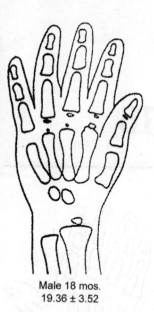

Male 18 mos.
19.36 ± 3.52

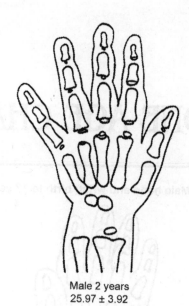

Male 2 years
25.97 ± 3.92

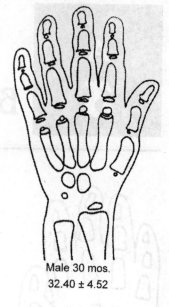

Male 30 mos.
32.40 ± 4.52

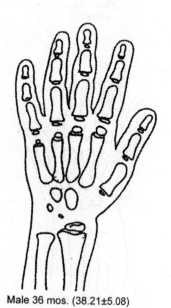

Male 36 mos. (38.21±5.08)

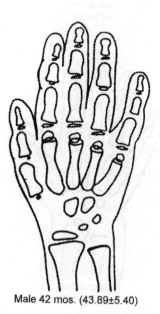

Male 42 mos. (43.89±5.40)

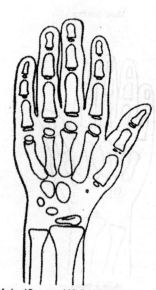

Male 48 mos. (49.04±6.66)

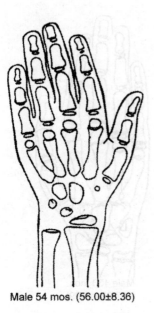

Male 54 mos. (56.00±8.36)

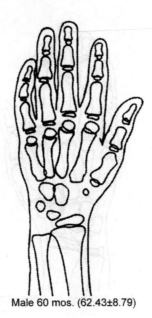

Male 60 mos. (62.43±8.79)

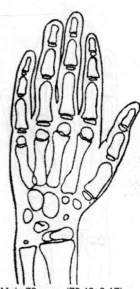

Male 72 mos. (75.46±9.17)

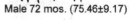

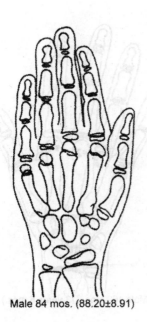

Male 84 mos. (88.20±8.91)

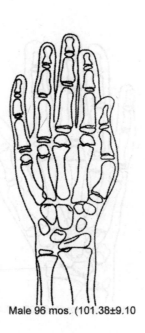

Male 96 mos. (101.38±9.10

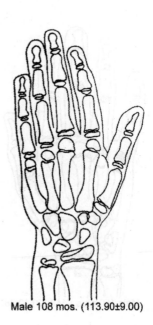

Male 108 mos. (113.90±9.00)

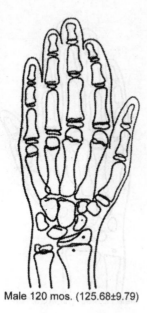

Male 120 mos. (125.68±9.79)

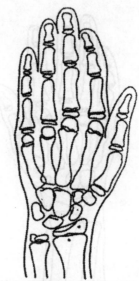

Male 120 mos. (125.68±9.79)

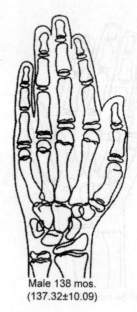

Male 138 mos. (137.32±10.09)

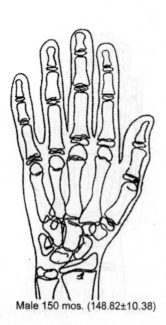

Male 150 mos. (148.82±10.38)

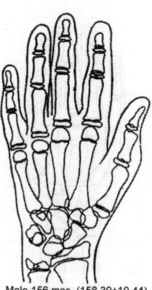

Male 156 mos. (158.39±10.44)

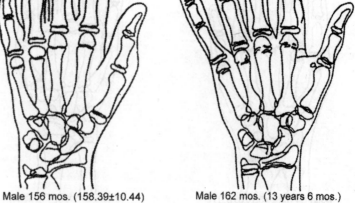

Male 162 mos. (13 years 6 mos.)

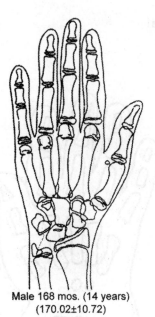

Male 168 mos. (14 years)
(170.02±10.72)

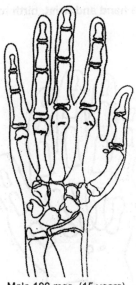

Male 180 mos. (15 years)
(182.72 ±11.32)

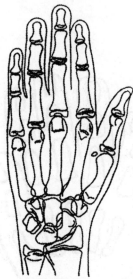

Male 186 mos.
(15 years 6 mos.)

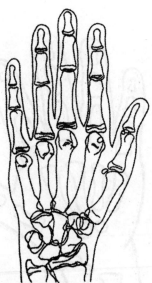

Male 192 mos. (16 years)
(195.32±12.86)

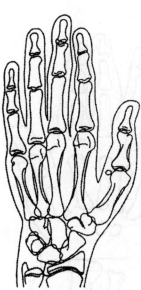

Male 204 mos. (17 years)
(206.21±13.05)

2. Female hand and wrist, birth to 18 years

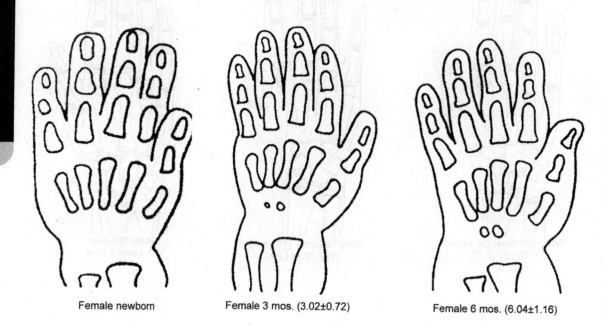

Female newborn

Female 3 mos. (3.02±0.72)

Female 6 mos. (6.04±1.16)

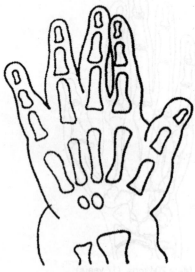

Female 9 mos. (9.05±1.36)

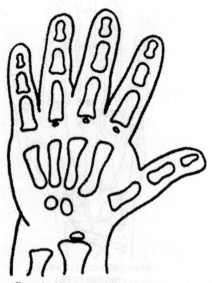

Female 12 mos. (12.04±1.77)

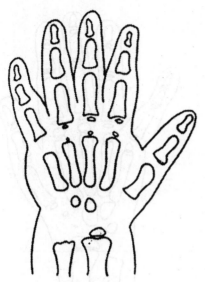

Female 15 mos.

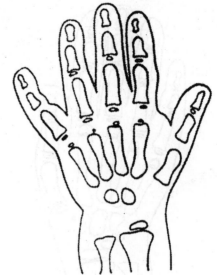

Female 18 mos. (18.2±3.49)

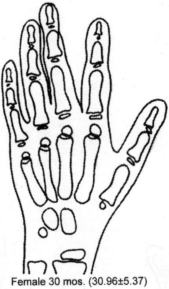

Female 30 mos. (30.96±5.37)

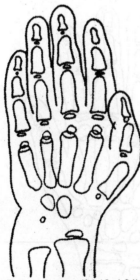

Female 2 years (24.16±4.64)

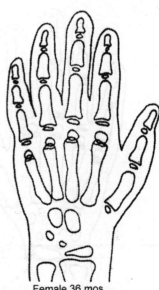

Female 36 mos.

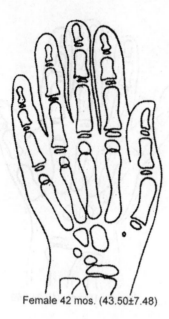

Female 42 mos. (43.50±7.48)

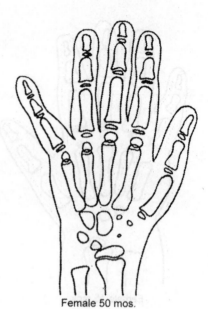

Female 50 mos.

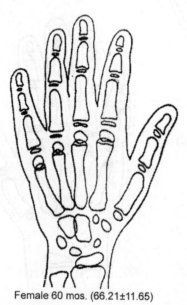

Female 60 mos. (66.21±11.65)

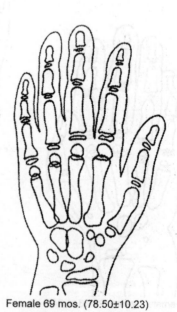

Female 69 mos. (78.50±10.23)

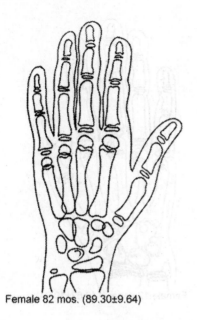

Female 82 mos. (89.30±9.64)

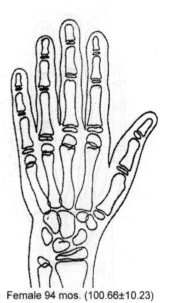

Female 94 mos. (100.66±10.23)

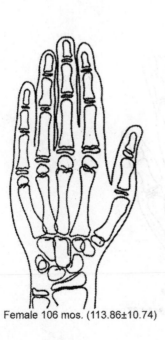

Female 106 mos. (113.86±10.74)

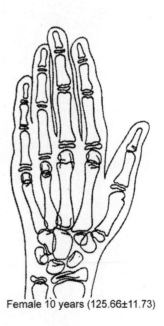

Female 10 years (125.66±11.73)

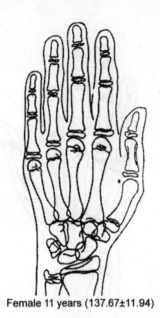

Female 11 years (137.67±11.94)

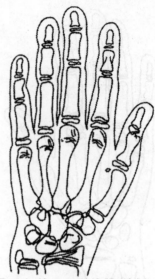

Female 12 years (149.62±10.24)

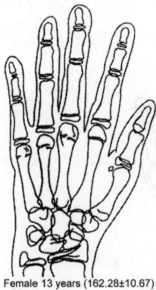

Female 13 years (162.28±10.67)

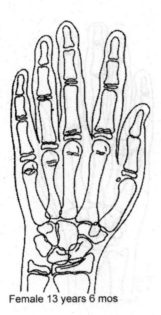

Female 13 years 6 mos

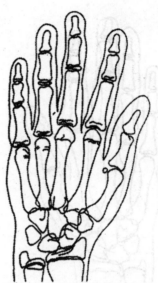

Female 14 years (174.25±11.30)

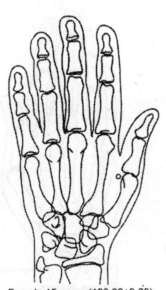

Female 15 years (183.62±9.23)

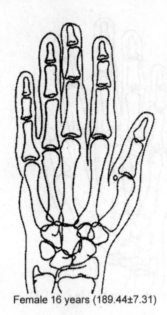

Female 16 years (189.44±7.31)

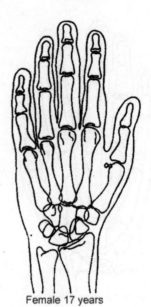

Female 17 years

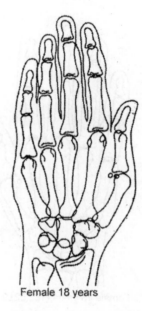

Female 18 years

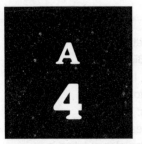

SPECIAL GROWTH CHARTS FOR SPECIFIC SYNDROME

Anthropometric assessment of the nutritional status of patients with genetic and other medical conditions can be difficult using the National Center for Health Statistics (NCHS) data. To help evaluate the growth patterns of these patients, special weight and height curves for several syndromes have been published. Weight and height curves for common syndromes as well as contact information for obtaining other curves for less common syndromes are given below:

Special Growth Charts*

Condition	Reference
Achondroplasia	Horton WA *et al.*
	Stature, growth velocity, head
	circumference, upper and lower segments.
	J Pediatr 1978;93:435.
Brachmann-de	Kline AD *et al.*
Lange syndrome	Length- and weight-for-age
	birth to 36 months, height- and weight-for-
	age 2 to 18 years, and head circumference-for-age birth
	to18 years.
	Am J Med Genet.1993;47:1042.
Cerebral palsy Krick J *et al.*	Stature and weight-for age and weight-for
(quadriplegia)	stature age birth to 10 years.
	J Am Diet Assoc 1996;96:680.
Down syndrome	Cronk CE *et al.*
	Length-for-age and weight-for-age birth to
	36 months. Pediatrics 1978;61:564.
	Cronk C, Crocker AC, Pueschel SM *et al.*
	Stature-for-age and weight-for-age 2 to 18 years. Pediatrics
	1988;81:102.
Marfan syndrome	Pyeritz RE. In: Emery AH, Rimoirn DL,
	editors. Principles and practice of medical
	genetics. New York: Churchill Livingstone; 1983.
	Pyeritz RE. In: Papadatos CJ, Bartsocas

Contd.

Contd.

	CS, editors. In: Endocrine genetics and genetics of growth (Prog Clin Biol Res v200). New York: Alan R. Liss, Inc; 1985. Stature- and weight-for-age 2 to 18 years, 20 to 24 years, and > 24 years. Upper and lower segment ratios 2 to 20 years and adult.
Myelomeningocele	Appendix 2. Ekvall S, editor. Pediatric nutrition in chronic disease and development disorders: Prevention, assessment and treatment. New York: Oxford University Press; 1993. (Preliminary charts) height- and weight-for-age 2 to 18 years.
Noonan's syndrome	Witt DR *et al.* Growth curves for height in Noonan syndrome. Clin Genet 1986;30:150-3.
Prader-Willi syndrome	Holm VA. Appendix A. In: Greeway LR, Alexander PC, editors. Management of Prader-Willi syndrome. New York: Springer Verlag; 1998. p. 317. Height-for-age 3 to 25 years. Butler, *et al.* Weight, height, sitting height, head circumference, triceps, and subscapular skinfold (plus other measure) for age 2 to 22 years. Pediatrics 1991;88:853.
Sickle cell disease	Phebus CK *et al.* Height- and weight-for-age birth to 18 years. J Pediatr 1984;105:28. Tanner JM *et al.* Height velocity (cm/yr) age 21/2 to 19 years. J Pediatr 1985;107:317-29.
Silver-Russell syndrome	Tanner JM *et al.* Height- and height velocity-for-age 2 to 19 years (includes periods of treatment with human growth hormone). Pediatr Res 1975;9:611.
Turner's syndrome	Lyon AJ *et al.* Height-for-age birth to 18 years (girls). Arch Dis Child 1985:60:932.
Williams syndrome	Morris CA *et al.* Natural history of Williams syndrome: Physical characteristics. J Pediatr 1988;113:318-26. Partsch CJ *et al.* Longitudinal evaluation of growth, puberty, and bone maturation in children with Williams syndrome. J Pediatr 1999;134:82-9.

*Unless otherwise specified, charts are available for both girls and boys.

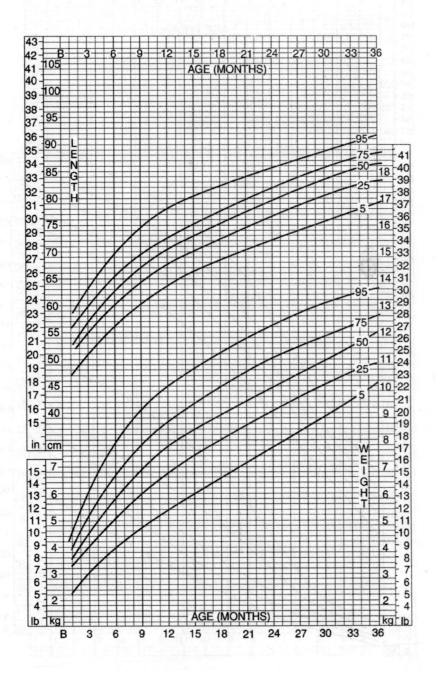

Figure 1: Physical growth of females with Down syndrome (1 to 36 months)

APPENDIX 4

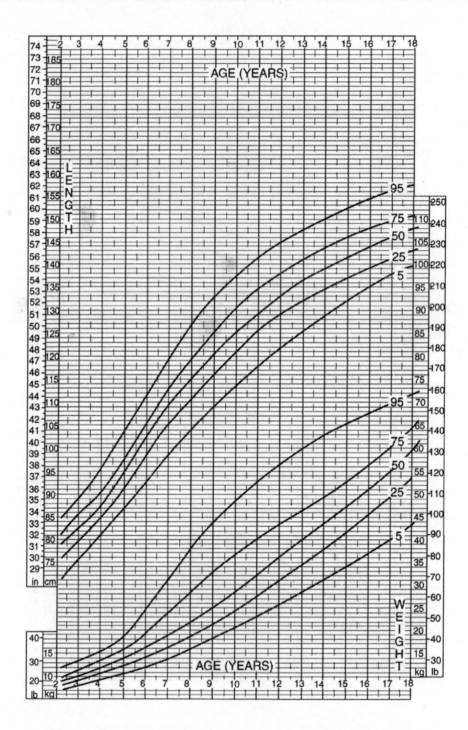

Figure 2: Physical growth of females with Down syndrome (2 to 18 years)

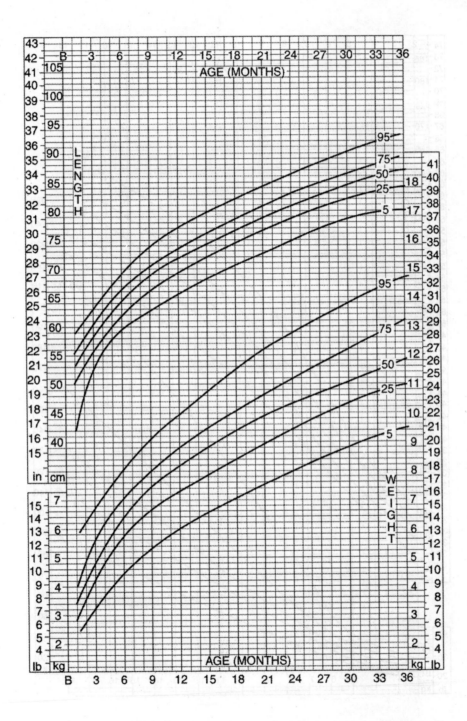

Figure 3: Physical growth of males with Down syndrome (1 to 36 months)

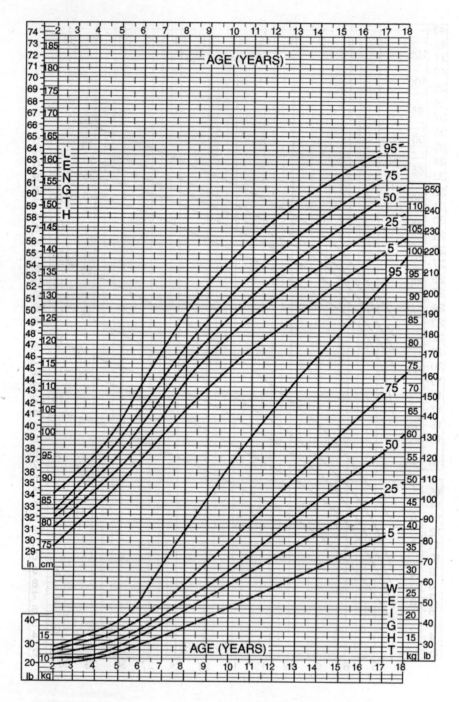

Figure 4: Physical growth of males with Down syndrome (2 to 18 years)

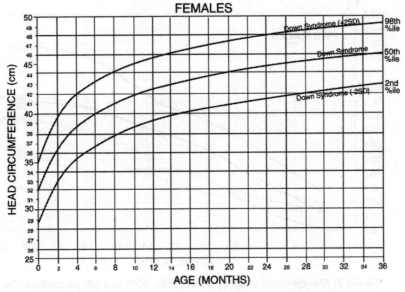

Figure 5: Head circumference of females with Down syndrome
(0 to 36 months)

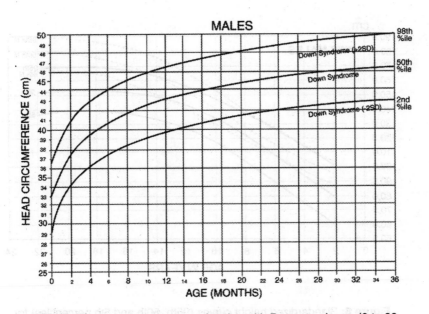

Figure 6: Head circumference of males with Down syndrome (0 to 36 months)

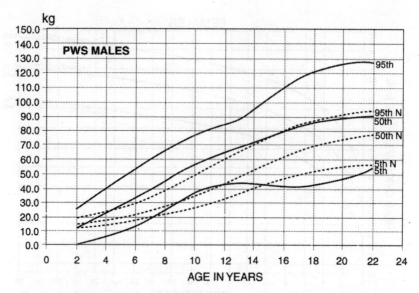

Figure 7: Standardized weight curves (95th, 50th and 5th percentiles) for Caucasian Prader-Willi syndrome males compared with normal controls

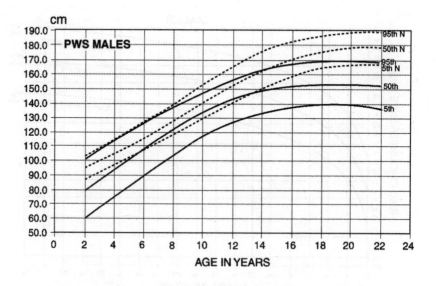

Figure 8: Standardized height curves (95th, 50th and 5th percentiles) for Caucasian Prader-Willi syndrome males compared with normal controls

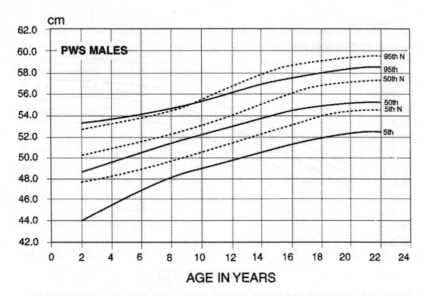

Figure 9: Standardized head circumference curves (95th, 50th and 5th percentiles) for Caucasian Prader-Willi syndrome males compared with normal controls

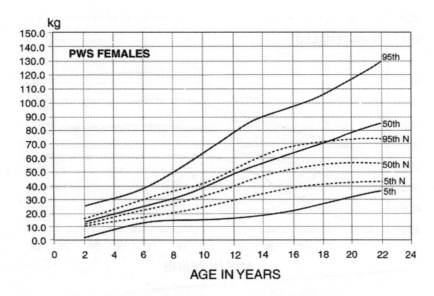

Figure 10: Standardized weight curves (95th, 50th and 5th percentiles) for Prader-Willi syndrome females compared with normal controls

APPENDIX 4

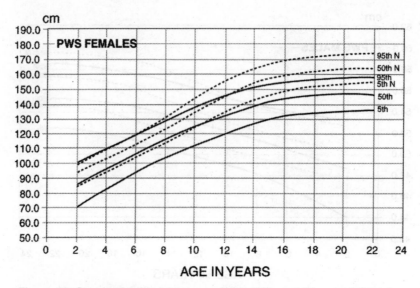

Figure 11: Standardized height curves (95th, 50th and 5th percentiles) for Prader-Willi syndrome females compared with normal controls

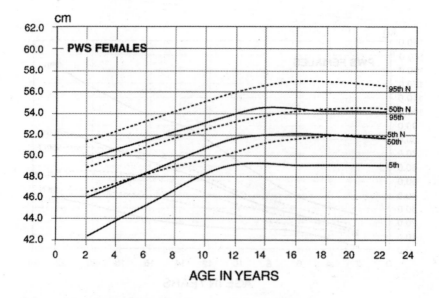

Figure 12: Standardized head circumference curves (95th, 50th and 5th percentiles) for Prader-Willi syndrome females compared with normal controls

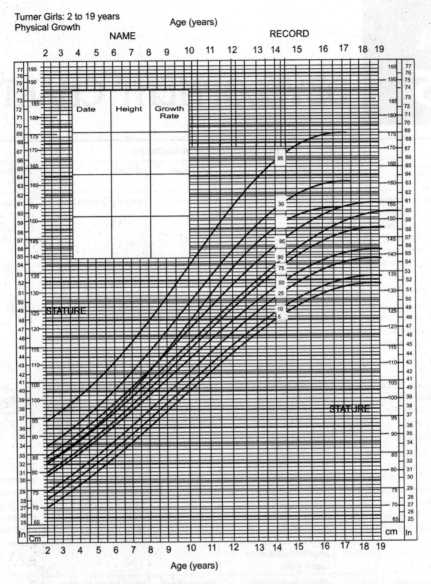

Figure 13: Physical growth of girls with Turner's syndrome aged 2 to 19 years. Normal girls' (top three lines) percentiles derived from National Center for Health Statistics. Untreated Turner's syndrome growth rates derived from Lyon AJ, Preece MA, Grant DB. Growth curve for girls with Turner's syndrome. Arch Dis Child 1985;60:932-5

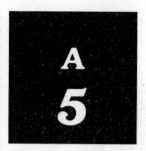

DEVELOPMENT CHARTS

1. Developmental milestones

Age (months)	Motor	Adaptive	Language	Social	Vision and hearing
1	Head lifts momentarily in the plane of body, ATNR predominates, complete head lag, momentarily holds chin of couch in prone position, sitting position holds head up momentarily,			Beginning to smile	Follows moving object, <u>less than 90°</u>, turns his head to rattle
2	Head in plane of body, head lag partial, sitting position–head bobs, plane of face at 45° by raising chin recurrently	<u>Hands predominantly closed</u>	Coos	Social smile +	Follows objects 180°
3	Lifts head and chest, head above plane of body, moderate head control, <u>bears weight on forearms</u>	Reaches toward object and misses, hands open, no more grasp reflex, <u>hand regard present</u>, pulls at his dress	Says aah or naah, vocalizes with pleasure	Sustained social contact	Binocular vision develops by 3-6 months
4	<u>No head lag, head steady</u>, enjoys sitting with full truncal support, when erect pushes with feet, ATNR gone, <u>holds head and chest of couch</u>	<u>Reaches and grasps object and brings to mouth</u>, approaches object and overshoots, <u>Hands in midline and plays with them</u>, pulls his dress over the face, plays with rattle when kept in hand		Laughs out loud, excited at sight of food and breast Laughs out loud, excited at sight of food and breast	Turns head towards a round at the same level at 3-4 months Turns head towards a sound at the same level at 3-4 months
5	Full head control	Able to grasp objects deliberately, <u>no more hand regard</u>, crumples paper, plays with toys, <u>bi dexterous grasp</u>	Smiles at self in the mirror	When he drops rattle looks to see where it has fallen	Truns head towards a sound below the level at 5-6 months
6	<u>Holds chest and abdomen of the couch</u>, weight bearing on extended arms<u>, rolls over from prone to supine</u>	<u>Grasps his feet and brings to mouth,</u> holds bottle if he has one cube in hand, drops it if another is offered	<u>Smiles and vocalizes at self in the mirror, monosyllabic babble</u>	When he drops the rattle he tries to recover it, may protrude tongue as imitation, may show stranger	

Contd.

Contd.

			anxiety, laughs when head is hidden in towel in peep-bo-game, beginning to show likes and dislikes of food	
7	Rolls over from supine to prone, sits briefly with support of pelvis, weight bearing present, bounces actively, weight bearing on 1 hand	Reaches out for large objects and grasps, transfers object, uses radial palm, rakes at pellet, if he has 1 cube in hand retains it even if another is offered, bangs object on table, takes all objects to mouth, feeds self with biscuit, palmar grasp	Polysyllabic sounds formed, says da ma ba	Prefers mother, enjoys mother, pats image of self in mirror, resists if toy is pulled from hand, gastro colic reflex weakens	Turns head towards a sound above the level at 7-9 months
8	Sits alone back straight, pulls to standing position, cruises	Grasps object with thumb and forefinger, picks up pellet with assisted pincer grasp, uncovers hidden toy, attempts to retrieve fallen toy, releases object grasped by another person	Says mama or dada by combining syllables	Responds to sound of name, plays peek a boo or pat a cake, waves bye-bye, reaches persistently to toys out of reach, responds to "no"	
9	Stands holding on to furniture, in trying to crawl may progress backwards, sitting—can lean forward	Brings 2 cubes together as if to compare the sizes and bangs them on the table		Puts arm in front of face to prevent mother from washing face	
10	Pulls self to standing position, pulls self to sitting position, crawls with abdomen on the couch	Let's go objects deliberately, picks up pellet neatly, coat sign	Can understand the meaning of some words	Pats a doll, can be placed on toilet seat	
11	Creeps – abdomen of ground, sitting–can lean sideways, walks with 2 hand held, sitting–can turn round to pick up object (pivots), walks sideways holding on to furniture	Will place object in examiner's hand but will not release it, rolls ball to examiner	Says 1 word with meaning	Let's go objects deliberately in order that they will be picked up, likes repetitive play	
12	Walks with one hand held, rises independently, bear walking	Unassisted pincer grasp, releases object to person on request, feeds with spoon with spilling	Few words besides mama or dada 2-3 words with meaning	Plays simple ball game, may kiss on request, mimicry	
15	Stand alone (13 months). Walks alone with broad base and high stepping gait; crawls upstairs, take several steps sideward	Makes tower of 2 cubes; makes a line with crayon; inserts a pellet into a bottle. Constantly throwing objects on the ground, takes of shoes, feeds with spoon without spilling, feeds self managing cup with slight spilling	Jargon; follows simple commands; may name an object	Indicate some needs by pointing; hugs parents. Asks for objects by pointing	

Contd.

Contd.

18	Runs stiffly, sits on a small chair, walks upstairs with one hand held, walks normally, <u>pulls toy as he walks, throws ball without falling</u>	Makes <u>tower of 4 cubes</u>, imitates scribbling, imitates <u>vertical stroke</u>, dumps pellet in the bottle, feeds self managing cup without spilling, turns 2-3 pages at a time	Average 10 words, names one or more parts of the body, points correctly to 1 picture, names 1 object	Feeds self, tells when wet or soiled, clean and dry with occasional accident, carries out 2 simple orders, uses stick to reach toy, dry by day
21	<u>Walks backwards</u> , picks up object without falling, <u>walks upstairs with 2 feet per step</u>	<u>Tower of 6 cubes</u>	Points correctly to 2 pictures, knows 4 parts of body, joins 2 words together, asks for food, drink and toilet	Obeys 3 simple orders
24	Runs well, <u>walks up and down stairs one step at a time 2 feet per step</u>, opens doors, jumps, climbs on furniture's	<u>Tower of 7 cubes, circular scribbling, imitates horizontal stroke, turns pages 1 at a time</u>, washes and dries hands	Puts 3 words together, talks incessantly, names 2 objects, tells a simple sentence	Handles spoon well, listens to stories with pictures, helps to undress, obeys 4 simple orders, dry at night, wears socks or shoes
30	Goes upstairs with alternating feet, jumps with both feet, <u>walks on tiptoe</u> when asked	<u>Tower of 9 cubes , makes vertical and horizontal stroke but generally not a cross , imitates circular stroke</u>, forming closed figure, holds pencil in hand	<u>Uses pronoun I , knows full name</u>, names 3 objects, repeats 2 digits	Helps put things away, pretends to play, beginning to take interest in sex organs
36	<u>Rides tricycle, stand momentarily on single foot, goes upstairs with 1 foot per step and downstairs with 2 feet per step, jumps off bottom step</u>	<u>Tower of 10 cubes, copies a circle and imitates a cross</u> (copies a cross by 3½ years), beginning to draw spontaneously or on request	Counts three objects, repeats 3 numbers or a sentence of 6 syllables, constantly asking questions, knows some nursery rhymes, vocabulary = 250 words	Knows age and sex, parallel play present, washes hands , helps in dressing and does by self if helped with the buttons, postpone toilet movement
48	<u>Hops on 1 foot</u>, throws ball overhand, climbs well, <u>goes downstairs with 1 foot per step</u>	Copies a <u>square</u>, draws a man with 2-4 parts, names longer of the 2 lines, uses scissors, <u>tripod grasp</u>	Counts 4 numbers correctly, tells a story, obeys 4 commands, tells tall stories	Plays with children, role playing present, goes to toilet alone, right-left discrimination, imaginative play with a doll, can button clothes fully
60	Skips	Names the heavier object, <u>copies a triangle</u>	Names 4 colors; counts to 10, distinguishes morning from afternoon, repeats 4 digits	Dresses and undresses; domestic role playing; asks questions regarding meaning of words
66		<u>Copies a diamond</u>	Repeats 5 digits	Knows number of fingers, names of week days, names 4 coins

2. Amiel Tison Angles

Age	Adductor angle	Popliteal	Dorsiflexion	Scarf sign
0-3	40-80	80-100	60-70	Elbow does not cross the midline
4-6	70-110	90-120	60-70	Elbow crosses the midline
7-9	110-140	110-160	60-70	Elbow goes beyond the anterior axillary line
10-12	140-160	150-170	60-70	Elbow goes beyond the anterior axillary line

3.

CDC grading	Head control (4 months)	Sitting (8 months)	Standing (12 months)
I	Head erect and steady momentarily	Sits momentarily	Stand momentarily holding on to furniture
II	Dorsal suspension—lifts head along with body	Sits 30 seconds or more leaning forward	Take few steps while both hands supported
III	Prone position—elevates on arms, lifting chest	Sit with child's back straight	Can stand alone with legs wide apart
IV	Holds head steady while mother moves around	While sitting can turn around	Come to standing position with support of stool
V	Head balanced at all times	Raises to sitting position without support	Without support can take few steps

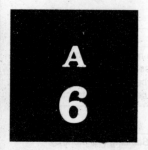

NUTRITION CHARTS

1. ICMR recommendations of RDA (1998)

Group	Particulars	Body wt (Kg)	Net energy (Kcal/d)	Protein (g/d)	Fat (g/d)	Calcium (mg/d)	Iron (mg/d)
Man	Sedentary work		2425				
	Moderate work	60	2875	60	20	400	28
	Heavy work		3800				
Woman	Sedentary work	50	1825				
	Moderate work		2225	50	20	400	30
	Heavy work		2925				
	Pregnant woman	50	+ 300	+15	30	1000	38
	Lactation						
	0-6 months	50	+550	+ 25	45	1000	30
	6-12 months		+400	+18			
Infants	0-6 months	5.4	118/kg	2.05/kg		500	
	6-12 months	8.6	108/kg	1.65/kg			
Children	1-3 years	12.2	1240	22			12
	4-6 years	19.0	1690	30	25	400	18
	7-9 years	26.9	1950	41			26
Boys	10-12 years	35.4	2190	54	22	600	34
Girls	10-12 years	31.5	1970	57			19
Boys	13-15 years	47.8	2450	70	22	600	41
Girls	13-15 years	46.7	2060	65			28
Boys	16-18 years	57.1	2640	78	22	500	50
Girls	16-18 years	49.9	2060	63			30

Age		Kilocal/Kg/day
1 year		110
1-3 years		100
4-6 years		90
7-9 years		80
Adult	male	45
	female	40

Average daily intake of energy

Age	Protein g/Kg
0-6 months	2.0
6-12 months	1.7
1-3 years	1.5
3-6 years	1.4
Adolescent	1.2
Adult	1.0

Average daily intake of protein

2. Recommended dietary allowances for Indians—ICMR 1998 (Vitamins)

Group	Particulars	Vit. A (μg/d) Retinol	β-carotene	Thiamine (mg/d)	Ribofla-vin (mg/d)	Nicotinic acid (mg/d)	Pyridoxine (mg/d)	Ascorbic acid (mg/d)	Folic acid (μg/d)	Vit. B$_{12}$ (μg/d)
Man	Sedentary work	600		1.2	1.4	16				
	Moderate work		2400	1.4	1.6	18	2.0	40	100	1
	Heavy work			1.6	1.9	21				
Woman	Sedentary work	600		0.9	1.1	12				
	Moderate work		2400	1.1	1.3	14	2.0	40	100	1
	Heavy work			1.2	1.5	16				
	Pregnant woman	600	2400	+0.2	+0.2	+2	2.5	40	400	1
	Lactation									
	0-6 months	950	3800	+0.3	+ 0.3	+4	2.5	80	150	1.5
	6-12 months			+0.2	+ 0.2	+3				
Infants	0-6 months	350	1200	55 μg/kg	65 μg/kg	710 μg/kg	0.1	25	25	0.2
	6-12 months			50 μg/kg	60 μg/kg	650 μg/kg	0.4			
Children	1-3 years	400	1600	0.6	0.7	8	0.9		30	
	4-6 years	400	2400	0.9	1.0	11		40	40	0.2-1.0
	7-9 years	600	2400	1.0	1.2	13	1.6		60	
Boys	10-12 years	600	2400	1.1	1.3	15	1.6	40	70	0.2-1.0
Girls	10-12 years			1.0	1.2	13				
Boys	13-15 years	600	2400	1.2	1.5	16	2.0	40	100	0.2-1.0
Girls	13-15 years			1.0	1.2	14				
Boys	16-18 years	600	2400	1.3	1.6	17	2.0	40	100	0.2-1.0
Girls	16-18 years			1.0	1.2	14				

3. Coefficient of calorie requirement

Age (years)	Co-unit	Energy (Kcal)
1-3	0.4	960
3-5	0.5	1200
5-7	0.6	1440
7-9	0.7	1680
9-12	0.8	1920
12-21	1.0	2400
Adult male		
Sedentary	1.0	2400
Moderate	1.2	2880
Heavy	1.6	3840
Adult female		
Sedentary	0.8	1920
Moderate	0.9	2160
Heavy	1.2	2880

Source: National Institute of Nutrition, Hyderabad.

4. Holliday and Segar formula for calculation of calories*

Holliday and Segar Formula		
Upto 10 kg	- 100	Kcal/kg
10-20 kg	- 1000 + 50	Kcal for each kg above 10 kg
Above 20 kg	- 1500 + 20	Kcal/each kg in excess above 20 kg

Age (years)	Expected weight (Kg)	Energy (Kcal)
1	10	1000
2	12	1100
3	14	1200
4	16	1300
5	18	1400
6	21	1520
7	24	1580
8	27	1640
9	30	1700
10	33	1760
11	36	1820
12	39	1880

* Also applicable for fluid calculation using observed weight instead of expected weight.

5. Bedside calculation energy and protein

Age (years)	Energy (Kcal)	Protein (g/Kg)
1	1000	22
2	1100	22
3	1200	22
4	1300	30
5	1400	30
6	1500	30
7	1600	41
8	1700	41
9	1800	41
10	1900	50-60
11	2000	50-60
12	2100	60-60
Adolescent boy	2400	60-80
Adolescent girl	2100	60-65

6. The approximate RDA of vitamins and minerals

1.	Vitamin A	1500 IU/day (500 µg)
2.	Vitamin D	400 IU/day (10 µg)
3.	Vitamin E	5-15 IU/day (5-15 mg)

Vitamin B complex

4.	B_1 (Thiamine)	0.5-1.5 mg/day (1 mg/1000 Kcal)
5.	B_2 (Riboflavin)	0.5-1.5 mg/day
6.	B_6 (Pyridoxine)	0.5-1.5 mg/day
7.	B_3 (Niacin)	5-15 mg/day
8.	B_{11} (Folic acid)	50-150 µg/day
9.	B_{12} (Cyanocobalamine)	0.5-1.5 µg/day
10.	Vitamin C	40 mg/day

Macro elements

11.	Calcium	500-1000 mg/day
12.	Phosphorus	800-1000 mg/day
13.	Magnesium	200-300 mg/day

Trace elements

14.	Iron	10-20 mg/day
15.	Iodine	50-150 µg/day
16.	Copper	1-2 mg/day
17.	Zinc	5-15 mg/day
18.	Fluroide	1-5 mg/day
19.	Manganese	1-5 mg/day
20.	Selenium	100 µg/day
21.	Molybdenum	200-500 µg/day
22.	Chromium	10 µg/day

7. Balanced diet for infants, children and adolescents—ICMR 1998 (Number of portions)

Food groups	g/Portion	Infants 6-12 months	Years			10-12		13-18	
			1-3	4-6	7-9	Girls	Boys	Girls	Boys
Cereals and millets	30	1.5	4	7	9	9	11	10	14
Pulses	30	0.5	1	1.5	2	2	2	2	2
Milk (mL)	100	5[a]	5	5	5	5	5	5	5
Roots and tubers	100	0.5	0.5	1	1	1	1	1	1
Green leafy vegetables	100	0.25	0.5	0.5	1	1	1	1	1
Other vegetables	100	0.25	0.5	0.5	1	1	1	1	1
Fruits	100	1	1	1	1	1	1	1	1
Sugar	5	5	5	6	6	6	7	6	7
Fats/oils (visible)	5	2	4	5	5	5	5	5	5

[a] Quantity indicates top milk. For breastfed infants, 200 mL top milk is required.

One portion of pulse may be exchanged with one portion (50 g) of egg/meat/chicken/fish.

For infants, introduced egg/meat/chicken/fish around 9 months.

Specific recommendations as compared to a sedentary woman.

Children:

1-6 years	-	1/2 to 3/4 the amount of cereals, pulses and vegetables and extra cup of milk.
7-12 years	-	Extra cup of milk.
Adolescent girls	-	Extra cup of milk.
Adolescent boys	-	Diet of sedentary man with extra cup of milk.

8. Nutritive value of common food items

	Protein (g)	Energy (Kcal)
Fish 1 oz (10 cm piece)	6	80
Mutton 1 oz (8 bits)	6	50
Bread 1 oz (1 slice)	2	70
Dosa 1	2	70
Idli 1	2	50
Chappathi 1	2	70
Puri 1	1	35
Vada/bonda 1	1	50
Upma 1 cup	6	250
Sugar 1 tsp	-	20
Jaggery 1 tsp	-	20
Ghee/Butter 1 tsp	-	36
Mashed potato 1 tsp	-	40
Plantain 1	0.5	50
Groundnut 10	1	20
Pappadam 1	0.5	20
Biscuit 1	0.5	20
Coffee 1 cup	1.8	80
Tea 1 cup	1.0	60

Balanced diet: A balanced diet is one which supplies all the nutrients in the right quantity and proportion. It is essential for growth, to maintain good health and to prevent deficiencies. Carbohydrate should yield 55-60 percent of the calories, protein should yield 10-15 per cent of the calories and fat should yield 30-35 per cent of the calories.

9. Balanced diet for an adult/adolescent boy (2400 Kcal/1 unit)

Food item	Quantity	Kilocalories
Cereal	400 g	1400
Legumes	60 g	230
Roots and tubers	50 g	50
Vegetables	50 g	50
Green leafy vegetables	50 g	50
Fruits	50 g	50
Milk/Curd	250 mL	150
Oil/Fats	30 g	270
Sugar	30 g	120
Total		**2370**

10. High energy isodense formula (100 mL=100 Kcal)

Item	Composition	Kilocalories
High energy milk	1/2 glass milk 1 teaspoon sugar 1/2 teaspoon oil	100 Kcal/100 ml
Cereal milk	1/2 glass milk 1 teaspoon sugar 1½ teaspoon cereal flour	100 Kcal/100 ml
Cereal pulse (SAT mix)	1/2 glass milk 2 teaspoon SAT mix	100 Kcal/100 ml
Fruit juice	1 orange, 2 teaspoon sugar, water upto 100 mL	100 Kcal/100 ml
Egg flip	One egg, 2 teaspoon sugar 3/4 glass milk	200 Kcal/200 ml
Curd/Lassee	1/2 glass curd 2 teaspoon sugar	100 Kcal/100 ml
SAT mix is roasted and powdered rice: wheat: blackgram: *powdered sugar in the ratio 1:1:1:2*		

11. Gomez's classification according to weight for age

Nutritional status		Weight for age (Harvard) (% of expected)
Normal	-	> 90
First degree PEM	-	75-90
Second degree PEM	-	60-75
Third degree PEM*	-	< 60

*All cases with oedema to be included in third degree PEM irrespective of weight for age.

12. Jelliffe's classification according to weight for age

Nutritional status		Weight for age (Harvard) (% of expected)
Normal	-	> 90
First degree PEM	-	80-90
Second degree PEM	-	70-80
Third degree PEM	-	60-70
Fourth degree PEM		< 60

13. Wellcome Trust classification of malnutrition

Weight for age (Boston) (% of expected)	Oedema	Clinical type of PEM
60-80	+	Kwashiorkor
60-80	-	Underweight
< 60	-	Marasmus
< 60	+	Marasmic Kwashiorkor

14. The IAP classification of malnutrition

Nutritional status*		Weight for age (% of expected)
Normal	-	> 80
Grade I PEM	-	71-80
Grade II PEM	-	61-70
Grade III PEM	-	51-60
Grade IV PEM	-	< 50

* If the patient has oedema of nutritional origin, the letter K is placed along with the grade of PEM in order to denote kwashiorkor.

Classification according to height for age: The calculation based on weight for age does not help to exclude other obvious syndromes with short stature. Moreover, it does not imply whether the PEM is of recent or past onset. Almost simultaneously two workers. Waterlow from London and McLaren from Beirut, independently came out with the height for age and weight for height concept to indicate stunting and wasting respectively in 1972. Height for age is used to grade stunting. It indicates past or chronic PEM. Classification based on height for age is given in the table below:

15. Classification according to height for age

Height for age (% of expected)	Waterlow's classification	McLaren's classification	Visweshwara Rao's classification
Normal	> 95	> 93	> 90
First degree stunting/short*	90-95	80-93	80-90
Second degree stunting	85-90	-	-
Third degree stunting/dwarf*	< 85	< 80	< 80
*Terminology used in McLaren's classification			

Classification according to weight for height: It is used to grade wasting. Wasting indicates recent or acute PEM. Classification based on weight for height is detailed in the following table:

16. Classification according to weight for height

Weight for height (% of expected)	Waterlow's classification	McLaren's classification
Normal	> 90	> 90
First degree wasting/mild wasting*	80-90	85-90
Second degree wasting/moderate wasting*	70-80	75-85
Third degree wasting/severe wasting*	< 70	< 75
*Terminology used in McLaren's classification		

A 7 FLUID AND ELECTROLYTE CHARTS

1. Composition of common IV fluids (m Eq/L)

IVF	Glucose (g/L)	Na (mEq/L)	K (mEq/L)	Cl (mEq/L)	Others (mEq/L)	
NS	-	154	-	154	-	
RL	-	131	5	111	HCO$_3$	29
					Ca	4
5% Dextrose	50	-	-	-	-	
3% Saline	-	510	-	510	-	
Maintenance fluid						
Isolyte P* with dextrose	50	27	19	19	HCO$_3$	27
Isolyte E** with dextrose	50	141	10	103	Citrate	8
					Mg	3
Isolyte G*** with dextrose	50	65	17	149	NH$_4$	70
Sancelyte P*	33	47	5	35	HCO$_3$	18
					Mg	1
Others					**mEq/mL**	
7.5% HCO$_3$	-	-	-	-	0.9	
10% Ca gluc	-	-	-	-	1.8	
15% KCl	-	-	-	-	2.0	

*For pediatric use ** For enteric loss *** For gastric loss

2. Practical tips on fluid therapy
Sodium concentration of IV fluids

I.V. fluids	NS/DNS	Isolyte-E	Ringer's Lactate	Isolyte-G	Isolyte-M	Isolyte-P	3% NaCl
Na (mEq/L)	154.0	140.0	130.0	63.0	40.0	25.0	513.0

Potassium concentration of IV fluids

IV fluids	Isolyte-M	Isolyte-P	Isolyte-G	Isolyte-E	Ringer's lactate
K (mEq/L)	35.0	20.0	17.0	10.0	4.0

3. Characteristics of IV fluids

Characteristics	Type of fluid
Most physiological	Ringer's lactate (RL)
Rich in sodium	Isotonic saline, DNS
Rich in chloride	NS, DNS, Isolyte-G
Rich in potassium	Isolyte-M-P and G
Corrects acidosis	RL, Isolyte-E, P and M
Corrects alkalosis	Isolyte-G
Cautiously in renal failure	RL, Isolyte-M, G, P and E
Avoid in liver failure	RL Isolyte-G
Glucose free	Saline, Ringer's lactate
Sodium free	Dextrose solutions
Potassium free	NS, DNS, Dextrose fluids

4. Selection of IV fluids

Clinical disorders	Ideal initial fluid
Hypovolemic shock	Saline, Ringer's lactate
Diarrhea	Ringer's lactate, Saline
Vomiting	Isolyte-G, Saline
Diabetic ketoacidosis	Saline (0.9% NaCl)
Burns	Ringer's lactate
Intra operative	Ringer's lactate
Starvation deficit	5% Dextrose
Adult maintenance	Isolyte-M
Paediatric maintenance	Isolyte-P
Stroke, Neurosurgery	NS avoid 5% Dextrose
Hypokalemia	Isolyte-M, KCl drip

5. Calculation of drop rate for IV fluid infusion

1. *For Routine IV set*

    A. 15 drops = 1 ml

    B. "Rule of Ten" for calculation of fluid infusion in 24 hours

    IV fluid in litre/24 hours × 10 = Drop rate/minute

    Drop rate per minute ÷ 10 = IV fluid in litre/24 hours.

    C. "Rule of four" for calculation of fluid infusion in one hour

    Volume in ml/hour ÷ 4 = Drop rate/minute

    Drop rate/min × 4 = Volume in ml/hour.

    D. Drop rate calculation for any parameters

$$\frac{\text{Volume to be infused (in ml)}}{\text{Duration of infusion in hours} \times 4} = \text{Drop rate/minute}$$

2. *For Micro Drip IV Set*

    A. 60 drops = 1 ml.

    B. Volume in ml/hour = Number of micro drops per minute.

6. Practical tips on parenteral nutrition (PN)

Basic indications of PN
- Inadequate oral or
  EN for at least 7-10 days.
- Pre-existing severe malnutrition with inadequate oral or EN.

Estimating energy need, Calculation of requirements
Resting energy expenditure—
REE (Kcal/day) = 25 × wt (Kg)
Total energy expenditure—TEE = REE x AF x DF x TF
AF = Activity factor
1.2   Bed rest
1.3   Out of bed
DF = Disease factor
1.25   General surgery
1.3   Sepsis
1.6   Multiorgan failure
1.7   30-50% Burns
1.8   50-70% Burns
2.0   70-90% Burns
TF = Thermal factor
1.1   38°C
1.2   39°C
1.3   40°C

Major nutrients in PN

Proportion of

50-70% Carbohydrate

20-30% Fat

15-20% Protein

Caloric value of

1 gram dextrose = 3.4 Kcal

1 gram lipid = 9.0 Kcal

1 gram protein = 4.0 Kcal

7. Composition of PN products available commercially

Solution	Volume ml	Calorie g	Dext g	AA g	Lipids g
Dextrose 10%	1000	400	100	–	–
Dextrose 20%	1000	800	200	–	–
Amino acid for peripheral PN					
Aminoven 5%	500	100	–	25	–
Aminoven infant 6%	100	24	–	6	–
Amino acid for central PN					
Aminoven 10%	500	200	–	50	–
Aminoven infant 10%	100	40	–	10	–
Amino acid + dextrose for peripheral PN					
Celemine 5S	500	400	25	50	–
Amino acid + dextrose for central PN					
Aminomix 1	1000	1000	200	50	–
PNA-10	1000	1200	250	50	–
Lipid emulsion for peripheral PN					
Cele/Intralipid 10%	500	450	–	–	50
Cele/Intralipid 20%	500	900	–	–	100
Intralipid 30%	333	900			100
Celepid M/L 20%	500	954	–	–	100
3 in 1 for peripheral PN					
Vitrimix	1000	1000	75	53	50
Celemix	1000	800	37.5	37.5	50
TNA Peri	2000	1525	159	60	68
3 in 1 for central PN					
Kabiven	1000	1000	110	34	40
Celemix G	1000	1040	60	75	50
TNA	2000	2044	240	80	80

Contd..

Contd.

Hepatic and renal Failure for peripheral PN

Aminosteril	500	160	–	40	–
Celemine Hepa	500	160	–	40	–
Nephrosteril 7%	500	140	–	35	–
Celemine Nephro	500	140	–	35	–

Immunomodulator solutions for peripheral PN

Dipeptiven 20% (glutamine), Omegaven 10% (omega 3 fatty acids)

8. Various types of ORS and ReSoMal

Item	WHO ORS	Hypoosmolar ORS	IAP Hypoosmolar ORS
NaCl	3.5 g	2.6 g	1.75 g
KCl	1.5 g	1.5 g	1.5 g
Na citrate	2.9 g	2.9 g	2.9 g
Glucose	20 g	13.5 g	15 g
Na	90 mEq/L	75 mEq/L	60 mEq/L
K	20 mEq/L	20 mEq/L	20 mEq/L
Cl	80 mEq/L	65 mEq/L	50 mEq/L
Citrate	10 mEq/L	10 mEq/L	10 mEq/L
Glucose	111 mEq/L	75 mEq/L	84 mEq/L
Osmolarity	311 mOsm/L	245 mOsm/L	224 mOsm/L

9. Composition of stool (mEq/L)

Cholera	Na	K	Cl	HCO$_3$
Child	101	27	92	32
Adult	140	13	104	44
Non cholera	56	25	55	14

10. ReSoMal

ORS	1 pkt	Na (mEq/L)	45
H$_2$O	2 L	K (mEq/L)	40
Sugar	50 g	Cl (mEq/L)	70
Electrolyte		Citrate (mEq/L)	7
Mineral		Mg (mEq/L)	3
Mixture (EMM)	40 ml	Zn (mEq/L)	0.3
Composition		Cu (mEq/L)	0.045
KCl	22.4g	Osmolarity	300
Tripot, citrate	81 g	(mOsm/L)	
MgCl	76 g		
Cu sulphate	1.4 g		
Zn acetate	8.2 g		
Water	2.5 L		

ReSoMal is rehydration solution for the malnourished. Mineral mixture has to be prepared as per the composition given and added to ORS.

11. ELIZ solution for potassium and magnesium supplementation

Indication

1. Malnutrition
2. Bartter's syndrome (Avoid Bicarbonate).
3. Gittleman syndrome (Avoid Bicarbonate).

Composition

	(Qty)
Glucose	50 g
NaCl	2 g
15% KCl	20 cc
7.5% NaHCO$_3$	20 cc
MgCl 6 H$_2$O	30 g
Water	1L

	(mEq/L)
Na	70
K	40
Cl	70
HCO$_3$	20
Mg	3
Glucose	278

PSYCHO-SOCIO-ECONOMIC STATUS SCALES

1. Socio-economic status according to revised Kuppuswamy's scale—2007

Item	Score
A. Education	
1. Professional degree/Hons., MA and above	7
2. BA, BSc degree	6
3. Intermediate/Post high school certificate	5
4. High school certificate	4
5. Middle school completion	3
6. Primary school/literate	2
7. Illiterate	1
B. Occupation	
1. Profession	10
2. Semi profession	6
3. Clerical, shop/farm owner	5
4. Skilled worker	4
5. Semi-skilled worker	3
6. Unskilled worker	2
7. Unemployed	1
C. Income*	
1. Rs. 19575 and above	12
2. Rs. 9788-19574	10
3. Rs. 7323-9787	6
4. Rs. 4894-7322	4
5. Rs. 2936-4893	3
6. Rs. 980-2935	2
7. Rs. 979 and below	1

Total score	Socio-economic status scale
26-29	Class I (upper)
16-25	Class II (upper middle)
11-15	Class III (lower middle)
5-10	Class IV (upper lower)
< 5	Class V (lower)

Source: * Kuppuswamy's SES Scale–Updating for 2007, IJP.2007;74:1131-1132.

2. Standards of sanitation according to Briscoe's scale

Behaviour	Points		
	3	2	1
1. Water:			
Drinking	Tube well/tap	Ring well	Pond
Washing	Tube well/tap	Ring well	Pond
Bathing	Tube well/tap	Ring well	Pond
2. Defecation children < 5 years	Latrine/disposed off	Open, within the compound	Anywhere
3. Hand washing by mother before handling/eating food	Yes	Occasional	No
4. Hand washing by mother after defecation	Yes with soap	Yes with sand/ash	Yes with water
5. Appearance of mother's hands and cloth	Clean	One clean	Unclean
6. Drinking water storage	Direct use	Clean, covered	Unclean, uncovered
7. Water for washing	Direct use	Clean, covered	Unclean, uncovered

Points	Behaviour
18-21	Good
13-17	Fair
7-12	Poor
Source: Briscoe, 1978	

APPENDIX 8

3. Colour coding and type of container for disposal of biomedical wastes

Colour coding	Waste category	Treatment options	Type of container
Yellow	**Cat. 1:** Human anatomical waste (These contain human tissues, organs and body parts). **Cat. 2:** Animal waste (This contains animal tissues, organs, body parts carcasses, bleeding parts, fluid, blood and experimental animals used in research, waste generated by veterinary hospitals and colleges, discharge from hospitals and animal houses). **Cat. 3:** Microbiology and biotechnology waste (Wastes from laboratory cultures, stocks or micro organisms live or vaccines, human and animal cell, culture used in research and infectious agents from research and industrial laboratories, wastes from production of biologicals, toxins, dishes and devices used for transfer of cultures). **Cat. 6:** Soiled waste (This contains items contaminated with blood, and body fluids including cotton, dressings, soiled plaster castes, linens, beddings, other material contaminated with blood)	Incineration/ deep burial	Plastic bag
Red	**Cat. 3,6 and 7:** Solid waste (Plastic) (This contains wastes generated from disposable items other than the waste sharps such as tubings, catheters, intravenous sets etc.)	Autoclaving/ Micro waving/ Chemical treatment	Disinfected container/ plastic bag
Blue/ White/ Translucent	**Cat. 4:** Waste sharps (This contains needles, syringes, scalpels, blades, glass etc. that may cause puncture and cuts. This includes both used usable sharps) and **Cat. 7**	Autoclaving/ Micro waving/ Chemical treatment and destruction/ Shredding	Plastic bag/ Puncture proof container
Black	**Cat. 5:** Discarded medicine and cytotoxic drugs (this cotnains waste comprising outdated, contaminated and discarded medicines). **Cat. 9:** Incineration Ash (This contains ash from incineration of any bio-medical waste) and **Cat. 10** (Solid)— Chemical waste (this contains chemical used in production of biologicals and chemicals used for disinfection, insecticides etc.)	Disposal in secured landfill	Plastic bag

Note: **Categories 8 and 10 (liquid) do not require containers/bags.**
Source: The Gazette of India, Annexure-A (1998).

4. Micro-Environment Scoring Scale, Elizabeth, 1994

Item	Score		
	3	2	1
A. Maternal attitude*			
1. Do you yell at your child when you are angry?	No	Occasionally yes	Yes
2. Do you punish your child you are angry?	No	Occasionally yes	Yes
3. Do you hit your child when you are angry?	No	Occasionally yes	Yes
4. Do you ignore your child when he/she asks for help?	No	Occasionally yes	Yes
B. Supportive system to the mother**			
1. Do your in-laws help in household work and child rearing?	Yes	Occasionally yes	No
2. Do you have someone to turn to during any difficulty?	Yes	Occasionally yes	No
3. Do your friends/ neighbours look after your child in your absence?	Yes	Occasionally yes	No
4. Are you happy about your life/fate?	Yes	Occasionally yes	No

Score	Micro-environment
19-24	Good
15-18	Fair
8-14	Poor

Source: Elizabeth, 1994
*Items selected from the Handbook of Parental Acceptance and Rejection (Rohner, 1980)
**Items selected from the Supportive System Scale (Vazir, 1983)

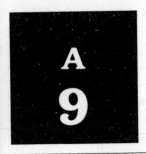

IMMUNIZATION CHARTS AND PEDIGREE SYMBOLS

1. IAP immunization record

Age	Vaccine	Due on	Given on	Batch
Birth	BCG			
	OPV_0			
	Hepatitis B_1			
6 weeks	$DTPw_1/DTPa_1$			
	OPV_1			
	Hepatitis B_2			
	Hib_1			
10 weeks	$DTPw_2/DTPa_2$			
	OPV_2			
	Hib_2			
14 weeks	$DTPw_3/DTPa_3$			
	OPV_3			
	Hepatitis B_3*			
	Hib_3			
9 months	Measles			
15-18 months	$DTPw B_1/DTPa B_1$			
	$OPV B_1$			
	$Hib B_1$			
	MMR			
2 years	Typhoid [+]			
5 years	$DTPw B_2/DTPa B_2$			
	$OPV B_2$			
10 years	$Td^#/TT$			
16 years	$Td^#/TT$			

Pregnant women 2 doses of $Td^#/TT$.

*3rd dose of Hepatitis B can be given at 6 months of age.

[+]Revaccination every 3-4 years.

[#]Td preferred over TT.

w-whole cell killed pertussis.

a-Acellular pertussis vaccine.

Vaccines that can be given after discussion with the parents

Age	Vaccine	Due on	Given on	Batch
> 15 months of age	Varicella Vaccine[#]			
> 18 months of age	Hepatitis A vaccine[+]			
> 6 weeks	Pneumococcal conjugated vaccine[*]			

[#] < 13 years of age: 1 dose; > 13 years of age: 2 doses at 4-8 weeks interval.

[+] 2 doses at 6-12 months interval.

[*] 3 primary doses at 6, 10 and 14 weeks followed by a booster dose at 15 months.

2. Cold Chain

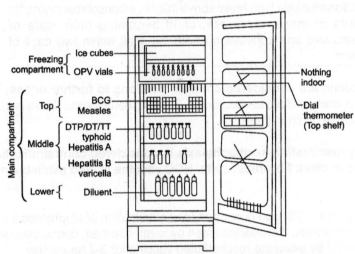

*Refrigerator showing correct storage of vaccines.
*Food items should not be stored along with vaccines.

Vaccine Vial Monitor (VVM)

It is a small square made of heat sensitive material and placed on an outer coloured circle printed on the label of OPV vial. Time and temperature cause the VVM to change colour and become darker. The darkening is irreversible and is compared with the outer coloured circle to check the potency of the vaccine.

Reverse Cold Chain

Reverse cold chain is the system of sending vaccines cold at the right temperature from the periphery to the laboratory for potency testing. OPV being most temperature sensitive, it is taken for potency testing.

Vaccine Requirements

The vaccine requirements are calculated based on the population and the number is beneficiaries. The calculated number is then multiplied by the *wastage multiplication factor* to get the estimated vaccine requirement. For BCG and measles, the number of doses required is multiplied by 2 and for all others it is multiplied by 1.33 to ensure allowance for wastage during administration.

Side Effects and Contraindications

The common **side effects** are fever, temporary swelling, redness, pain and induration at the site of injection. Rarely anaphylaxis may occur. Mild reactions are associated with pruritus, flush, urticaria and angiooedema. Serious reactions include bronchospasm, laryngeal oedema, shock and cardiovascular collapse. **All the vaccinated children should be asked to stay for at least 15-20 minutes to watch for reaction.**

> *Reactions* include high fever above 105° F, inconsolable crying for 3 hours or more, dizziness, child becoming blue, pale or unresponsive and convulsion or staring spell within two days of injection.

Such severe reactions are considered contraindications to further doses: High fever and severe infections are contraindications to vaccination. Evolving neurological illness is a contraindication to DPT vaccine. DT can be given in them.

Severe egg allergy manifesting as anaphylaxis is considered contraindication to measles vaccination prepared in chick fibroblast cells. HDC vaccine is also available now which can be given in them.

Toxic Shock Syndrome (TSS) can occur due to contamination of staphylococcus aureus in the multidose measles vaccine vials. It is characterised by fever, diarrhea, coma, convulsion and septic shock. It can be prevented by using the reconstituted vaccine for 3-4 hours only.

3. Symbols for pedigree charting

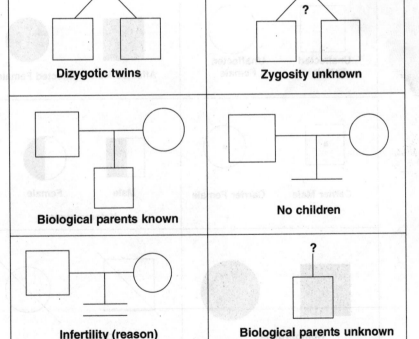

Non-consanguinous mating	Consanguinous mating
Separated	Monozygotic twins
Dizygotic twins	Zygosity unknown
Biological parents known	No children
Infertility (reason)	Biological parents unknown

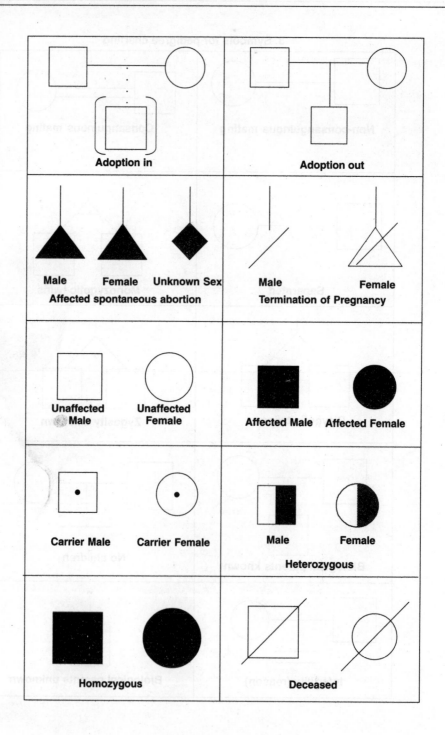

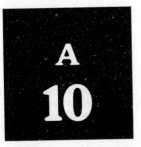

DRUGS AND DOSAGES

Drugs and Dosages

Drug	Preparations	Dose	Side Effects
ACETOZOLAMIDE	T.125 mg, 250 mg INJ: 500mg vial	10-30mg/kg/day in 3-4 div doses PO	Acidosis, Hypokalemia, Stevens-Johnson Syndrome
ACETYL CYSTEINE	Solution as Sodium 10% 100 mg/ml (4 ml, 10 ml, 30 ml) 20% 200 mg/ml (4 ml, 10 ml,30 ml, 100 ml)	Infants 2-4 ml as inhalation, Children 6-10 ml, Adolescents: 10ml **Acetaminophen over dose—** 140mg/kg loading followed by 70 mg/kg Q 4 H x17 doses PO 150mg/kg IV in 5% Glucose or 15-30 min followed by 50mg/kg over 4 hrs then 100mg/kg over 16 hrs 20-40 units IM OD x 2 weeks	Stomatitis, Urticaria Rapid IV push may cause Hypotension
ACTH	Inj 5ml vials 60 IU/ml Human ACTH 0.125 to 0.25 mg		
ACYCLOVIR	T.200 mg Inj 250 mg solution 400 mg/5 ml	10mg/kg/dose over 1 hr I/V as infusion in D_5 or NS Q_8H	Nephrotoxicity, Rashes, Thrombocytosis
ADENOSINE	INJ: 3 mg/ml	0.05mg/kg I/V push along 3ml Saline simultaneously by a 3-way increase the bolus by 0.05mg/kg every 2 units until clinical response occurs. MAX: 0. 25mg/kg	Use peripheral I/V site may cause bronchoconstriction, heart block, Bradycardia, hypertension needs continuous ECG monitoring
ADRENALINE	1ml amp of 1:1000 solution	0.01ml/kg/dose slow S/C. Do not exceed 0.5ml/dose may repeat after 5 mts. Nebulisation: Same dose diluted in 3cc NS.	Ventricular premature contraction, Atrial arrhythmias prolonged QT interval
ALBENDAZOLE	T.400mg Suspension: 400 mg in 10 ml	**1-2 years** 200mg single dose 400 mg PO single dose >2 years	High doses can cause sore throat and fever, worm migration in heavy infestation
ALBUMIN	10,50,100 ml vials of 20% human albumin	1g/kg/dose I/V infusion over 1-2 hr at rate of 0.1g/min	Rapid infusion may cause volume overload and CCF: Hypersensitivity reactions
AMIKACIN	INJ: 100,250 mg 500 mg/2 ml	7.5 mg/kg/dose I/V x 2-3 doses	Ototoxicity, Nephrotoxicity
AMINO CAPROIC ACID	T: 500 mg 100 mg/kg/dose Not available freely 250 mg/5ml	200 mg/kg/day PO	Hypertension, Bradycardia, Arrhythmias

Contd.

Contd.

AMINOPHYLLINE	T. 100 mg INJ: 250 mg In 10 ml amp.	5 mg/kg/dose I/V dilution. With double volume of Dextrose I/V push or added to 5% Dextrose drip to run over 6 hrs x 4 doses Total daily dose should not exceed 20 mg/kg/day	Arrhythmias, seizures
AMIODARONE	CORDARONE T: 200mg INJ: 50mg/5ml	**ORAL** <1yr. 600-800 mg/2.7m^2/day in 2 div doses >1year: 10-15 mg/kg/dy in 2 div doses **I/V Doses** Load –5 mg/kg over 1 hour, then continuous infusion of 5-15 microgram/kg/min	Pro arrhythmia, hyperglycemia, hypothyroidism, pulmonary toxicity, hepatotoxicity, hypersensitivity, pneumonitis
AMOXICILLIN	DT: 125 mg, 250 mg. Dry syp or readymade suspension 125, 250 mg/5ml drops100 mg/ml suspension and COAMOXYCLAV T/Inj T.250 mg Amoxicillin+ 125 mg clavulanic acid Dry syp: 125 mg Amoxycillin +31.25 mg clavulanic acid in 5 ml	30-50mg/kg/day/2 or 3 PO	Diarrhea, skin rash
AMPHOTERICIN- B **AMPICILLIN**	C: 250, 500 DT: 125, 250 Dry syp: 125, 250 mg/5 ml INJ: 500mg, 1g	2.5-5mg/kg I/V infusion over 1-2 hrs 50-100 mg/kg/day—4 Po I/V, I/M	Hypotension, fever, chills Pruritus, maculo papular rashes Rashes in 1min
AMPICILLIN + SULBACTAM	INJ: 1.5g vial 1gm Ampicillin + 500 mg Sulbactam	150mg/kg/24hrs I/V, I/M—3-4 doses	
ANTI HEMOPHILIC FACTOR		25U/kg/dose every 12-24 hrs. Units required → wt in kg x 0.5 x desired % increase in factor	Tachycardia, blood borne diseases
ASPIRIN	T. 75 mg, 100 mg, 150 mg, 350 mg	Rheumatic fever 75-100 mg/kg/ 24 hours PO anti platelet dose 5mg/kg / 24hrs ODPO Analgesic 10mg/kg/dose x 4PO	Angioedema, Urticaria, anaphylactoid reaction Risk of stone formation in higher doses
ASCORBIC ACID	T.100/500 mg;drops 100 mg/ml	10mg/kg/day;2-3 doses	
ARTEMETHER	INJ: 80mg/ 1ml/amp C.40 mg	Not standardized in children 1.6mg I/M BD X day one followed by 1.6 mg I/M once daily x next 4 days	
ATENOLOL	T: 25mg, 50mg	1mg/kg/24 hrs OD DO	Bradycardia, Headache, wheezing and hypoglycemia
ATROPINE	INJ: 1ml/amp	0.01mg/kg I/V or I/M higher doses for organophosphorous poisoning	Dry mouth, blurred vision, urinary retention, tachycardia, mydriasis Gastric upset
AZITHROMYCIN	Dry Syp: 100mg, 200mg/5ml	10mg/kg upto 500mg on first day. Then 5mg/kg/day upto 250 mg on days 2 through five	

Contd.

AZTREONAM	INJ: 500,750mg,1.5gm	100mg/kg/day;newborn 30mg/kg/dose Q12H.Can be given IM (diluted)	Dose correction in renal failure
BACLOFEN	T: 10mg, 20mg INJ: 2mg/8ml	15mg/day–Q8H max 40mg/kg/day PO	Drowsiness vertigo, hypotonia, ataxia
BECLOME-THASONE	Inhaler 100 or 200 mcg/puff. Also available as rotocaps and as nasal spray for allergic rhinitis	100-200mcg x 4 in 24 hours and titrate depending on response	Oral candidiasis, irritation of nasal mucosa
BETAMETHA-SONE	T. 0 5 mg, inj, 4 mg/ml, 0.1% eye drops, skin cream and oral drops containing 0.5 mg/ml	0.2 mg/kg/24 hr div into 2 to 3 PO	
BUDESONIDE	MDI/RESP Solution 50μg/puff 100, 200 ug/puff	**>6 years** 1-2 puffs BD Acute Asthma 3-4 puffs every 20mts x 3 doses	Oral thrush, dysphonia etc.
CALCIUM GLUCONATE	10ml amps of 10% INJ	I/V only 0.5ml 10% solution 1kg/dose slow I/V dil: NS	Bradycardia on rapid infusion
CALCITRIOL	C.0.25 mcg, 0.5 mcg INJ: 1mcg/ml	Premature infants 0.05 mcg/kg/day I/V Children 0.01-0.08 mcg/kg/day	Hypercalcemia, Vitamin D toxicity
CAPTOPRIL	T.25 and 50 mg	Start with 0.5 mg/ kg/24 hr div x 3 PO may increase to 0.5 mg/kg/dose. Maximum doses is 5 mg/kg/ 24 hr. Neonates 0.1 mg /kg/ dose every 8-12 hours	Hyperkalemia, altered taste, rashes, neutropenia, cough, oliguria etc.
CARBAMA-ZEPINE	T. 100 200 mg. susp. 100, mg/5 ml	10mg/kgs/day–2PO may increase up to 20 mg/kg/day	Sedation, Blurred vision, Bone marrow depression, Stevens-Johnson syndrome
CARNITINE	C: 250 mg INJ: 1g/5ml	50-100mg/kg/dose div into 2-3 PO 50mg/kg/dose Q4-6H IV	
CEFACLOR	C 250 mg Dry syp or readymade susp 125 or 187 mg/ 5 ml. Drops 50 mg/ml	30 mg/kg/24 hr div into 2-3 PO	Abdominal cramps, body odor
CEFADROXIL	DT 125 mg and 250 mg, susp 125 or 250 mg/5 ml and Drops 100 mg / ml	30 mg/kg/24 hr div into 2 PO	Nausea, epigastric distress, vomiting, skin rashes
CEFAZOLIN	Vials of 125 mg, 250 mg, 500 and 1 G	50-100 mg/kg/24 hrs div into 4 IM, IV for intramuscular use, add 2 ml of sterile water for injection or 0.9 percent sodium chloride injection to each 250 or 500 mg vial, or 2.5 ml of diluent to 1- gram vial. For IV use add 10 ml of sterile water for injection to each 500 mg or 1 gram vial, administered over 3-5 minutes period	Skin rashes pruritus, diarrhea, drug fever
CEFOPERA-ZONE	INJ. 250 mg, 500 mg and 1 g vials	100-200 mg/kg / 24 hr. div into 4 IV IM	Skin rash, drug fever, anaphylaxis, diarrhea
CEFOTAXIME	INJ: 250,500mg 1g vials	100-200mg/kg/day -4 doses I/V or I/M Newborn: 50mg/kg/dose Q12H	Skin rash, drug fever, anaphylaxis, diarrhea
CEFTAZIDIME	INJ: 250, 500mgs, 1gm vial	100-150mg/kg/day – 3 I/V or I/M	Skin rash, eosinophilia, urticaria, local pain

Contd.

Contd.

CEFPODOXIME	T: 100 mg 200 mg Dry: Syp: 50/ 100mg/ 5ml	10mg/kg/day- 2 doses PO	Diarrhea, nausea, vomiting
CEFTRIAXONE	INJ: 250mg, 1g	50-100 mg/kg/day div into 2 I/V, I/M	Diarrhea, skin rash, urticaria, eosinophilia
CEFUROXIME	T. 250mg, 500 mg, Inj. Vials 250 mg/750 mg and dry syp 125 mg/5 ml.	IM/ IV 50-100 mg/kg/24 hr. div into 3. In meningitis 240 mg/kg/day div into 3 IV PO 30 mg/kg/day div. Into 2-3	Skin rash, eosinophilia
CEPHALEXIN	C.250MG DT: 125mg /5ml 1gm vials	50-100 mg/kg/day: 4 PO	Renal function impairment
CHLORAM- PHENICOL	C.250MG, 500MG Susp.125mg/5ml 1gm vials	50-100mg/kg/day in 4 divided doses PO/I/V	Skin rashes, Epigastric diseases, Bone marrow depression
CHLOROQUINE	250mg T contains 150mg of chloroquine base INJ: vial contains 64.5mg of chloroquine base	**PO:** 10mg/kg of base per kg followed by 5mg/kg 6hrs later and to be repeated on day 2 and day 3	Hypotension, GI upset, rash, peripheral neuropathy
CIPROFLOXACIN	T.250 mg, 500 mg, 750 mg and IV infusion 200 mg in 100 ml	20–30 mg/kg/24 hrs div into 2 PO 20 mg/kg/24 hr div into 2 IV	Nausea epigastric distress, dizziness
CHORIONIC GONADOTROPIN	INJ: 200, 500,1000, 2000 Units/ml	Children: Prepubertal cryptorchidism 1000-2000 units/m^2/dose 3 times/wk 500-1000 units dose 3 times/week x 3 weeks	Hypogonadotropic hypogonadism Mental depression, tiredness, precocious puberty, premature closure of epiphysis
CISAPRIDE	Syp 1mg/ml T: 10mg	0.1-0.2 mg/kg/dose 3-4 times a day 20 min before feeds	QT prolongation, Cardiac arrhythmias
CLARITHROMYCIN	T: 250mg Dry Syp: 125mg/5ml	15mg/kg/day-2 PO	GI upset, dyspepsia, nausea, abdominal cramps
CLOBAZAM		0.25-1mg/kg/day BD PO	Dizziness, fatigue, weight gain, ataxia
CLOXACILLIN	C.250, 500 MG Dry syp. 125mg/5ml Inj: 250mg, 500mg	100mg/kg/day up to 200mg/kg/day PO, I/V, I/M	Thrombophlebitis Anaphylaxis, rash
COTRIMOXAZOLE	(Trimethoprim + Sulphamethoxazole) T.80 mg TMP+400 mg Ped T. 20+100 Syp: 40+200	In terms of Trimethoprim 6-10 mg/kg/day-2 PO	Skin rashes, Stevens-Johnson syndrome, fixed drug eruption
CYCLOSPORINE	C.25, 50, 100MG Inj: 100MG/ML	3-6mg/kg/day	Hypertension,diabetes Nephrotoxicity, gingival hypertrophy, hirsutism
DESFERRIOXA- MINE	INJ: 500mg	Acute iron overload: IV-15mg/kg/hr Chronic iron overload: I/V-15 mg/kg/hr. S/C-20-40 mg/kg over 8-12 min	Local pain and induration, flushing
DESMOPRESSIN	INJ: 4mg/ml Nasal solution: 0.1 mg/ml	Diabetes insipidus 3 months-12years 0.05 mcg PO initially, IV- 5 mcg/day in 1-2 div doses Hemophilia >3/12 I/V 0.3 mcg/kg Nocturnal enuresis >6 years 20 mcg at bed time	Monitor S electrolytes, plasma and urine osmolality, urine output

APPENDIX 10

Contd.

DEXAMETHASONE	INJ: 4 mg/ml T.0.5mg Drops 0.5mg/ml	**Cerebral edema**—1mg/kg/day – div into 4→anti inflammatory 0.2 mg/1kg/day	Hyperglycemia, fatigue, glycosuria, Cushing's disease
DIAZEPAM	T.2, 5,10mg INJ: mg/ml SYP: 2mg/5ml	0.1-0.3 mg/kg/day→3 PO status 0.3mg/kg/dose repeated after 3-5 minutes Max dose 5-10mg I/V infusion, NS 0.3 mg/kg/hr	Respiratory depression, sedation, nausea
DIETHYL CARBAMAZINE	T.50 mg 100mg, syp.50 mg/5ml	6mg/kg/day-3 PO X 14 – 21 days Tropical eosinophilia→10mg/kg/day	Drowsiness, anorexia, vomiting Nausea, cardiac arrhythmias
DIGOXIN	T.0.25mg INJ: 0.5mg/2ml pediatric Elixir 0.05 mg/ml	Loading dose: 0.02mg/kg start 0.01mg/kg at 8 hrs; 0.01mg/kg at 16 hrs and 0.01mg/kg OD Dose of pediatric elixir: If weight of infant is *n* kg–dose is *0.n* ml BD i.e. for 8 kg child it is 0.8 ml BD	Vomiting, ECG changes
DOBUTAMINE	200mg/5ml inj	Start with 6 mcg/kg/minute and titrate infusion	Tachycardia, ectopic heart beats
DOPAMINE	200mg/5ml	6-20 mcg/kg/minute 6 X Body wt mg of Dopamine is taken in 100ml 5% dextrose and this can be given as *n* micro drops /minute = *n* mcg//kg/minute	Tachycardia, ventricular arrhythmias tissue necrosis
ERYTHROMYCIN	T.250mg, 500mg Susp: 125mg and 250 mg /5ml Drops: 100mg/ml	40mg/kg/day—4 doses PO	Abdominal pain, vomiting
ETHAMBUTOL	T.200, 400mg, 800mg	25mg/kg/day OD PO for the first 2 months followed by 15mg/kg/day OD	Optic neuritis, Color blindness, Rash
FLUOROCORTI- SONE	T0.1 mg	0.05- 0.1mg/kg/ 24 hr PO, OD	Hypertension, Edema, Congestive heart failure, headache
FRUSEMIDE	T.40mg INJ: 20mg/2ml	1-2 mg/kg/dose PO 0.5-1 mg/kg/dose I/V, I/M (MAX: 5-10 mg/kg/dose)	Electrolyte imbalance, may precipitate hepatic coma if used during pre coma
FLUTICASONE	MDI: 110, 220 mcg/spray Nasal spray: 50mcg/spray	MDI:88-880 mcg BD	Dysphonia, oral thrush, adrenal suppression
GENTAMYCIN	INJ: 10mg/ml 40mg/ml 0.3% eye/ear drops	5-7.5 mg/kg/day—2-3 dose I/V I/M Newborn: 2-5 mg/kg/dose Q12H	Skin rashes, Nephrotoxicity, Ototoxicity
GLUCAGON		Neonates 0.3mg/kg/dose I/V, I/M, S/C Children 0.02-0.03 mg/kg/dose	Nausea, Vomiting, Hypersensitivity
G-CSF	Inj:300mcg/ml	5-10mcg/kg/day OD, SC/IV till count improves for 1-2 weeks	
HALOPERIDOL	T.0.25 mg, 1.5 mg Syp: 2 mg/ml Inj: 5 mg/ml	0.1mg/kg/day -3 or 4 doses In Chorea >5 years 0.25 mg x 3 PO	Use carefully in children with epilepsy and in less than 3 years
HYALURONIDASE	INJ: 150u/ml	150 U S/C or I/D at 5 times (Q.2 ml to each) at the leading edge of extravasations	Tachycardia, Hypotension, Erythema

Contd.

Contd.

Drug	Formulation	Dose	Side Effects
HYDROCORTISONE	Vial 100 mg T.20 mg	Shock-10mg/kg I/V bolus go up to 50mg/kg followed by same dose Q6H x 2-4 days Status Asthmatics 4mg/kg/dose Q6H Physiologic-replacement →20mg/m²PO (0.75mg/kg/day) 2/3 in the morning 1/3 in the evening	Hyperglycemia, Hypertension, Peptic ulcer, Cushing's syndrome
IBUPROFEN	T.200mg, 400mg Susp: 100mg/5ml	8-10mg/kg/dose x 3 or 4 PO	Abdominal pain, nausea, vomiting
ISONIAZID	T.100mg 300mg Syp: INH 300mg/5ml	5mg/kg/day OD PO	Hepatitis, Peripheral neuritis, GI upset
LEUPROLIDE	Inj:5mg/ml	I/M Depot 0.15-0.3mg/kg/dose every 28 days.	Weight gain, hot flashes, depression, nausea, vomiting, myalgia
LEVAMISOLE	T.50, 150mg Susp: 50mg/5ml	3mg/kg/day PO single dose	Neutropenia in prolonged use
LINEZOLID	Newer anti staphylococcal against resistant gram +ve organisms, skin infections	**Adults** 400-600 mg I/V, oral in 2 div doses Children Ltd use 10mg/kg/day div into 2 doses x 10-14 days	Myelosuppression, Rash, Headache, Thrombocytopenia
LORAZEPAM	INJ: 1mg, 2mg/1ml	0.1mg/kg I/V bolus can be repeated after 15-20 mts	Sedation, anorexia, amnesia
MANNITOL	20% IN 100, 250, 350ml	2.5-5 ml/kg/dose I/V infusion over 30 mts lower doses used frequently (4-6 hrly) avoid rebound	Headache, nausea, vomiting
MEBENDAZOLE	T.100mg Susp: 100mg/5ml	100mg Bd x 3 days Irrespective of age	Migration of worms, urticaria
METHYL PREDNISOLONE	INJ: vial 500mg, 1g	1-30 mg/kg/day as infusion in 5% Dextrose	
METOCLOPROMIDE	T.10mg, Syp 5mg/5ml Inj:5mg/5ml	0.1mg/kg/dose	Extra pyramidal reaction
MEFLOQUINE	T 250mg	15-25mg/kg as a single dose (Dose above 15mg/kg may be split into 2 doses) 15mg/kg followed 8 hours later by 10mg/kg	Nausea, Dizziness
METRONIDAZOLE	T. 200,400 Syp: 200mg/5ml I/V infusion 500mg in 100ml	30-50mg/kg/day-3 PO Rate: 5ml/mt	Metallic taste, vomiting, diziness
MIDAZOLAM	Inj 1mg/ml Or 5mg/ml	I/V loading dose of 0.15 mg/kg followed by continuous infusion of 1mg/kg/mt (in 5%D or 9% NaCl) step up as per response	Respiratory depression
NALIDIXIC ACID	T-500mg Syp 300mg/5ml	50-55mg/kg/day div x - 3-4 doses PO	Pseudo tumour cerebri, skin rashes
NAPROXEN	T.250, 500mg	10-15 mg/kg/day-2-3 doses	GI irritation
NIFEDIPINE	C-5, 10mg SR:T-10,20,30mg	Start with 0.5 mg/kg/dose S/L or PO x 4 doses/day	Tachycardia, Flushing and Odema
OCTREOTIDE	Inj:0.05,0.1,0.2,0.5, 1 mg/ml vials	1-10 mcg/kg/hr (Dilute in 100 ml NS or 5% D) given over 3 mts	Mild transient hypo or hyper glycemia

Contd.

Contd.

PENCILLAMINE	C.125 mg, 250 mg, T.250 mg	**WILSON DISEASE** 20mg/kg/day Po Q6-Q12H (Max 1g/day) **LEAD INTOXICATION** 30-40 mg/kg/day Q8H/Q12H (Max 1.5 g/day) **RHEUMATOID ARTHRITIS** 3mg/kg/day PO 12 hrly increasing by 3 mg/kg every 2-3 months to max 10 mg/kg/day	Rash, Pruritus, SLE like syndrome, nephrotic syndrome
PENICILLIN-G	5 lakhs, 10 lakhs	50,000 unit/kg/day x 4 upto 50,000U/kg/dose x six times a day I/M, I/V	Anaphylaxis
PENTAZOCINE	INJ: 30 mg/ml	0.5mg/kg/dose I/V 1mg/kg/dose IM,SC	CNS depression and vomiting
PHENO BARBITONE	T. 15, 30, 60 mg Inj: 200 mg/ml Elix: 20 mg/5ml	5-8mg/kg/day OD or → 2 doses PO Loading dose 15-20 mg/kg Slow I/V is needed for acute seizure	Sedation, Hyperactivity, ataxia
PHENYTOIN	T: 100 mg Syp: 30 or 125mg/5ml Inj: 50mg/ml	5-8 mg/kg/day- 1-2 PO dose Loading 15-20 mg/kg slow I/V at a rate 1mg/kg per mt	Bradycardia, Arrhythmia, Extravasation, Hirsuitism, Gum hypertrophy
PIPERACILLIN	INJ. 1,2 and 4 gm	200-300 mg/kg/day in 4 divided doses	Rash, eosinophilia, transient rise of liver enzymes
PIPERAZINE CITRATE	SYP: 750 mg/5ml ,T.500 mg	75-100mg/kg OD at bed times x 2d	Nausea, vomiting, skin rashes
PIROXICAM	DT: 20mg ,C.10,20 mg Inj: 20 mg/ml	0.2mg/kg as a single oral dose max not more than 15mg/kg/day	G.I. upset
PRALIDOXIME	INJ: 25 mg/ml T.500 mg	20-50 mg/kg slow I/V repeat after 1-2 hours if muscle weakness has not improved, then continue 12 hrly. I/V injection add 20ml of sterile water to each 1g vial	Higher doses may cause neuromuscular blockade
PREDNISOLONE	T.5, 10, 20 mg Syp:5 mg/ml	2mg/kg/day X 2-4 div doses	Gastric upset, Hypertension, Psychosis
PRIMAQUINE	T.2.5, 7.5 and 15 mg	0.55mg/kg/dose or 0.3 mg/kg/dose of base OD x 5-14 days	Nausea, vomiting, abdominal pain
PROMETHAZINE	T.10, 25 mg Pediatric Elixir: 5 mg/5ml Inj: 25 mg/ml	0.25-1mg/kg dose I/M, I/V 1mg/kg/dose PO	Dizziness, dry mouth
PROPRANOLOL	T.10, 20,40, 80 mg Inj 1mg/ml	1-2 mg/kg/day-3-4PO I/V 0.01-0.1 mg/kg/dose over 10-15 min	Bradycardia
PYRANTEL PAMOATE	T.250mg Susp: 250 mg/5ml	11 mg/kg/day single dose PO x 1 day	Skin rash
PYRAZINAMIDE	T.500mg, 750 mg Susp: 300mg/5ml	15-40 mg/kg/day PO single dose or div into 2	Hepatotoxicity, GI upset
QUININE	T.100mg, 300mg, 600mg Inj: 300 mg/ml	10mg/kg/dose x 3 PO x 7-10 days. I/V loading dose infusion 20mg/kg over 4 hrs in 10ml/kg of DNS followed by infusion 10mg/kg after 12 hrs	Vertigo, tinnitus, blurred vision, cardiac arrhythmia

Contd.

APPENDIX 10

Contd.

RANITIDINE	T.150, 300 mg INJ: 50 mg/2ml	2mg/kg/dose PO 1-2mg/kg/dose I/V x 2-3 doses	Skin rashes
RIBAVIRIN	SYP: 50 mg/5 ml C:100,200mg	10mg/kg/24hours	
RIFAMPICIN	C.150, 300, 450g, 600 mg Syp: 100 mg/5ml OD PO on empty stomach	10mg/kg/day	Hepatotoxicity, Flu like syndrome
ROXITHROMYCIN	DT.50 mg T.150 mg Syp.50 mg/5ml	5-8 mg/kg/24 hrs into 2 PO	Nausea, Vomiting, Skin rashes
SALBUTAMOL	T. 2 mg, 4 mg Syp: 2 mg/5ml Rotacap: 200 mg Aerosol: 100 mg/ Repulses: 2.5 mg Respirator solution 5mg/ml	0.1mg/kg/dose x 4 PO Nebulisation: 0.03ml respirator solution/kg/dose with equal volume NS 4-6 hourly Aerosol: 2 puff x 4	Fine tremor, Palpitation, Tachycardia
SALMETROL	25mcg/puff Rotacaps 50 mcg/puff	1-2 puff: 12 hourly	Tachycardia
SILVER SULPHA OINTMENT	1% Cream		Burning at the site of application
SODIUM VALPROATE	T.200, 300,500 mg Syp: 200mg/5ml	20 mg/kg/day PO/IV Rectal infusion of syp. 15-20mg/kg/dose diluted with equal volume of tap water	Hepatotoxicity
SPIRONOLACTONE	T.25,50, 100 mg	2-3 mg/kg/day into 2 or 3	Hyperkalemia, gynaecomastia
STREPTOMYCIN	INJ: 0.75g, 1g vials	20-40mg/kg/day X 1-2 I/M	8th N damage and nephrotoxicity
TEICOPLANIN	INJ: 200, 400mg vials	10mg/kg/dose OD I/M or I/V twice daily on 1st day	Pain, phlebitis at the site of injection
THEOPHYLLINE	C.125,250mg Syp:100 mg/5ml	5mg/kg/dose not to exceed 20mg/kg/day	GI disturbances, nausea, vomiting
THYROXIN	T:0.1mg (100 mcg)	Newborn10mcg/kg Child 4-6 mcg/kg PO OD	Palpitation, Loss of weight
TRICLOFOS	SYP: 500 mg/5 ml	0.5ml/kg/dose	Skin rash
TRANEXAMIC ACID	INJ: 100 mg/ml T.500 mg	10mg/kg I/V immediately before surgery then oral 25 mg/kg/dose 3-4 times	Hypotension, Thromboembolic complications
URSO DEOXY CHOLIC ACID	C.300 mg	Neonates 10-15 mg/kg/day PO Infants 30mg/kg/day 8-12 hourly	Dyspepsia, diarrhea, biliary pain, headache
VANCOMYCIN	INJ: 500 mg vial	45-60 mg/kg/day div into 3 or 4 I/V infusion over 1hour NS or 5% Dextrose	Ototoxicity, Nephrotoxicity

INDEX

INDEX

INDEX

INDEX

INDEX

NOTES

NOTES

NOTES

NOTES

NOTES